Comorbidities in Chronic Kidney Disease (CKD)

Comorbidities in Chronic Kidney Disease (CKD)

Special Issue Editors

Joachim Jankowski
Heidi Noels

MDPI • Basel • Beijing • Wuhan • Barcelona • Belgrade

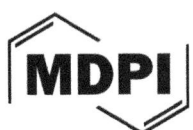

Special Issue Editors
Joachim Jankowski
Institute of Molecular
Cardiovascular Research (IMCAR),
University Hospital Aachen,
RWTH Aachen University,
Germany
Cardiovascular Research Institute
Maastricht (CARIM),
Maastricht University,
The Netherlands

Heidi Noels
Institute of Molecular
Cardiovascular Research (IMCAR),
University Hospital Aachen,
RWTH Aachen University,
Germany
Cardiovascular Research Institute
Maastricht (CARIM),
Maastricht University,
The Netherlands

Editorial Office
MDPI
St. Alban-Anlage 66
4052 Basel, Switzerland

This is a reprint of articles from the Special Issue published online in the open access journal *Toxins* (ISSN 2072-6651) in 2020 (available at: https://www.mdpi.com/journal/toxins/special_issues/Kidney_Comorbidities).

For citation purposes, cite each article independently as indicated on the article page online and as indicated below:

LastName, A.A.; LastName, B.B.; LastName, C.C. Article Title. *Journal Name* **Year**, *Article Number*, Page Range.

ISBN 978-3-03936-668-2 (Pbk)
ISBN 978-3-03936-669-9 (PDF)

Cover image courtesy of Joachim Jankowski.

© 2021 by the authors. Articles in this book are Open Access and distributed under the Creative Commons Attribution (CC BY) license, which allows users to download, copy and build upon published articles, as long as the author and publisher are properly credited, which ensures maximum dissemination and a wider impact of our publications.

The book as a whole is distributed by MDPI under the terms and conditions of the Creative Commons license CC BY-NC-ND.

Contents

About the Special Issue Editors vii

Heidi Noels and Joachim Jankowski
Editorial on the Special Issue "Comorbidities in Chronic Kidney Disease"
Reprinted from: *Toxins* 2020, 12, 384, doi:10.3390/toxins12060384 1

Nadine Kaesler, Anne Babler, Jürgen Floege and Rafael Kramann
Cardiac Remodeling in Chronic Kidney Disease
Reprinted from: *Toxins* 2020, 12, 161, doi:10.3390/toxins12030161 6

Thomas Ebert, Sven-Christian Pawelzik, Anna Witasp, Samsul Arefin, Sam Hobson, Karolina Kublickiene, Paul G. Shiels, Magnus Bäck and Peter Stenvinkel
Inflammation and Premature Ageing in Chronic Kidney Disease
Reprinted from: *Toxins* 2020, 12, 227, doi:10.3390/toxins12040227 22

Britt Opdebeeck, Patrick C. D'Haese and Anja Verhulst
Molecular and Cellular Mechanisms that Induce Arterial Calcification by Indoxyl Sulfate and P-Cresyl Sulfate
Reprinted from: *Toxins* 2020, 12, 58, doi:10.3390/toxins12010058 43

Yu-Hsien Lai, Chih-Hsien Wang, Chiu-Huang Kuo, Yu-Li Lin, Jen-Pi Tsai and Bang-Gee Hsu
Serum P-Cresyl Sulfate Is a Predictor of Central Arterial Stiffness in Patients on Maintenance Hemodialysis
Reprinted from: *Toxins* 2020, 12, 10, doi:10.3390/toxins12010010 55

Anika Himmelsbach, Carina Ciliox and Claudia Goettsch
Cardiovascular Calcification in Chronic Kidney Disease—Therapeutic Opportunities
Reprinted from: *Toxins* 2020, 12, 181, doi:10.3390/toxins12030181 64

Merita Rroji, Andreja Figurek and Goce Spasovski
Should We Consider the Cardiovascular System While Evaluating CKD-MBD?
Reprinted from: *Toxins* 2020, 12, 140, doi:10.3390/toxins12030140 82

Juan Rafael Muñoz-Castañeda, Cristian Rodelo-Haad, Maria Victoria Pendon-Ruiz de Mier, Alejandro Martin-Malo, Rafael Santamaria and Mariano Rodriguez
Klotho/FGF23 and Wnt Signaling as Important Players in the Comorbidities Associated with Chronic Kidney Disease
Reprinted from: *Toxins* 2020, 12, 185, doi:10.3390/toxins12030185 105

Eduardo J. Duque, Rosilene M. Elias and Rosa M. A. Moysés
Parathyroid Hormone: A Uremic Toxin
Reprinted from: *Toxins* 2020, 12, 189, doi:10.3390/toxins12030189 122

Pieter Evenepoel, Sander Dejongh, Kristin Verbeke and Bjorn Meijers
The Role of Gut Dysbiosis in the Bone–Vascular Axis in Chronic Kidney Disease
Reprinted from: *Toxins* 2020, 12, 285, doi:10.3390/toxins12050285 138

Sol Carriazo, Adrián M Ramos, Ana B Sanz, Maria Dolores Sanchez-Niño, Mehmet Kanbay and Alberto Ortiz
Chronodisruption: A Poorly Recognized Feature of CKD
Reprinted from: *Toxins* 2020, 12, 151, doi:10.3390/toxins12030151 156

About the Special Issue Editors

Joachim Jankowski is Director of the Institute of Molecular Cardiovascular Research (IMCAR) at the University Hospital Aachen and RWTH Aachen University, Germany. This institute strives for scientific excellence in the field of cardiovascular diseases with a particular focus on patients with chronic renal insufficiency. Research is performed in close collaboration with the Cardiovascular Research Institute of the partner University of Maastricht (CARIM) in the Netherlands. Prof. Dr. Jankowski is the Speaker of the Transregional Collaborative Research Consortium SFB/TRR219 funded by the German Research Foundation (2018–2021). He is the Coordinator of the Marie Skłodowska-Curie International Training Network "CaReSyAn" (2018–2021).

Heidi Noels is leading the research group "Experimental Cardiovascular Pathophysiology" in the Institute of Molecular Cardiovascular Research (IMCAR) at the RWTH Aachen University, Germany. Her group is focusing on the identification and characterization of pathological mechanisms and mediators underlying cardiovascular and cardiorenal disease. Dr. Noels is Managing Director of the Transregional Collaborative Research Consortium SFB/TRR219 funded by the German Research Foundation (2018–2021) and Program Manager of the Marie Skłodowska-Curie International Training Network "CaReSyAn" (2018–2021).

This Special Issue was created in the context of the SFB/TRR219 Research Consortium funded by the German Research Foundation (Project-ID 322900939) and the European Union's Horizon 2020 research and innovation programme under the Marie Skłodowska-Curie grant agreement No 764474 (CaReSyAn).

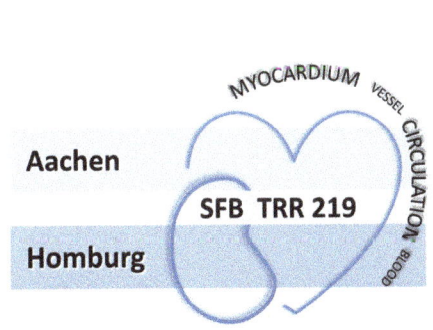

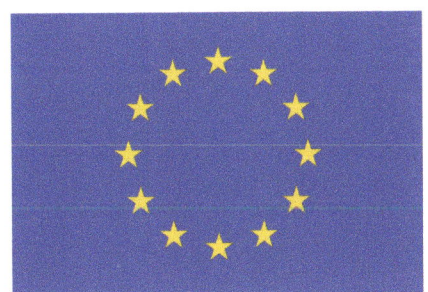

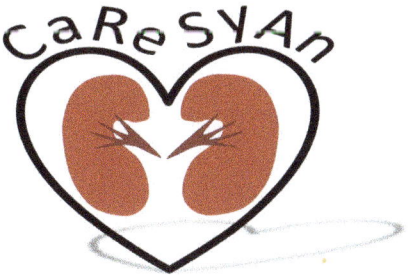

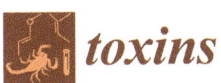

Editorial

Editorial on the Special Issue "Comorbidities in Chronic Kidney Disease"

Heidi Noels [1,*] **and Joachim Jankowski** [1,2,*]

1. Institute of Molecular Cardiovascular Research (IMCAR), RWTH Aachen, University Hospital Aachen, 52074 Aachen, Germany
2. Department of Pathology, Cardiovascular Research Institute Maastricht, Maastricht University Medical Centre, 6200 Maastricht, The Netherlands
* Correspondence: hnoels@ukaachen.de (H.N.); jjankowski@ukaachen.de (J.J.)

Received: 8 June 2020; Accepted: 9 June 2020; Published: 11 June 2020

Keywords: chronic kidney disease; cardiovascular; CKD–MBD; comorbidity; inflammation; fibrosis; calcification; senescence; uremic toxin

---

With a mean worldwide prevalence of 13.4% [1], chronic kidney disease (CKD) imposes a massive health burden on our society. In addition to a reduced kidney function, patients with CKD suffer increasingly from **cardiovascular disease** (CVD) [2–4], with CVD accounting for around half of the deaths of patients in CKD stages 4–5 [3]. In fact, CKD has been identified as an independent risk factor for CVD [5], but therapeutic options are highly inadequate. In addition to traditional cardiovascular risk factors, CKD-specific pathological mechanisms are expected to contribute to increased cardiovascular risk in this patient group, especially with progressing CKD [6–8]. However, detailed insights into the underlying pathophysiology of CKD-driven CVD largely remain to be unveiled [9,10].

Inflammation and **fibrosis** are increased in CKD patients [11–13], and the Chronic Renal Insufficiency Cohort (CRIC) study recently revealed that inflammation biomarkers are independently associated with atherosclerotic cardiovascular events and death in CKD patients [14]. Moreover, **vascular calcification** is highly prevalent in CKD patients, increases with declining kidney function [15] and is associated with increased risk of cardiovascular events and death in CKD [16–19]. As one aspect, **uremic retention solutes**, also referred to as uremic toxins, accumulate in the circulation of CKD patients due to a failing kidney filtration function [20]. Many of these solutes have been associated with pathophysiological effects, including inflammation, oxidative stress and calcification. As a consequence, they are expected to contribute to increased cardiovascular risk in CKD patients [21].

Furthermore, patients with CKD often present with enhanced bone demineralization along with extraosseous calcification, a condition clinically referred to as **CKD-mineral and bone disorder** (CKD–MBD). CKD–MBD highly coincides with increased vascular calcification and correlates with cardiovascular events, underlining the importance of identifying and characterizing CKD–MBD biomarkers as well as mediators of this pathological bone–vascular axis [22]. Moreover, patients with CKD present **disturbances of gut microbiota** [23], which too are expected to contribute to both reduced bone and cardiovascular health in CKD patients.

This Special Issue aims to provide insights into comorbidities in CKD patients with a main focus on increased cardiovascular risk and summarizes the current knowledge of underlying pathophysiological mechanisms.

1. Increased Cardiovascular Risk in CKD

Patients with CKD have an increased risk of atherosclerosis-related cardiovascular events, such as myocardial infarction and stroke [3,24]. However, with declining renal function, CKD patients are also becoming more prone to non-atherosclerotic cardiovascular events. Underlying cardiac remodeling involves left-ventricular hypertrophy, fibrosis and capillary rarefaction, and is often referred to as uremic cardiomyopathy. In this Special Issue, Kaesler et al. [25] provide detailed insights into cardiac remodeling in CKD and provide an update on the current knowledge of the cellular and molecular mechanisms of pathophysiological kidney–heart crosstalk in CKD patients. This includes alterations in relation to phosphate homeostasis, uremic toxins, growth factors, metabolic and oxidative stress, inflammation as well as fibrosis. Moreover, an overview of current mouse models to study cardiac remodeling in CKD is provided and potential therapeutic targets are being discussed in the context of current knowledge. This underlines the urgent need to further invest in closely studying the pathological crosstalk between kidney and heart in order to guide the development of effective therapies.

2. Inflammation and Vascular Calcification in CKD Impact on Cardiovascular Health

Chronic low-grade inflammation is a hallmark of CKD and is closely associated with cellular senescence and accelerated ageing. In this Special Issue, Ebert et al. [26] elaborate on this so-called "inflammageing" in CKD. They address the phenotype of inflammation and premature ageing in CKD patients as well as their mutual activation. Underlying cellular and molecular mechanisms are summarized with a focus on cellular senescence, uremic toxins, the phosphate–FGF23–Klotho axis and the CKD-mediated downregulation of NRF2 as a key transcription factor protecting from mitochondrial dysfunction and oxidative stress. Promising therapeutic candidates to reduce inflammageing in CKD are discussed.

Uremia and uremic toxins not only trigger inflammation, but also accelerate vascular calcification in CKD. This was recently shown for the protein-bound uremic toxins indoxyl sulfate and p-cresyl sulfate, with underlying cellular and molecular mechanisms discussed in detail in this Special Issue by Opdebeeck et al. [27]. Along this line, Lai. et al. [28] reveals within this Special Issue that p-cresyl sulfate is a predictor of arterial stiffness in patients on hemodialysis, with arterial stiffness known to be associated with increased cardiovascular risk and mortality in CKD patients [29,30].

Although vascular calcification has been associated with increased cardiovascular risk, there are currently no therapies available that adequately tackle this pathological axis. This is being discussed by Himmelsbach et al. [31]: a detailed overview of new potential therapeutic strategies to reduce cardiovascular calcification in CKD is provided, covering findings from in vitro molecular studies and animal models to observational and interventional studies in CKD patients.

3. CKD–MBD as a Major Complication in CKD Affects Cardiovascular Health

Vascular calcification and bone demineralization often coincide in CKD patients, which is often referred to as the bone–vascular axis or "calcification paradox". In this Special Issue, Rroji et al. [32] discuss the pathophysiology of CKD–MBD and its association with increased cardiovascular risk. Insights are provided for how vitamin D deficiency, secondary hyperparathyroidism and hyperphosphatemia, as classical CKD-MBD biomarkers, could impact cardiac remodeling in uremic cardiomyopathy. Furthermore, accumulating data supporting a role for FGF23, Klotho-deficiency and sclerostin as new CKD-MBD biomarkers in early cardiovascular risk assessment are discussed in detail, and a role beyond biomarker function and as mediators of cardiovascular risk in CKD is being elaborated on.

Muñoz-Castañeda et al. [33] further elaborate on the FGF23–Klotho axis, its regulation by the Wnt/β-catenin signaling pathway and vice versa. Starting from their deregulation in CKD, the impact of these axes on pathophysiological processes underlying CKD progression as well as cardiovascular disease and bone disorders are being discussed in detail.

Duque et al. [34] specifically focused on secondary hyperparathyroidism as a complication of CKD, with its causes as well as its impact on the bone–vascular axis being discussed. In extension, current literature in relation to a potential impact of secondary hyperparathyroidism on CKD progression, cardiac remodeling, muscle weakness as well as glucose metabolism is summarized.

Furthermore, with CKD patients presenting with gut dysbiosis, Evenepoel et al. [35] provide detailed insights into the increasing evidence that CKD-associated gut dysbiosis contributes to the pathophysiology of the bone-vascular axis. This may include pathophysiological processes such as increased exposure to protein fermentation metabolites, decreased systemic levels of specific short-chain fatty acids by reduced carbohydrate fermentation, vitamin K deficiency as well as a leaky gut triggering a pro-inflammatory environment in CKD.

4. Chronodisruption in CKD: Implications for Kidney and Cardiac Health?

Finally, the concept of chronodisruption as a chronic disturbance of circadian rhythms with a negative impact on health is being discussed in the context of CKD. **Carriazo et al**. [36] review current evidence for chronodisruption in CKD as well as its potential impact on kidney and cardiac pathology. Among others, diet, inflammatory factors and uremic toxins are being discussed as potential chronodisrupters in CKD, and the main challenges and open questions regarding the underlying mechanisms, implications for kidney–cardiac health, as well as therapeutic opportunities are summarized.

5. Conclusions

Altogether, this Special Issue summarizes current knowledge on the pathophysiological mechanisms underlying the development of comorbidities in CKD, with a main focus on CVD. This reveals the urgent need to further invest efforts in uncovering CKD-specific cardiovascular pathological mechanisms and mediators of disease in order to pave the way for new therapeutic strategies, tailored specifically to the CKD patient.

Author Contributions: All authors listed have made substantial, direct and intellectual contribution to the work, and approved it for publication. All authors have read and agreed to the published version of the manuscript.

Funding: This work and associated APC were funded by the German Research Foundation (DFG) SFB/TRR219 (S-03, C-04, M-05), Project-ID 403224013-SFB 1382 (A-04), by the CORONA foundation, the Interreg V-A EMR program (EURLIPIDS, EMR23) and by a grant from the Interdisciplinary Centre for Clinical Research within the faculty of Medicine at the RWTH Aachen University (project E8-3). In addition, this work has received funding from the European Union's Horizon 2020 research and innovation program under the Marie Skłodowska-Curie grant agreement No 764474 (CaReSyAn).

Acknowledgments: We thank all scientists who contributed to this Special Issue.

Conflicts of Interest: The authors declare that this work was conducted in the absence of any commercial or financial relationships that could present a potential conflict of interest.

References

1. Hill, N.R.; Fatoba, S.T.; Oke, J.L.; Hirst, J.A.; O'Callaghan, C.A.; Lasserson, D.S.; Hobbs, F.R. Global prevalence of chronic kidney disease—A systematic review and meta-analysis. *PLoS ONE* **2016**, *11*, e0158765. [CrossRef] [PubMed]
2. Gansevoort, R.; Correa-Rotter, R.; Hemmelgarn, B.; Jafar, T.H.; Heerspink, H.J.L.; Mann, J.F.; Matsushita, K.; Wen, C.P. Chronic kidney disease and cardiovascular risk: Epidemiology, mechanisms, and prevention. *Lancet (Lond. Engl.)* **2013**, *382*, 339–352. [CrossRef]
3. Thompson, S.; James, M.; Wiebe, N.; Hemmelgarn, B.; Manns, B.; Klarenbach, S.; Tonelli, M. Cause of death in patients with reduced kidney function. *J. Am. Soc. Nephrol.* **2015**, *26*, 25042–25511. [CrossRef] [PubMed]
4. Valholder, R.; Massy, Z.; Argiles, A.; Spasovski, G.; Verbeke, F.; Lameire, N. Chronic kidney disease as cause of cardiovascular morbidity and mortality. *Nephrol. Dial. Transplant. Off. Publ. Eur. Dial. Transpl. Assoc. Eur. Ren. Assoc.* **2005**, *20*, 1048–1056. [CrossRef]
5. Tonelli, M.; Muntner, P.; Lloyd, A.; Manns, B.; Klarenbach, S.; Pannu, N.; James, M.T.; Hemmelgarn, B.R. Risk of coronary events in people with chronic kidney disease compared with those with diabetes: A population-level cohort study. *Lancet (Lond. Engl.)* **2012**, *380*, 807–814. [CrossRef]
6. Fleischmann, E.H.; Bower, J.D.; Salahudeen, A.K. Are conventional cardiovascular risk factors predictive of two-year mortality in hemodialysis patients? *Clin. Nephrol.* **2001**, *56*, 2212–2230.

7. Alani, H.; Tamimi, A.; Tamimi, N. Cardiovascular co-morbidity in chronic kidney disease: Current knowledge and future research needs. *World J. Nephrol.* **2014**, *3*, 1561–1568. [CrossRef]
8. Ortiz, A.; Covic, A.; Fliser, D.; Fouque, D.; Goldsmith, D.; Kanbay, M.; Mallamaci, F.; Massy, Z.A.; Rossignol, P.; Vanholder, R.; et al. Epidemiology, contributors to, and clinical trials of mortality risk in chronic kidney failure. *Lancet (Lond. Engl.)* **2014**, *383*, 18311–18843. [CrossRef]
9. Marx, N.; Noels, H.; Jankowski, J.; Floege, J.; Fliser, D.; Böhm, M. Mechanisms of cardiovascular complications in chronic kidney disease: Research focus of the transregional research consortium SFB TRR219 of the University Hospital Aachen (RWTH) and the Saarland University. *Clin. Res. Cardiol. Off. J. Ger. Card. Soc.* **2018**, *107*, 1201–1226. [CrossRef] [PubMed]
10. Noels, H.; Boor, P.; Goettsch, C.; Hohl, M.; Jahnen-Dechent, W.; Jankowski, V.; Kindermann, I.; Kramann, R.; Lehrke, M.; Linz, D.; et al. The new SFB/TRR219 research centre. *Eur. Heart J.* **2018**, *39*, 9759–9777. [CrossRef] [PubMed]
11. Zoccali, C.; Vanholder, R.; Massy, Z.A.; Ortiz, A.; Sarafidis, P.; Dekker, F.J.; Fliser, D.; Fouque, D.; Heine, G.H.; on behalf of the European Renal and Cardiovascular Medicine (EURECA-m) Working Group of the European Renal Association—European Dialysis Transplantation Association (ERA-EDTA); et al. The systemic nature of CKD. *Nat. Rev. Nephrol.* **2017**, *13*, 3443–3458. [CrossRef]
12. Stenvinkel, P.; Wanner, C.; Metzger, T.; Heimbürger, O.; Mallamaci, F.; Tripepi, G.; Malatino, L.; Zoccali, C. Inflammation and outcome in end-stage renal failure: Does female gender constitute a survival advantage? *Kidney Int.* **2002**, *62*, 1791–1798. [CrossRef] [PubMed]
13. Ruiz-Ortega, M.; Rayego-Mateos, S.; Lamas, S.; Ortiz, A.; Rodrigues-Diez, R.R. Targeting the progression of chronic kidney disease. *Nat. Rev. Nephrol.* **2020**, *16*, 269–288. [CrossRef] [PubMed]
14. Amdur, R.L.; Feldman, H.I.; Dominic, E.A.; Anderson, A.H.; Beddhu, S.; Rahman, M.; Wolf, M.; Reilly, M.; Ojo, A.; Townsend, R.R.; et al. Use of measures of inflammation and kidney function for prediction of atherosclerotic vascular disease events and death in patients with CKD: Findings from the CRIC study. *Am. J. Kidney Dis. Off. J. Natl. Kidney Found.* **2019**, *73*, 3443–3453. [CrossRef] [PubMed]
15. Budoff, M.J.; Rader, D.J.; Reilly, M.P.; Mohler, E.R.; Lash, J.; Yang, W.; Rosen, L.; Glenn, M.; Teal, V.; Feldman, H.I.; et al. Relationship of estimated GFR and coronary artery calcification in the CRIC (Chronic Renal Insufficiency Cohort) study. *Am. J. Kidney Dis. Off. J. Natl. Kidney Found.* **2011**, *58*, 519–526. [CrossRef]
16. Raggi, P. Cardiovascular disease: Coronary artery calcification predicts risk of CVD in patients with CKD. *Nat. Rev. Nephrol.* **2017**, *13*, 324–326. [CrossRef]
17. Schlieper, G.; Schurgers, L.; Brandenburg, V.; Reutelingsperger, C.; Floege, J. Vascular calcification in chronic kidney disease: An update. *Nephrol. Dial. Transpl.* **2016**, *31*, 313–319. [CrossRef]
18. Okuno, S.; Ishimura, E.; Kitatani, K.; Fujino, Y.; Kohno, K.; Maeno, Y.; Maekawa, K.; Yamakawa, T.; Imanishi, Y.; Inaba, M.; et al. Presence of abdominal aortic calcification is significantly associated with all-cause and cardiovascular mortality in maintenance hemodialysis patients. *Am. J. Kidney Dis. Off. J. Natl. Kidney Found.* **2017**, *49*, 417–425. [CrossRef]
19. Claes, K.; Heye, S.; Bammens, B.; Kuypers, D.; Meijers, B.K.; Naesens, M.; Vanrenterghem, Y.; Evenepoel, P. Aortic calcifications and arterial stiffness as predictors of cardiovascular events in incident renal transplant recipients. *Transpl. Int. Off. J. Eur. Soc. Organ Transplant.* **2013**, *26*, 9739–9781. [CrossRef]
20. Vanholder, R.; de Smet, R.; Glorieux, G.; Argilés, A.; Baurmeister, U.; Brunet, P.; Clark, W.; Cohen, G.; De Deyn, P.P.; for the European Uremic Toxin Work Group (EUTox); et al. Review on uremic toxins: Classification, concentration, and interindividual variability. *Kidney Int.* **2003**, *63*, 19341–19943. [CrossRef]
21. Lekawanvijit, S. Cardiotoxicity of uremic toxins: A driver of cardiorenal syndrome. *Toxins* **2018**, *10*, 352. [CrossRef] [PubMed]
22. Covic, A.; Vervloet, M.; Massy, Z.A.; Torres, P.U.; Goldsmith, D.; Brandenburg, V.M.; Mazzaferro, S.; Evenepoel, P.; Bover, J.; Apetrii, M.; et al. Bone and mineral disorders in chronic kidney disease: Implications for cardiovascular health and ageing in the general population. *Lancet Diabetes Endocrinol.* **2018**, *6*, 319–331. [CrossRef]
23. Vaziri, N.; Wong, J.; Pahl, M.; Piceno, Y.; Yuan, J.; DeSantis, T.Z.; Ni, Z.; Nguyen, T.-H.; Andersen, G. Chronic kidney disease alters intestinal microbial flora. *Kidney Int.* **2013**, *83*, 308–315. [CrossRef] [PubMed]
24. Lindner, A.; Charra, B.; Sherrard, D.J.; Scribner, B.H. Accelerated atherosclerosis in prolonged maintenance hemodialysis. *N. Engl. J. Med.* **1974**, *290*, 697–701. [CrossRef] [PubMed]

25. Kaesler, N.; Babler, A.; Floege, J.; Kramann, R. Cardiac remodeling in chronic kidney disease. *Toxins* **2020**, *12*, 161. [CrossRef]
26. Ebert, T.; Pawelzik, S.-C.; Witasp, A.; Arefin, S.; Hobson, S.; Kublickiene, K.; Shiels, P.; Bäck, M.; Stenvinkel, P. Inflammation and premature ageing in chronic kidney disease. *Toxins* **2020**, *12*, 227. [CrossRef]
27. Opdebeeck, B.; D'Haese, P.C.; Verhulst, A. Molecular and cellular mechanisms that induce arterial calcification by indoxyl sulfate and P-cresyl sulfate. *Toxins* **2020**, *12*, 58. [CrossRef]
28. Lai, Y.-H.; Wang, C.-H.; Kuo, C.-H.; Lin, Y.-L.; Tsai, J.-P.; Hsu, B.-G. Serum P-cresyl sulfate is a predictor of central arterial stiffness in patients on maintenance hemodialysis. *Toxins* **2019**, *12*, 10. [CrossRef]
29. Blacher, J.; Guerin, A.; Pannier, B.; Marchais, S.J.; Safar, M.E.; London, G.M. Impact of aortic stiffness on survival in end-stage renal disease. *Circulation* **1999**, *99*, 24342–24439. [CrossRef]
30. Vlachopoulos, C.; Aznaouridis, K.; Stefanadis, C. Prediction of cardiovascular events and all-cause mortality with arterial stiffness: A systematic review and meta-analysis. *J. Am. Coll. Cardiol.* **2010**, *55*, 13181–13327. [CrossRef]
31. Himmelsbach, A.; Ciliox, C.; Goettsch, C. Cardiovascular calcification in chronic kidney disease-therapeutic opportunities. *Toxins* **2020**, *12*, 181. [CrossRef] [PubMed]
32. Rroji, M.; Figurek, A.; Spasovski, G. Should we consider the cardiovascular system while evaluating CKD-MBD? *Toxins* **2020**, *12*, 140. [CrossRef] [PubMed]
33. Muñoz-Castañeda, J.R.; Rodelo-Haad, C.; De Mier, M.V.P.-R.; Martin-Malo, A.; Santamaria, R.; Rodríguez, M. Klotho/FGF23 and wnt signaling as important players in the comorbidities associated with chronic kidney disease. *Toxins* **2020**, *12*, 185. [CrossRef]
34. Duque, E.J.; Elias, R.M.; Moysés, R.M.A. Parathyroid hormone: A uremic toxin. *Toxins* **2020**, *12*, 189. [CrossRef]
35. Evenepoel, P.; Dejongh, S.; Verbeke, K.; Meijers, B. The role of gut dysbiosis in the bone-vascular axis in chronic kidney disease. *Toxins* **2020**, *12*, 285. [CrossRef]
36. Carriazo, S.; Ramos, A.; Sanz, A.; Sanchez-Niño, M.D.; Kanbay, M.; Ortiz, A. Chronodisruption: A poorly recognized feature of CKD. *Toxins* **2020**, *12*, 151. [CrossRef] [PubMed]

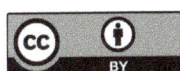

© 2020 by the authors. Licensee MDPI, Basel, Switzerland. This article is an open access article distributed under the terms and conditions of the Creative Commons Attribution (CC BY) license (http://creativecommons.org/licenses/by/4.0/).

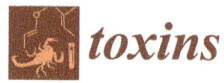

Review

Cardiac Remodeling in Chronic Kidney Disease

Nadine Kaesler [1,†], Anne Babler [1,†], Jürgen Floege [1] and Rafael Kramann [1,2,*]

1. Clinic for Renal and Hypertensive Disorders, Rheumatological and Immunological Disease, University Hospital of the RWTH Aachen, 52074 Aachen, Germany; nkaesler@ukaachen.de (N.K.); ababler@ukaachen.de (A.B.); jfloege@ukaachen.de (J.F.)
2. Department of Internal Medicine, Nephrology and Transplantation, Erasmus Medical Center, 3015 GD Rotterdam, The Netherlands
* Correspondence: rkramann@gmx.net
† These authors contributed equally.

Received: 17 February 2020; Accepted: 3 March 2020; Published: 5 March 2020

Abstract: Cardiac remodeling occurs frequently in chronic kidney disease patients and affects quality of life and survival. Current treatment options are highly inadequate. As kidney function declines, numerous metabolic pathways are disturbed. Kidney and heart functions are highly connected by organ crosstalk. Among others, altered volume and pressure status, ischemia, accelerated atherosclerosis and arteriosclerosis, disturbed mineral metabolism, renal anemia, activation of the renin-angiotensin system, uremic toxins, oxidative stress and upregulation of cytokines stress the sensitive interplay between different cardiac cell types. The fatal consequences are left-ventricular hypertrophy, fibrosis and capillary rarefaction, which lead to systolic and/or diastolic left-ventricular failure. Furthermore, fibrosis triggers electric instability and sudden cardiac death. This review focuses on established and potential pathophysiological cardiorenal crosstalk mechanisms that drive uremia-induced senescence and disease progression, including potential known targets and animal models that might help us to better understand the disease and to identify novel therapeutics.

Keywords: uremia; uremic cardiomyopathy; organ crosstalk; cardiorenal syndrome; chronic kidney disease; left-ventricular hypertrophy; heart failure; cardiac fibrosis

Key Contribution: Here, we provide a most recent overview on the proposed mechanisms in organ crosstalk from kidney disease to myocardium, underlying cellular mechanisms and available mouse models. We thereby aim to offer potential therapeutic target sites in this understudied disease condition.

---

1. Chronic Kidney Disease

Chronic kidney disease (CKD) affects an increasing number of patients worldwide and is associated with dramatically increased morbidity and mortality [1,2]. Recent data suggest that CKD currently affects more than 10% of the population in the developed world [3,4].

Diabetes mellitus and high blood pressure are among the most prevalent risk factors for the development of CKD and are responsible for the majority of cases. Other conditions that affect the kidneys are glomerulonephritis, the third most common type of kidney disease, inherited diseases, such as polycystic kidney disease, and loss of renal tissue due to infections, malformations or urinary tract obstruction. Repeated episodes of acute kidney injury and certain therapeutics, such as non-steroidal anti-inflammatory drugs (NSAIDs) can also contribute to CKD [2].

In end-stage renal failure, dialysis and subsequent kidney transplantation are the only available treatment options apart from palliative care. However, not all patients qualify for kidney transplantation and transplant waiting times are often long. Thus, patients usually undergo many years of dialysis treatment. Longstanding uremia in turn promotes cardiovascular disease. Consequently, the leading causes of death in dialysis patients are sudden cardiac death and recurrent heart failure due to cardiac and vascular remodeling [5].

Cellular Crosstalk in the Heart

The mammalian heart is a highly interactive complex of cardiac muscle cells, extracellular matrix (ECM) and vessels. Other essential cell types include endothelial cells, fibroblasts, vascular smooth muscle cells and perivascular cells [6,7]. Studies, using state-of-the-art methods such as single-cell transcriptomics, suggest that all cardiac cell types communicate vigorously with one another in homeostasis and disease [8–10]. Each cardiomyocyte is in physical contact with at least one capillary, allowing mechanical and paracrine crosstalk between at least four key cell types, namely, cardiomyocytes, endothelial cells, vascular smooth muscle cells (VSMCs) and pericytes/fibroblasts [11]. Cardiomyocytes crosstalk with endothelial cells and fibroblasts by secreting various specific growth factors [7]. Various lines of evidence suggest that endothelial cells crosstalk with cardiomyocytes and are key players in angiogenesis and vasomotor tone control by secreting angiocrine factors such as nitric oxide or endothelin-1 [12]. One example of paracrine intercellular crosstalk inside the myocardium is vasomotion. Endothelial cells are directly exposed to shear stress, contrary to VSMCs. To facilitate vasomotion, endothelial cells release nitric oxide in response to shear stress, thus signaling to the VSMCs to dilate. The cardiac morphology and function can be affected by further external and internal stimuli.

2. Pathology and Pathophysiology of the Cardiorenal Syndrome

Kidney and cardiac health are highly linked to each other, with diseases of either organ affecting the other organ. In the following, we aim to give an overview of the mechanisms and relevant factors that have been reported to be involved in cardiac remodeling due to kidney injury, i.e., cardiorenal syndrome.

The presence of CKD and end-stage renal disease (ESRD) leads to cardiac remodeling with hypertrophy, fibrosis and capillary loss [13]. Uremic cardiomyopathy affects about 80% of hemodialysis patients [14] and is the main cause of death in this cohort. A similar prevalence has even been reported in pediatric uremic patients [15] who presumably lack traditional atherosclerotic risk factors. The comorbidities in CKD patients that contribute to cardiovascular remodeling are atherosclerosis, hyperlipidemia, diabetes and/or hypertension, but also include a plethora of so-called non-traditional cardiovascular risk factors such as those discussed below and summarized in Table 1. These stimuli exacerbate the pathophysiological cardiac changes, including left-ventricular hypertrophy (LVH), diffuse interstitial fibrosis and capillary rarefaction leading to systolic and diastolic dysfunction. In this review, we consider these cardiac abnormalities that frequently occur in patients with CKD as uremic cardiomyopathy.

2.1. Left-Ventricular Hypertrophy in CKD

LVH is an independent predictor of cardiac death in dialysis patients. LVH can occur early in the course of CKD, even when the glomerular filtration rate (GFR) is still normal [16]. Once GFR is reduced, myocytes enlarge and cardiomyocytes expand, leading to LVH [17]. Cardiomyocytes are the major cell type, comprising about 70–85% of the total volume. They generate contractility by cyclic calcium fluxes [17,18]. Fibroblasts secrete collagen precursors and matrix metalloproteinases (MMPs) and thereby actively remodel the ECM [17–19]. The ECM embeds the myocytes and non-myocytes. Collagen is the most abundant protein here [19]. These structural changes are closely related to a functional impairment of the left ventricle causing diastolic dysfunction [20] while systolic function may, at least initially, remain normal [21]. LVH can be a consequence of increased preload due to hypervolemia or increased afterload due to increased peripheral resistance or hypertension, which are both very common in CKD. Further factors involved in the pathogenesis of LVH might be high cardiac output due to anemia or large arteriovenous fistulas for dialysis access [18,21].

2.2. Cardiac Fibrosis

In CKD patients, myocardial fibrosis is a pathologic process that occurs together with LVH. One hallmark of myocardial fibrosis is a marked increase in the production of extracellular matrix, especially collagens, which impair diastolic filling due to increased stiffness of the left ventricle, but they may also affect systolic function since functional myocytes are replaced by fibrotic scar tissue [22,23].

The main causes of myocardial fibrosis are hemodynamic alterations and disturbed secretion of various systemic soluble factors. A primary factor leading to myocardial fibrosis in CKD patients is hypertension, which is mainly associated with pressure overload. Factors related to hemodynamic alterations in CKD patients like senescence, ischemia, catecholamines, angiotensin II and aldosterone further promote the development of cardiac fibrosis [21]. Arterial stiffening is accelerated in the presence of CKD and is caused by a loss of elastic fibers and vascular calcification [24]. Increased vascular stiffness leads to increased cardiac afterload, which promotes cardiac hypertrophy and fibrosis [21,25].

However, during CKD progression, left ventricular remodeling has been found to occur even earlier than changes in large arteries [26]. This might be explained by a range of factors and mechanisms including uremic toxins, TGF-β and other growth factors. In addition to the role of hemodynamic changes in the development of cardiac fibrosis, non-hemodynamic factors related to the uremic milieu, such as overactivity of the renin-angiotensin-aldosterone system, FGF-23, parathyroid hormone, endothelin, increased sympathetic nerve discharge and increased plasma catecholamines might also play an important role [21,27].

Perivascular mesenchymal cells surround the VSMC layer in the so-called adventitia of larger arteries but are also present as pericytes around the vasa vasorum and in direct contact with endothelial cells of both the large arteries and micro-vessels. They play a role in vasomotion, homeostasis and permeability of the vasculature [11]. The heterogeneity of perivascular cells has been unclear for many years, but recent single-cell RNA-sequencing data suggest that various, previously unknown, perivascular mesenchymal populations exist [28,29]. We have reported that Gli1 marks a specific perivascular cell type that drives cardiac fibrosis and vascular calcification [30,31]. Gli1+ cells are a subset of cardiac interstitial PDGFRβ+ cells, but are mostly distinct from cardiac NG2+ pericytes [31]. However, the complex system of the cardiac perivascular cell types remains unclear, and single-cell experiments are needed to shed light on their heterogeneity and the role they play in homeostasis and disease.

2.3. Capillary Rarefaction

Endothelial cells line blood or lymphatic vessels and are the most abundant cells of the non-myocyte fraction in murine hearts [6,7]. The medial layer of small and large vessels consists of vascular smooth muscle cells (VSMCs). Endothelial dysfunction is frequent in CKD [32] and can be considered an early manifestation of coronary vascular disease [33]. Endothelial dysfunction leads to disturbed microcirculation and is considered an independent risk factor for cardiovascular events [33,34]. CKD-induced microangiopathy has been shown to lead to tissue hypoxia and dysfunctional angiogenesis [33].

2.4. Oxidative Stress

Oxidative stress in CKD results from an imbalance in reactive oxygen species production and impaired antioxidant defense [35]. Various oxidation products have been shown to be overabundant in CKD. Increased ROS production has been reported to contribute to myocardial hypertrophy and fibrosis by lipid peroxidation, proinflammatory cytokines and DNA damage [35,36]. A marker of oxidative stress, 8-isoprostane, increases as CKD progresses [37]. Furthermore, NADPH oxidase generates reactive oxygen species, and this in turn leads to endothelial dysfunction [38]. Another effect of elevated oxidative stress is the oxidation of plasma proteins, which causes activation of phagocytes and increases inflammation [39]. Advanced oxidation protein products promote cardiomyocyte apoptosis. This process is mediated by upregulation of c-Jun N-terminal kinase (JNK) signaling and enhanced endoplasmic reticulum stress [40].

2.5. Inflammation

CKD can be seen as a state of increased systemic inflammation with various cytokines being among the recognized uremic toxins. The Chronic Renal Insufficiency Cohort Study (CRIC) study found that elevated plasma levels of high-sensitivity C-reactive protein (hs-CRP) and IL-6 were associated with LVH and systolic dysfunction in CKD patients [41]. Freise et al. stated that, amongst others, inflammatory processes involving tumor necrosis factor (TNF) and IL-10 impact pathobiological responses in arteries from children with CKD, and are thus associated with tissue remodeling and cardiovascular disease [42]. Furthermore, CKD patients develop endotoxemia, characterized by elevated levels of endotoxin, IL-6, CRP and lipopolysaccharide-binding protein (LBP), which contributes to chronic inflammation and has been associated with higher left-ventricular mass index (LVMI) and subsequently left-ventricular dysfunction [43]. Most of the soluble factors mentioned here are described as being secreted by cells of the heart (cardiomyocytes, endothelial cells, fibroblasts, VSMCs and pericytes) but also resident immune cells (e.g., macrophages, dendritic cells) and/or circulating cells might contribute to this. Thus, the contribution of inflammatory cells to the described mechanisms cannot be excluded.

2.6. Advanced Glycation end Products

The soluble receptor for advanced glycation end-products (sRAGE) seems to play an important role in cardiac remodeling in CKD patients. sRAGE has been described as a prognostic factor for mortality in diabetic dialysis patients [43,44]. Elevated sRAGE concentrations could represent a protective mechanism against the increased risk of cardiovascular complications resulting from AGEs and inflammation, although the underlying mechanisms need to be further confirmed [45]. It has also been shown that AGEs are involved in the upregulation of fibroblast growth factor 23 (FGF23).

In addition, cardiomyocytic FGF23 expression has been shown to be induced by activated renin-angiotensin aldosterone system (RAAS) [46]. In turn, FGF23-mediated activation of local RAAS in the heart promotes cardiac hypertrophy and fibrosis [47]. This finding underlines the organ crosstalk between the kidney and heart in CKD-CVD.

2.7. Growth Factors

In addition to the above-mentioned metabolic and inflammatory pathways, several growth factors might play important roles in cardiac fibrosis in CKD. One of the profibrotic modulators that stimulates fibroblast proliferation is FGF2. FGF2 binds to FGF-receptor (FGFR) 1, which is expressed in human cardiomyocytes. Additionally, FGF2 has been shown to promote growth of isolated cardiomyocytes [47,48] and cardiac hypertrophy in rats following myocardial infarction [49], thus further contributing to the cardiac phenotype in the cardiorenal syndrome. Another important growth factor-based mechanism of cardiac fibrosis development was found by analyzing human heart specimens. A marked reduction in cardiac Klotho, often found in CKD patients, was associated with increased TGF-β signaling. This in turn upregulated Wnt signaling, a major pathway in fibrosis. This was confirmed by in vitro studies with cardiomyocytes, where upregulation of endogenous Klotho inhibited Wnt/β-catenin signaling [50].

2.8. FGF23

FGF23 is a phosphaturic hormone primarily secreted by osteocytes. Its main actions are maintaining phosphate and mineral homeostasis. Furthermore, FGF23 decreases the synthesis of calcitriol. Its level rises early and dramatically with the decline of kidney function [51]. FGF23 has effects on various organs. Numerous studies have shown a correlation between serum FGF23 and cardiac alterations in CKD patients [52–58]. FGF23 directly induces LVH independent of preserved or reduced renal function; this has been shown in vitro in cultured cardiomyocytes and by in vivo studies in mice, as well as by correlations of circulating FGF23 levels with LVH in CKD patients [55]. FGF23 stimulates pro-fibrotic and pro-hypertrophic factors in cardiomyocytes and induces fibrosis-related pathways in fibroblasts [55,59,60]. In addition to its direct effects on cardiac remodeling, FGF23 has also been shown to increase blood pressure [61], inflammation [62] and CKD progression itself [63], and may thus promote the development of LVH also by indirect mechanisms. FGF23 signaling in the liver causes production of inflammatory cytokines. In the bone, FGF23 inhibits mineralization, leading to increased circulating phosphorus levels while reducing the production of erythropoietin (EPO) in the bone marrow [64]. All of the above-mentioned actions affect the outcome of CKD patients, and thus directly or indirectly lead to progression of cardiovascular disease.

2.9. Klotho

Membrane-bound Klotho serves as a co-receptor for FGF23 signaling and is synthesized in the kidney and bone. Soluble Klotho shows endocrine actions correlated with anti-aging effects [65]. Soluble Klotho levels are decreased in CKD [65]. Using Klotho-deficient mice, it could be shown that the Klotho-FGF23 axis plays a key role in pathologic cardiac remodeling in CKD, but also in phosphotoxicity and aging [66]. In pediatric CKD patients, serum FGF23 levels increased and Klotho levels decreased with progressing renal failure, while phosphorus levels were maintained in the normal range [67]. In those patients, high FGF23 and low Klotho levels were strongly associated with impaired left ventricular diastolic function [67]. In addition to this finding, FGF23 signaling via fibroblast growth factor receptor 4 (FGFR4) activates the phospholipase Cγ/calcineurin/nuclear factor of the activated T-cell pathway, and thus promotes cardiac myocyte hypertrophy, independent of its co-receptor Klotho [60,67]. Furthermore, FGFR4 signaling is responsible for FGF23-mediated increased cardiac contractility [68]. Correspondingly, aging mice lacking FGFR4 were protected from LVH. Thus, FGF23/FGFR4 signaling plays an important role in the regulation of cardiac remodeling and function [68]. Additionally, pharmacological blockade of the FGF receptor improved cardiac structure and function in 5/6 nephrectomy rats, thus underlining the role of FGFR activation as a mechanism of LVH in CKD [59].

2.10. Uremic Toxins

The role of uremic toxins in the development of cardiac remodeling is less well established. Recent work sheds light on the potential roles of asymmetric dimethylarginine (ADMA), advanced glycation end-products (AGE), trimethylamine N-oxide (TMAO) and indoxyl sulfate [69]. ADMA has been reported to be involved in regulation of nitric oxide, reactive oxygen species and renal anemia [69,70]. The AGE/RAGE axis is responsible for cell damage in CVD [69], driving cardiac fibrosis. TMAO, a metabolite derived from choline, is linked with left-ventricular diastolic dysfunction [71] and cardiac fibrosis [69].

In addition, several other uremic toxins are also thought to promote the cardiorenal syndrome by direct cardiotoxicity, including indoxyl sulfate and p-cresyl sulfate [71,72]. Indoxyl sulfate is a product of the intestinal catabolism of tryptophan with insufficient dialytic removal, as it is bound to albumin in the blood. In uremia, it increases up to 88-fold [73] and has been shown to mediate immune dysfunction and cytotoxic effects on endothelial cells in patients with end-stage renal disease [74]. Indoxyl sulfate stimulates the cannabinoid receptor type 1 and was associated with fibrotic effects via modulation of Akt signaling in myofibroblasts [75].

Table 1. Some systemic factors that have been reported to be involved in uremic cardiomyopathy.

	Factor	References
Phosphate Homeostasis		
	FGF23/Klotho	[46,47,50,52–60,67,68,76]
	Vit D receptor agonists	[77,78]
Uremic Toxins		
	p-Cresylsulfate	[72]
	Indoxylsulfate	[72,75]
	ADMA	[69,70]
Growth Factors		
	TGF-β	[50]
	FGF2	[48,49]
	EPO	[64,79,80]
Metabolic Stress		
	AGE	[44,45,69]
	ROS	[36,38,40,81–83]
	PPARα	[84]
	TMAO	[69,71]
Inflammation		
	S100/calgranulin	[85,86]
	Interleukin 6	[43]
	Interleukin 10	[42]
	CRP	[41]
	TNF	[42]

Several studies have pointed towards a role of uremic toxins in cardiac remodeling, however, the complex mechanisms of cell-type activation that drive cardiac fibrosis, hypertrophy and capillary loss are still unclear. Further studies using state-of-the-art single-cell technologies may shed more light on this important disease that affects numerous CKD/ESRD patients.

3. Mouse Models of Cardiac Remodeling in CKD

To date, most animal studies investigating mechanisms and interventions in the cardiorenal syndrome have been performed in rats. The models employed (5/6 nephrectomy, adenine nephropathy, ischemia reperfusion injury, etc.) are well established and cause reliable cardiac remodeling. However, mouse models do offer some advantages, the most important of which is the possibility of generating genetic modifications, which enable the analysis of specific pathways and molecular mechanisms. Thus, improving mouse models of CKD-CVD is one important goal in order to clarify the pathogenesis of the cardiorenal syndrome and develop novel therapies for patients. Several attempts have been made to establish CKD-CVD in mice. They can be divided into three approaches: surgical interventions, chemical interventions and genetic interventions. Table 2 summarizes the kidney parameters and functional and structural cardiac parameters of murine CKD-CVD studies.

Table 2. Functional and structural cardiac parameters in mouse models of chronic kidney disease (CKD). GFR—glomerular filtration rate, sCr—serum creatinine, BUN—blood urea nitrogen, EF—ejection fraction, FS—fractional shortening, SV—stroke volume, CO—cardiac output, BP—blood pressure, LVH—left-ventricular hypertrophy, Nx—nephrectomy, AT1—angiotensin II type-1A receptor, UUO—unilateral ureteral obstruction, hBAC-S100—bacterial artificial chromosome of the human S100/calgranulin gene cluster, Col4a3—collagen type IV alpha 3 chain, n.d.—not determined, wk—week.

Model	Mouse Strain	Duration (Weeks)	Kidney				Heart (Functional)					Heart (Structural)		References
			GFR	sCr	BUN	EF/FS	SV/CO	BP	LVH		Fibrosis	Capillary Loss	
surgically induced														
5/6 Nx (2-step)	C57BL/6	8	n.d.	↑	↑	-	↓	n.d.	↑		↑	n.d.	[75]
5/6 Nx (2-step)	C57BL/6	12	n.d.	↑	↑	↓	n.d.	n.d.	↑		↑	↑	[87]
AT1 knockout, 5/6 Nx (2-step)	C57BL/7	12	n.d.	↑	↑	↓	n.d.	n.d.	↑		↑	-	[87]
5/6 Nx (2-step)	C57BL/6	12	n.d.	↑	↑	↓	n.d.	-	↑		↑	↑	[79]
5/6 Nx (2-step)	129X1/SvJ	16	n.d.	n.d.	↑	-	n.d.	↑	↑		↑	n.d.	[88]
5/6 Nx (2-step, pole ligation)	C57BL/6	4	n.d.	↑	↑	n.d.	n.d.	n.d.	↑		↑	n.d.	[89]
5/6Nx (1-step)	BALB/c	8, 16 and 24	n.d.	n.d.	↑ (8, 16, 24 wk)	↓ (24 wk)	n.d.	↑ (16, 24 wk)	n.d.		↑ (24 wk)	n.d.	[90]
5/6Nx (1-step)	CD1	4, 6 and 8	n.d.	n.d.	n.d.	↑	n.d.	↑	↑		↑	n.d.	[91]
UUO	C57BL/6	3	n.d.	↑	↑	-	n.d.	↑	↑		↑	-	[92]
hBAC-S100, UO	C57BL/6	10	n.d.	n.d.	↑	-	n.d.	↑	↑		n.d.	n.d.	[85]
	129sv	10	↓	↑	↑	↓	↓	↑	-		↑	n.d.	
chemically induced														
0.15% adenine	C57BL/6	20	↓	↑	↑	↓	n.d.	n.d.	↑		↑	n.d.	[86]
10 mg/kg cisplatin + high phosphate diet	129sv	20	↓	↑	↑	n.d.	n.d.	n.d.	↑		↑	n.d.	[93]
genetically induced														
Col4a3 knockout	C57BL/6	10 and 20	↓	↑	↑	-	↓ (only 20 wk)	↑ (only 10 wk)	↑ (only 20 wk)		↑ (only 20 wk)	n.d.	[94]

↓: reduced in comparison to control animals ↑: increased in comparison to control animals.

3.1. Surgically Induced Models

The most well-characterized surgical model is the subtotal nephrectomy model, also called 5/6 nephrectomy. There are different methods for performing this surgery; all involve unilateral nephrectomy. Reduction of the remaining kidney mass is then performed either by cauterization, ligation or slicing off the two poles, or by occlusion of the branches of the main kidney artery. Unilateral nephrectomy and reduction of the remaining kidney mass are either performed on the same day (1-step) or with a 7- to 14-day recovery phase after the unilateral nephrectomy (2-step). Various studies describe a cardiac phenotype resulting from CKD in these mice, which is aggravated with the time elapsed since surgery (see Table 2). The surgically induced model has been reported to mimic most phenotypic changes observed in the human disease. However, the resulting phenotype is highly dependent on the genetic background of the mice.

A study performed in nephrectomized C57BL/6 mice showed impaired renal function, anemia, cardiac hypertrophy, cardiac fibrosis and decreased systolic and diastolic heart function compared to sham-operated mice [75,89]. In addition, there was increased expression of natriuretic peptides, another marker of progressive heart failure, in nephrectomized male 129X1/SvJ mice [88]. Subtotal nephrectomy in male CD1 mice resulted in physiological and morphological changes that also mimicked the cardiac phenotype in patients with CKD [91]. In a study with male BALB/c mice, analyzed for up to 24 weeks after 5/6 nephrectomy, cardiac and arterial structure and function showed signs of fibrosis, oxidative damage and endothelial dysfunction [90,91].

RAAS is a key player in blood-pressure control and has been described as being highly relevant in the cardiorenal syndrome. Subtotal nephrectomy in angiotensin II type 1A receptor (AT1) knockout mice resulted in significantly reduced cardiac hypertrophy, fibrosis and capillary rarefaction compared to their wildtype littermates [87]. Other widely used cardioprotective and antihypertensive treatments such as β1-receptor blockers have also been shown to reduce cardiac hypertrophy in CKD [95].

CKD patients suffer from reduced erythropoietin (EPO) levels, and it has been shown that besides causing anemia, EPO reduction had direct effects on the cardiovascular system of these patients. In line with this, 5/6 nephrectomized mice receiving recombinant human erythropoietin (rhEPO) had a better outcome compared to saline-treated controls in terms of cardiac function and remodeling. These effects were independent of anemia. Thus, a control group that received an EPO derivate (asialo-EPO) still suffered from anemia but showed the same beneficial effects on cardiac remodeling [79,95]. Both compounds similarly attenuated LVH, indicating that EPO receptor signaling protected the hearts of CKD mice through mechanisms independent of erythropoiesis. The production of erythrocytes requires continuous stimulation of EPO receptors, whereas a brief stimulation is described to be sufficient for neuroprotection. The same mechanism might explain the cardioprotective effect in this model [79].

In addition, unilateral ureteral obstruction (UUO) can induce some cardiac hypertrophy and fibrosis [79,92]. However, since UUO does not cause renal failure in the presence of a non-injured contralateral kidney, the model is probably not suitable to induce a severe cardiac phenotype.

By performing a graded ureter obstruction model in combination with a systemic expression of humanized S100A8, S100A12, and S100A9 in C57BL/6 mice, the association between S100/RAGE/FGF23 and cardiac hypertrophy was revealed [85]. Elevated serum concentrations of S100A12 are associated with inflammatory diseases, and thus might accelerate pathological cardiac remodeling in CKD patients. As mice do not express S100A12 [34,96], a humanized model was generated and CKD was induced via reversible unilateral ureteral obstruction. For this method, the right ureter was obstructed using a clip that was relocated every other day to prevent irreversible obstruction. After 7 days, the clip was removed to allow recovery of the right kidney, followed by irreversible ligation of the left ureter. A potential mechanism to explain the results of the study was presented with the finding that in addition to osteocyte expression, in CKD patients, FGF23 is also expressed in the heart by cardiomyocytes, cardiac fibroblasts, vascular smooth muscle cells and endothelial cells in coronary arteries, and by inflammatory macrophages [60]. It was suggested that S100/RAGE-mediated chronic sustained systemic inflammation caused cardiac fibroblasts to upregulate FGF23 synthesis, and in turn, increased cardiac FGF23 levels were linked to pathological cardiac remodeling [86].

3.2. Chemically Induced Models

Surgical methods to induce CKD associated with cardiovascular changes are often accompanied by a high mortality and require well-trained surgeons. Thus, efforts have been made to establish non-surgical techniques for CKD induction. One option is to apply orally administered adenine, which is metabolized to 2,8-dihydroxyadenine, and which in turn precipitates as crystals in the renal proximal tubular epithelium causing inflammation and fibrosis, ultimately leading to CKD. Indeed, mice treated with adenine developed symptoms of the cardiorenal syndrome, in particular cardiac hypertrophy, impaired cardiac function, as well as increased fibrosis [97].

An additional chemically induced model for murine CKD-CVD was achieved in mice via a single injection of cisplatin and subsequent feeding of a high-phosphate diet. CKD was confirmed by decreased creatinine clearance, development of interstitial kidney fibrosis, hyperphosphatemia, high plasma levels of PTH and FGF23 and low levels of plasma calcitriol and αKlotho. The mice developed LVH and cardiac fibrosis. This model resembles the transition from acute kidney injury to chronic renal failure and thus displays a promising approach to study underlying mechanisms in humans [93].

3.3. Genetically Induced Models

In addition to the above-mentioned models for CKD induction, CVD has also been reported in genetic mouse models of CKD. One example is the Alport mouse model, i.e., murine Col4a3 deficiency. The phenotype of C57BL/6 Col4a3 knockout mice was milder than that of 129Sv mice, which correlated with prolonged survival of the C57BL/6 mice. After 20 weeks, the C57BL/6 mice developed CKD associated with functional and structural symptoms of cardiac remodeling [94]. This emphasizes the importance of the genetic background of the mice used in relation to the severity of cardiac disease. For example, C57BL/6 mice usually have much milder phenotypes compared to 129Sv mice.

4. Potential Therapeutic Targets of Cardiac Remodeling in CKD

Reduction or inhibition of LVH might be achieved by non-specific treatments such as reduction of hypervolemia, lowering of blood pressure and treatment with angiotensin-converting enzyme inhibitors or angiotensin receptor blockers that exhibit potential direct effects on the myocardium [16,94]. Further strategies to prevent left-ventricular remodeling in patients with mild-to-moderate CKD comprise of reducing overweightness and avoiding hemoglobin concentrations that are too high [98].

Paricalcitol, a vitamin D receptor agonist, has shown a beneficial effect on myocardial fibrosis in rats [77,78]. However, in CKD patients, paricalcitol administration failed to improve diastolic function [99,100].

As oxidative stress triggers cardiovascular remodeling, antioxidative therapies have been proposed to protect endothelial cells from reactive oxygen species, thereby preventing endothelial dysfunction. Quercetin and antioxidant enzyme mimetics were shown to inhibit the NFkB pathway and reduce ROS generation in an in vitro assay using endothelial cells [101]. Several studies have attempted to reduce imbalances caused by oxidative stress in cardiac remodeling in CKD. Accordingly, Liu et al. demonstrated that antagonism of the Na/K-ATPase ameliorates uremic cardiomyopathy in 5/6 nephrectomized mice [81,82]. Na/K-ATPase activation leads to increased ROS production and acts as a signal transducer inside cardiomyocytes [81]. In activated Na/K-ATPase signaling, microRNA 29b-3b is downregulated, and thus fails to inhibit collagen expression, which has been shown in cardiac fibroblasts [81,83]. Na/K-ATPase is also known to stimulate mTOR signaling, thereby activating pro-fibrotic pathways. Moreover, the mTOR inhibitor rapamycin has been shown to inhibit cardiac fibrosis in rats [102].

As some of the uremic toxins are derived from intestinal bacteria, the microbiome could be another potential target in the cardiorenal syndrome. Thus, indoxyl sulfate and para-Cresyl sulfate serum levels were reduced by antibiotic therapy in ESRD patients [103,104]. Indoxyl sulfate binds to the cannabinoid receptor [75]. Interestingly, inhibition of this receptor has also been shown to reduce cardiac fibrosis in 5/6 nephrectomized mice [75].

FGF23 promotes cardiac fibrosis and LVH. Additionally, FGF23 signaling in the liver causes the production of inflammatory cytokines. In the bone, FGF23 inhibits mineralization, leading to increased circulating phosphorus levels and a reduction in the production of EPO [64,75]. Thus, the identification of FGF23 receptors in the respective organs will be crucial in future research since their selective blockade could be considered as a therapeutic target [64]. On the other hand, FGF23 antibody treatment caused mineral disturbances, in particular hyperphosphatemia and was associated with increased mortality in a CKD rat model [105]. Recombinant Klotho was used in an experimental mouse model to attenuate cardiac remodeling and reduce cardiac and renal fibrosis [105,106]. A positive correlation between FGF23 and cardiac hypertrophy exists in a Klotho-deficient state, but not in a Klotho-repleted state [76,105,106]. In addition, pharmacological interference with cardiac FGF23/FGFR4 signaling might have a protective effect on CKD- and age-related LVH [68]. First studies in rats report that pharmacological inhibition of FGFR might be a potent blood pressure-independent mechanism to prevent LVH in CKD [59].

CKD patients have low EPO levels, which are associated with cardiac fibrosis. A study in 5/6 nephrectomized rats showed that EPO in combination with enalapril reduced cardiac fibrosis and capillary rarefaction. The underlying mechanisms are likely multifactorial but may encompass decreased myocardial oxidative stress [81]. In CKD patients, there is better survival in those treated with EPO to a hemoglobin level of 10-12 g/dl, whereas normalization of hemoglobin levels was not beneficial [80,107].

Calò et al. identified rho kinase (ROCK) activation as a potential LVH marker in CKD patients, which indicates that inhibition of ROCK activation might serve as a target to treat cardiac remodeling in those patients [108].

A study performed in 5/6 nephrectomized rats treated with the PPARα agonist clofibrate did indeed reveal improved cardiac function and prevention of LVH [84].

Finally, restoring kidney function can at least partially reverse cardiac changes. It has been shown by echocardiography that a kidney transplantation improves left-ventricular function [103].

In conclusion, to date, few specific therapies exist that can inhibit cardiac remodeling in CKD. A better understanding of the cell types involved and their mechanisms of activation, e.g., by crosstalk or presumed uremic toxins, will guide the development of urgently needed novel therapeutics.

Author Contributions: A.B. and N.K. drafted the manuscript and contributed equally. J.F. and R.K. revised the manuscript. All authors have read and agreed to the published version of the manuscript.

Funding: This work was supported by Deutsche Forschungsgemeinschaft Grant SFB/TRR 219.

Conflicts of Interest: The authors declare no conflict of interest.

References

1. Luyckx, V.A.; Tonelli, M.; Stanifer, J.W. The global burden of kidney disease and the sustainable development goals. *Bull. World Health Organ.* **2018**, *96*, 414–422. [CrossRef]
2. Wang, H.; Naghavi, M.; Allen, C.; Barber, R.M.; Bhutta, Z.A.; Carter, A.; Coggeshall, M. GBD 2015 Mortality and Causes of Death Collaborators Global, regional, and national life expectancy, all-cause mortality, and cause-specific mortality for 249 causes of death, 1980–2015: A systematic analysis for the Global Burden of Disease Study 2015. *Lancet* **2016**, *388*, 1459–1544. [CrossRef]
3. Bikbov, B.; Perico, N.; Remuzzi, G. On behalf of the GBD Genitourinary Diseases Expert Group Disparities in Chronic Kidney Disease Prevalence among Males and Females in 195 Countries: Analysis of the Global Burden of Disease 2016 Study. *Nephron* **2018**, *139*, 313–318. [CrossRef]
4. Hill, N.R.; Fatoba, S.T.; Oke, J.L.; Hirst, J.A.; O'Callaghan, C.A.; Lasserson, D.S.; Richard Hobbs, F.D. Global Prevalence of Chronic Kidney Disease—A Systematic Review and Meta-Analysis. *PLoS ONE* **2016**, *11*, e0158765. [CrossRef] [PubMed]

5. Shamseddin, M.K.; Khaled Shamseddin, M.; Parfrey, P.S. Sudden cardiac death in chronic kidney disease: Epidemiology and prevention. *Nat. Rev. Nephrol.* **2011**, *7*, 145–154. [CrossRef] [PubMed]
6. Zhou, P.; Pu, W.T. Recounting Cardiac Cellular Composition. *Circ. Res.* **2016**, *118*, 368–370. [CrossRef] [PubMed]
7. Pinto, A.R.; Ilinykh, A.; Ivey, M.J.; Kuwabara, J.T.; D'Antoni, M.L.; Debuque, R.; Chandran, A.; Wang, L.; Arora, K.; Rosenthal, N.A.; et al. Revisiting Cardiac Cellular Composition. *Circ. Res.* **2016**, *118*, 400–409. [CrossRef] [PubMed]
8. Massaia, A.; Chaves, P.; Samari, S.; Miragaia, R.J.; Meyer, K.; Teichmann, S.A.; Noseda, M. Single Cell Gene Expression to Understand the Dynamic Architecture of the Heart. *Front. Cardiovasc. Med.* **2018**, *5*, 167. [CrossRef]
9. Wagner, J.U.G.; Dimmeler, S. Cellular cross-talks in the diseased and aging heart. *J. Mol. Cell. Cardiol.* **2020**, *138*, 136–146. [CrossRef]
10. Wang, L.; Yu, P.; Zhou, B.; Song, J.; Li, Z.; Zhang, M.; Guo, G.; Wang, Y.; Chen, X.; Han, L.; et al. Single-cell reconstruction of the adult human heart during heart failure and recovery reveals the cellular landscape underlying cardiac function. *Nat. Cell Biol.* **2020**, *22*, 108–119. [CrossRef]
11. Perbellini, F.; Watson, S.A.; Bardi, I.; Terracciano, C.M. Heterocellularity and Cellular Cross-Talk in the Cardiovascular System. *Front. Cardiovasc. Med.* **2018**, *5*, 143. [CrossRef] [PubMed]
12. Talman, V.; Kivelä, R. Cardiomyocyte-Endothelial Cell Interactions in Cardiac Remodeling and Regeneration. *Front. Cardiovasc. Med.* **2018**, *5*, 101. [CrossRef] [PubMed]
13. Kramann, R.; Erpenbeck, J.; Schneider, R.K.; Röhl, A.B.; Hein, M.; Brandenburg, V.M.; van Diepen, M.; Dekker, F.; Marx, N.; Floege, J.; et al. Speckle tracking echocardiography detects uremic cardiomyopathy early and predicts cardiovascular mortality in ESRD. *J. Am. Soc. Nephrol.* **2014**, *25*, 2351–2365. [CrossRef] [PubMed]
14. Rasić, S.; Kulenović, I.; Haracić, A.; Catović, A. Left ventricular hypertrophy and risk factors for its development in uraemic patients. *Bosn. J. Basic Med. Sci.* **2004**, *4*, 34–40. [CrossRef]
15. Mitsnefes, M.M.; Daniels, S.R.; Schwartz, S.M.; Meyer, R.A.; Khoury, P.; Strife, C.F. Severe left ventricular hypertrophy in pediatric dialysis: Prevalence and predictors. *Pediatr. Nephrol.* **2000**, *14*, 898–902. [CrossRef]
16. Amann, K.; Rychlík, I.; Miltenberger-Milteny, G.; Ritz, E. Left ventricular hypertrophy in renal failure. *Kidney Int. Suppl.* **1998**, *68*, S78–S85. [CrossRef]
17. Izumaru, K.; Hata, J.; Nakano, T.; Nakashima, Y.; Nagata, M.; Fukuhara, M.; Oda, Y.; Kitazono, T.; Ninomiya, T. Reduced Estimated GFR and Cardiac Remodeling: A Population-Based Autopsy Study. *Am. J. Kidney Dis.* **2019**, *74*, 373–381. [CrossRef]
18. Fearnley, C.J.; Roderick, H.L.; Bootman, M.D. Calcium signaling in cardiac myocytes. *Cold Spring Harb. Perspect. Biol.* **2011**, *3*, a004242. [CrossRef]
19. Kisling, A.; Lust, R.M.; Katwa, L.C. What is the role of peptide fragments of collagen I and IV in health and disease? *Life Sci.* **2019**, *228*, 30–34. [CrossRef]
20. Rudenko, T.E.; Kamyshova, E.S.; Vasilyeva, M.P.; Bobkova, I.N.; Solomakhina, N.I.; Shvetsov, M.Y. Risk factors for diastolic left ventricular myocardial dysfunction in patients with chronic kidney disease. *Ter. Arkh.* **2018**, *90*, 60–67. [CrossRef]
21. London, G.M. Left ventricular alterations and end-stage renal disease. *Nephrol. Dial. Transplant.* **2002**, *17*, 29–36. [CrossRef] [PubMed]
22. Speiser, B.; Riess, C.F.; Schaper, J. The extracellular matrix in human myocardium: Part I: Collagens I, III, IV, and VI. *Cardioscience* **1991**, *2*, 225–232. [PubMed]
23. Weber, K.T. Cardiac interstitium in health and disease: The fibrillar collagen network. *J. Am. Coll. Cardiol.* **1989**, *13*, 1637–1652. [CrossRef]
24. Chen, M.; Arcari, L.; Engel, J.; Freiwald, T.; Platschek, S.; Zhou, H.; Zainal, H.; Buettner, S.; Zeiher, A.M.; Geiger, H.; et al. Aortic stiffness is independently associated with interstitial myocardial fibrosis by native T1 and accelerated in the presence of chronic kidney disease. *IJC Heart Vasc.* **2019**, *24*, 100389. [CrossRef]
25. Nitta, K.; Akiba, T.; Uchida, K.; Otsubo, S.; Otsubo, Y.; Takei, T.; Ogawa, T.; Yumura, W.; Kabaya, T.; Nihei, H. Left ventricular hypertrophy is associated with arterial stiffness and vascular calcification in hemodialysis patients. *Hypertens. Res.* **2004**, *27*, 47–52. [CrossRef] [PubMed]

26. Pluta, A.; Stróżecki, P.; Krintus, M.; Odrowąż-Sypniewska, G.; Manitius, J. Left ventricular remodeling and arterial remodeling in patients with chronic kidney disease stage 1–3. *Ren. Fail.* **2015**, *37*, 1105–1110. [CrossRef]
27. Pateinakis, P.; Papagianni, A. Cardiorenal Syndrome Type 4—Cardiovascular Disease in Patients with Chronic Kidney Disease: Epidemiology, Pathogenesis, and Management. *Int. J. Nephrol.* **2011**, *2011*, 938651. [CrossRef]
28. Vanlandewijck, M.; He, L.; Mäe, M.A.; Andrae, J.; Ando, K.; Del Gaudio, F.; Nahar, K.; Lebouvier, T.; Laviña, B.; Gouveia, L.; et al. A molecular atlas of cell types and zonation in the brain vasculature. *Nature* **2018**, *554*, 475–480. [CrossRef]
29. Gu, W.; Ni, Z.; Tan, Y.-Q.; Deng, J.; Zhang, S.-J.; Lv, Z.-C.; Wang, X.-J.; Chen, T.; Zhang, Z.; Hu, Y.; et al. Adventitial Cell Atlas of wt (Wild Type) and ApoE (Apolipoprotein E)-Deficient Mice Defined by Single-Cell RNA Sequencing. *Arterioscler. Thromb. Vasc. Biol.* **2019**, *39*, 1055–1071. [CrossRef]
30. Kramann, R.; Goettsch, C.; Wongboonsin, J.; Iwata, H.; Schneider, R.K.; Kuppe, C.; Kaesler, N.; Chang-Panesso, M.; Machado, F.G.; Gratwohl, S.; et al. Adventitial MSC-like Cells Are Progenitors of Vascular Smooth Muscle Cells and Drive Vascular Calcification in Chronic Kidney Disease. *Cell Stem Cell* **2016**, *19*, 628–642. [CrossRef]
31. Kramann, R.; Schneider, R.K.; DiRocco, D.P.; Machado, F.; Fleig, S.; Bondzie, P.A.; Henderson, J.M.; Ebert, B.L.; Humphreys, B.D. Perivascular Gli1+ progenitors are key contributors to injury-induced organ fibrosis. *Cell Stem Cell* **2015**, *16*, 51–66. [CrossRef] [PubMed]
32. Pannier, B.; Guerin, A.P.; Marchais, S.J.; Metivier, F.; Safar, M.E.; London, G.M. Postischemic vasodilation, endothelial activation, and cardiovascular remodeling in end-stage renal disease. *Kidney Int.* **2000**, *57*, 1091–1099. [CrossRef] [PubMed]
33. Prommer, H.-U.; Maurer, J.; von Websky, K.; Freise, C.; Sommer, K.; Nasser, H.; Samapati, R.; Reglin, B.; Guimarães, P.; Pries, A.R.; et al. Chronic kidney disease induces a systemic microangiopathy, tissue hypoxia and dysfunctional angiogenesis. *Sci. Rep.* **2018**, *8*, 5317. [CrossRef]
34. Bonetti, P.O.; Lerman, L.O.; Lerman, A. Endothelial dysfunction: A marker of atherosclerotic risk. *Arterioscler. Thromb. Vasc. Biol.* **2003**, *23*, 168–175. [CrossRef]
35. Duni, A.; Liakopoulos, V.; Rapsomanikis, K.-P.; Dounousi, E. Chronic Kidney Disease and Disproportionally Increased Cardiovascular Damage: Does Oxidative Stress Explain the Burden? *Oxid. Med. Cell. Longev.* **2017**, *2017*, 9036450. [CrossRef] [PubMed]
36. Sárközy, M.; Kovács, Z.Z.A.; Kovács, M.G.; Gáspár, R.; Szűcs, G.; Dux, L. Mechanisms and Modulation of Oxidative/Nitrative Stress in Type 4 Cardio-Renal Syndrome and Renal Sarcopenia. *Front. Physiol.* **2018**, *9*, 1648. [CrossRef] [PubMed]
37. Dounousi, E.; Papavasiliou, E.; Makedou, A.; Ioannou, K.; Katopodis, K.P.; Tselepis, A.; Siamopoulos, K.C.; Tsakiris, D. Oxidative stress is progressively enhanced with advancing stages of CKD. *Am. J. Kidney Dis.* **2006**, *48*, 752–760. [CrossRef] [PubMed]
38. DuPont, J.J.; Ramick, M.G.; Farquhar, W.B.; Townsend, R.R.; Edwards, D.G. NADPH oxidase-derived reactive oxygen species contribute to impaired cutaneous microvascular function in chronic kidney disease. *Am. J. Physiol. Renal Physiol.* **2014**, *306*, F1499–F1506. [CrossRef]
39. Himmelfarb, J.; McMonagle, E. Manifestations of oxidant stress in uremia. *Blood Purif.* **2001**, *19*, 200–205. [CrossRef]
40. Feng, W.; Zhang, K.; Liu, Y.; Chen, J.; Cai, Q.; He, W.; Zhang, Y.; Wang, M.-H.; Wang, J.; Huang, H. Advanced oxidation protein products aggravate cardiac remodeling via cardiomyocyte apoptosis in chronic kidney disease. *Am. J. Physiol. Heart Circ. Physiol.* **2018**, *314*, H475–H483. [CrossRef]
41. Gupta, J.; Dominic, E.A.; Fink, J.C.; Ojo, A.O.; Barrows, I.R.; Reilly, M.P.; Townsend, R.R.; Joffe, M.M.; Rosas, S.E.; Wolman, M.; et al. Association between Inflammation and Cardiac Geometry in Chronic Kidney Disease: Findings from the CRIC Study. *PLoS ONE* **2015**, *10*, e0124772. [CrossRef] [PubMed]
42. Freise, C.; Schaefer, B.; Bartosova, M.; Bayazit, A.; Bauer, U.; Pickardt, T.; Berger, F.; Rasmussen, L.M.; Jensen, P.S.; Laube, G.; et al. Arterial tissue transcriptional profiles associate with tissue remodeling and cardiovascular phenotype in children with end-stage kidney disease. *Sci. Rep.* **2019**, *9*, 10316. [CrossRef] [PubMed]

43. Hassan, M.O.; Duarte, R.; Dix-Peek, T.; Vachiat, A.; Naidoo, S.; Dickens, C.; Grinter, S.; Manga, P.; Naicker, S. Correlation between volume overload, chronic inflammation, and left ventricular dysfunction in chronic kidney disease patients. *Clin. Nephrol.* **2016**, *86*, 131–135. [CrossRef] [PubMed]
44. Dozio, E.; Ambrogi, F.; de Cal, M.; Vianello, E.; Ronco, C.; Corsi Romanelli, M.M. Role of the Soluble Receptor for Advanced Glycation End Products (sRAGE) as a Prognostic Factor for Mortality in Hemodialysis and Peritoneal Dialysis Patients. *Mediat. Inflamm.* **2018**, *2018*, 1347432. [CrossRef]
45. Dozio, E.; Corradi, V.; Vianello, E.; Scalzotto, E.; de Cal, M.; Corsi Romanelli, M.M.; Ronco, C. Increased Levels of sRAGE in Diabetic CKD-G5D Patients: A Potential Protective Mechanism against AGE-Related Upregulation of Fibroblast Growth Factor 23 and Inflammation. *Mediat. Inflamm.* **2017**, *2017*, 9845175. [CrossRef]
46. Leifheit-Nestler, M.; Kirchhoff, F.; Nespor, J.; Richter, B.; Soetje, B.; Klintschar, M.; Heineke, J.; Haffner, D. Fibroblast growth factor 23 is induced by an activated renin-angiotensin-aldosterone system in cardiac myocytes and promotes the pro-fibrotic crosstalk between cardiac myocytes and fibroblasts. *Nephrol. Dial. Transplant.* **2018**, *33*, 1722–1734. [CrossRef]
47. Böckmann, I.; Lischka, J.; Richter, B.; Deppe, J.; Rahn, A.; Fischer, D.-C.; Heineke, J.; Haffner, D.; Leifheit-Nestler, M. FGF23-Mediated Activation of Local RAAS Promotes Cardiac Hypertrophy and Fibrosis. *Int. J. Mol. Sci.* **2019**, *20*, 4634. [CrossRef]
48. Corda, S.; Mebazaa, A.; Gandolfini, M.P.; Fitting, C.; Marotte, F.; Peynet, J.; Charlemagne, D.; Cavaillon, J.M.; Payen, D.; Rappaport, L.; et al. Trophic effect of human pericardial fluid on adult cardiac myocytes. Differential role of fibroblast growth factor-2 and factors related to ventricular hypertrophy. *Circ. Res.* **1997**, *81*, 679–687. [CrossRef]
49. Scheinowitz, M.; Kotlyar, A.; Zimand, S.; Ohad, D.; Leibovitz, I.; Bloom, N.; Goldberg, I.; Nass, D.; Engelberg, S.; Savion, N.; et al. Basic fibroblast growth factor induces myocardial hypertrophy following acute infarction in rats. *Exp. Physiol.* **1998**, *83*, 585–593. [CrossRef]
50. Liu, Q.; Zhu, L.-J.; Waaga-Gasser, A.M.; Ding, Y.; Cao, M.; Jadhav, S.J.; Kirollos, S.; Shekar, P.S.; Padera, R.F.; Chang, Y.-C.; et al. The axis of local cardiac endogenous Klotho-TGF-β1-Wnt signaling mediates cardiac fibrosis in human. *J. Mol. Cell. Cardiol.* **2019**, *136*, 113–124. [CrossRef]
51. Isakova, T.; Wahl, P.; Vargas, G.S.; Gutiérrez, O.M.; Scialla, J.; Xie, H.; Appleby, D.; Nessel, L.; Bellovich, K.; Chen, J.; et al. Fibroblast growth factor 23 is elevated before parathyroid hormone and phosphate in chronic kidney disease. *Kidney Int.* **2011**, *79*, 1370–1378. [CrossRef]
52. Xue, C.; Yang, B.; Zhou, C.; Dai, B.; Liu, Y.; Mao, Z.; Yu, S.; Mei, C. Fibroblast Growth Factor 23 Predicts All-Cause Mortality in a Dose-Response Fashion in Pre-Dialysis Patients with Chronic Kidney Disease. *Am. J. Nephrol.* **2017**, *45*, 149–159. [CrossRef]
53. Mirza, M.A.I.; Larsson, A.; Melhus, H.; Lind, L.; Larsson, T.E. Serum intact FGF23 associate with left ventricular mass, hypertrophy and geometry in an elderly population. *Atherosclerosis* **2009**, *207*, 546–551. [CrossRef]
54. Nakano, C.; Hamano, T.; Fujii, N.; Obi, Y.; Matsui, I.; Tomida, K.; Mikami, S.; Inoue, K.; Shimomura, A.; Nagasawa, Y.; et al. Intact fibroblast growth factor 23 levels predict incident cardiovascular event before but not after the start of dialysis. *Bone* **2012**, *50*, 1266–1274. [CrossRef] [PubMed]
55. Faul, C.; Amaral, A.P.; Oskouei, B.; Hu, M.-C.; Sloan, A.; Isakova, T.; Gutiérrez, O.M.; Aguillon-Prada, R.; Lincoln, J.; Hare, J.M.; et al. FGF23 induces left ventricular hypertrophy. *J. Clin. Investig.* **2011**, *121*, 4393–4408. [CrossRef] [PubMed]
56. Jovanovich, A.; Ix, J.H.; Gottdiener, J.; McFann, K.; Katz, R.; Kestenbaum, B.; de Boer, I.H.; Sarnak, M.; Shlipak, M.G.; Mukamal, K.J.; et al. Fibroblast growth factor 23, left ventricular mass, and left ventricular hypertrophy in community-dwelling older adults. *Atherosclerosis* **2013**, *231*, 114–119. [CrossRef] [PubMed]
57. Leifheit-Nestler, M.; Große Siemer, R.; Flasbart, K.; Richter, B.; Kirchhoff, F.; Ziegler, W.H.; Klintschar, M.; Becker, J.U.; Erbersdobler, A.; Aufricht, C.; et al. Induction of cardiac FGF23/FGFR4 expression is associated with left ventricular hypertrophy in patients with chronic kidney disease. *Nephrol. Dial. Transplant.* **2016**, *31*, 1088–1099. [CrossRef]
58. Mitsnefes, M.M.; Betoko, A.; Schneider, M.F.; Salusky, I.B.; Wolf, M.S.; Jüppner, H.; Warady, B.A.; Furth, S.L.; Portale, A.A. FGF23 and Left Ventricular Hypertrophy in Children with CKD. *Clin. J. Am. Soc. Nephrol.* **2018**, *13*, 45–52. [CrossRef]

59. Di Marco, G.S.; Reuter, S.; Kentrup, D.; Grabner, A.; Amaral, A.P.; Fobker, M.; Stypmann, J.; Pavenstädt, H.; Wolf, M.; Faul, C.; et al. Treatment of established left ventricular hypertrophy with fibroblast growth factor receptor blockade in an animal model of CKD. *Nephrol. Dial. Transplant.* **2014**, *29*, 2028–2035. [CrossRef]
60. Leifheit-Nestler, M.; Haffner, D. Paracrine Effects of FGF23 on the Heart. *Front. Endocrinol.* **2018**, *9*, 278. [CrossRef]
61. Andrukhova, O.; Slavic, S.; Smorodchenko, A.; Zeitz, U.; Shalhoub, V.; Lanske, B.; Pohl, E.E.; Erben, R.G. FGF23 regulates renal sodium handling and blood pressure. *EMBO Mol. Med.* **2014**, *6*, 744–759. [CrossRef]
62. David, V.; Martin, A.; Isakova, T.; Spaulding, C.; Qi, L.; Ramirez, V.; Zumbrennen-Bullough, K.B.; Sun, C.C.; Lin, H.Y.; Babitt, J.L.; et al. Inflammation and functional iron deficiency regulate fibroblast growth factor 23 production. *Kidney Int.* **2016**, *89*, 135–146. [CrossRef] [PubMed]
63. Santamaría, R.; Díaz-Tocados, J.M.; Pendón-Ruiz de Mier, M.V.; Robles, A.; Salmerón-Rodríguez, M.D.; Ruiz, E.; Vergara, N.; Aguilera-Tejero, E.; Raya, A.; Ortega, R.; et al. Increased Phosphaturia Accelerates The Decline in Renal Function: A Search for Mechanisms. *Sci. Rep.* **2018**, *8*, 13701. [CrossRef] [PubMed]
64. Rodelo-Haad, C.; Santamaria, R.; Muñoz-Castañeda, J.R.; Pendón-Ruiz de Mier, M.V.; Martin-Malo, A.; Rodriguez, M. FGF23, Biomarker or Target? *Toxins* **2019**, *11*, 175. [CrossRef] [PubMed]
65. Zou, D.; Wu, W.; He, Y.; Ma, S.; Gao, J. The role of klotho in chronic kidney disease. *BMC Nephrol.* **2018**, *19*, 285. [CrossRef]
66. Hu, M.C.; Shi, M.; Cho, H.J.; Adams-Huet, B.; Paek, J.; Hill, K.; Shelton, J.; Amaral, A.P.; Faul, C.; Taniguchi, M.; et al. Klotho and phosphate are modulators of pathologic uremic cardiac remodeling. *J. Am. Soc. Nephrol.* **2015**, *26*, 1290–1302. [CrossRef]
67. Tranæus Lindblad, Y.; Olauson, H.; Vavilis, G.; Hammar, U.; Herthelius, M.; Axelsson, J.; Bárány, P. The FGF23-Klotho axis and cardiac tissue Doppler imaging in pediatric chronic kidney disease—A prospective cohort study. *Pediatr. Nephrol.* **2018**, *33*, 147–157. [CrossRef]
68. Grabner, A.; Schramm, K.; Silswal, N.; Hendrix, M.; Yanucil, C.; Czaya, B.; Singh, S.; Wolf, M.; Hermann, S.; Stypmann, J.; et al. FGF23/FGFR4-mediated left ventricular hypertrophy is reversible. *Sci. Rep.* **2017**, *7*, 1993. [CrossRef]
69. Taguchi, K.; Elias, B.C.; Brooks, C.R.; Ueda, S.; Fukami, K. Uremic Toxin-Targeting as a Therapeutic Strategy for Preventing Cardiorenal Syndrome. *Circ. J.* **2019**, *84*, 2–8. [CrossRef]
70. Yokoro, M.; Nakayama, Y.; Yamagishi, S.-I.; Ando, R.; Sugiyama, M.; Ito, S.; Yano, J.; Taguchi, K.; Kaida, Y.; Saigusa, D.; et al. Asymmetric Dimethylarginine Contributes to the Impaired Response to Erythropoietin in CKD-Anemia. *J. Am. Soc. Nephrol.* **2017**, *28*, 2670–2680. [CrossRef]
71. Tang, W.H.W.; Wang, Z.; Shrestha, K.; Borowski, A.G.; Wu, Y.; Troughton, R.W.; Klein, A.L.; Hazen, S.L. Intestinal microbiota-dependent phosphatidylcholine metabolites, diastolic dysfunction, and adverse clinical outcomes in chronic systolic heart failure. *J. Card. Fail.* **2015**, *21*, 91–96. [CrossRef] [PubMed]
72. Lekawanvijit, S. Cardiotoxicity of Uremic Toxins: A Driver of Cardiorenal Syndrome. *Toxins* **2018**, *10*, 352. [CrossRef] [PubMed]
73. For the European Uremic Toxin Work Group (EUTox); Vanholder, R.; De Smet, R.; Glorieux, G.; Argilés, A.; Baurmeister, U.; Brunet, P.; Clark, W.; Cohen, G.; De Deyn, P.P.; et al. Review on uremic toxins: Classification, concentration, and interindividual variability. *Kidney Int.* **2003**, *63*, 1934–1943. [CrossRef]
74. Kim, H.Y.; Yoo, T.-H.; Hwang, Y.; Lee, G.H.; Kim, B.; Jang, J.; Yu, H.T.; Kim, M.C.; Cho, J.-Y.; Lee, C.J.; et al. Indoxyl sulfate (IS)-mediated immune dysfunction provokes endothelial damage in patients with end-stage renal disease (ESRD). *Sci. Rep.* **2017**, *7*, 3057. [CrossRef] [PubMed]
75. Lin, C.-Y.; Hsu, Y.-J.; Hsu, S.-C.; Chen, Y.; Lee, H.-S.; Lin, S.-H.; Huang, S.-M.; Tsai, C.-S.; Shih, C.-C. CB1 cannabinoid receptor antagonist attenuates left ventricular hypertrophy and Akt-mediated cardiac fibrosis in experimental uremia. *J. Mol. Cell. Cardiol.* **2015**, *85*, 249–261. [CrossRef] [PubMed]
76. Xie, J.; Yoon, J.; An, S.-W.; Kuro-o, M.; Huang, C.-L. Soluble Klotho Protects against Uremic Cardiomyopathy Independently of Fibroblast Growth Factor 23 and Phosphate. *J. Am. Soc. Nephrol.* **2015**, *26*, 1150–1160. [CrossRef]
77. Panizo, S.; Barrio-Vázquez, S.; Naves-Díaz, M.; Carrillo-López, N.; Rodríguez, I.; Fernández-Vázquez, A.; Valdivielso, J.M.; Thadhani, R.; Cannata-Andía, J.B. Vitamin D receptor activation, left ventricular hypertrophy and myocardial fibrosis. *Nephrol. Dial. Transplant.* **2013**, *28*, 2735–2744. [CrossRef]

78. Gluba-Brzózka, A.; Franczyk, B.; Ciałkowska-Rysz, A.; Olszewski, R.; Rysz, J. Impact of Vitamin D on the Cardiovascular System in Advanced Chronic Kidney Disease (CKD) and Dialysis Patients. *Nutrients* **2018**, *10*, 709. [CrossRef]
79. Ogino, A.; Takemura, G.; Kawasaki, M.; Tsujimoto, A.; Kanamori, H.; Li, L.; Goto, K.; Maruyama, R.; Kawamura, I.; Takeyama, T.; et al. Erythropoietin receptor signaling mitigates renal dysfunction-associated heart failure by mechanisms unrelated to relief of anemia. *J. Am. Coll. Cardiol.* **2010**, *56*, 1949–1958. [CrossRef]
80. Gut, N.; Piecha, G.; Aldebssi, F.; Schaefer, S.; Bekeredjian, R.; Schirmacher, P.; Ritz, E.; Gross-Weissmann, M.-L. Erythropoietin combined with ACE inhibitor prevents heart remodeling in 5/6 nephrectomized rats independently of blood pressure and kidney function. *Am. J. Nephrol.* **2013**, *38*, 124–135. [CrossRef]
81. Kennedy, D.J.; Malhotra, D.; Shapiro, J.I. Molecular insights into uremic cardiomyopathy: Cardiotonic steroids and Na/K ATPase signaling. *Cell. Mol. Biol.* **2006**, *52*, 3–14.
82. Liu, J.; Tian, J.; Chaudhry, M.; Maxwell, K.; Yan, Y.; Wang, X.; Shah, P.T.; Khawaja, A.A.; Martin, R.; Robinette, T.J.; et al. Attenuation of Na/K-ATPase Mediated Oxidant Amplification with pNaKtide Ameliorates Experimental Uremic Cardiomyopathy. *Sci. Rep.* **2016**, *6*, 34592. [CrossRef]
83. Drummond, C.A.; Hill, M.C.; Shi, H.; Fan, X.; Xie, J.X.; Haller, S.T.; Kennedy, D.J.; Liu, J.; Garrett, M.R.; Xie, Z.; et al. Na/K-ATPase signaling regulates collagen synthesis through microRNA-29b-3p in cardiac fibroblasts. *Physiol. Genom.* **2016**, *48*, 220–229. [CrossRef] [PubMed]
84. Chuppa, S.; Liang, M.; Liu, P.; Liu, Y.; Casati, M.C.; Cowley, A.W.; Patullo, L.; Kriegel, A.J. MicroRNA-21 regulates peroxisome proliferator-activated receptor alpha, a molecular mechanism of cardiac pathology in Cardiorenal Syndrome Type 4. *Kidney Int.* **2018**, *93*, 375–389. [CrossRef] [PubMed]
85. Yan, L.; Mathew, L.; Chellan, B.; Gardner, B.; Earley, J.; Puri, T.S.; Hofmann Bowman, M.A. S100/Calgranulin-mediated inflammation accelerates left ventricular hypertrophy and aortic valve sclerosis in chronic kidney disease in a receptor for advanced glycation end products-dependent manner. *Arterioscler. Thromb. Vasc. Biol.* **2014**, *34*, 1399–1411. [CrossRef] [PubMed]
86. Yan, L.; Bowman, M.A.H. Chronic sustained inflammation links to left ventricular hypertrophy and aortic valve sclerosis: A new link between S100/RAGE and FGF23. *Inflamm. Cell Signal.* **2014**, *1*, e279.
87. Li, Y.; Takemura, G.; Okada, H.; Miyata, S.; Maruyama, R.; Esaki, M.; Kanamori, H.; Li, L.; Ogino, A.; Ohno, T.; et al. Molecular signaling mediated by angiotensin II type 1A receptor blockade leading to attenuation of renal dysfunction-associated heart failure. *J. Card. Fail.* **2007**, *13*, 155–162. [CrossRef]
88. Winterberg, P.D.; Jiang, R.; Maxwell, J.T.; Wang, B.; Wagner, M.B. Myocardial dysfunction occurs prior to changes in ventricular geometry in mice with chronic kidney disease (CKD). *Physiol. Rep.* **2016**, *4*, e12732. [CrossRef]
89. Wang, X.; Chaudhry, M.A.; Nie, Y.; Xie, Z.; Shapiro, J.I.; Liu, J. A Mouse 5/6th Nephrectomy Model That Induces Experimental Uremic Cardiomyopathy. *J. Vis. Exp.* **2017**, e55825. [CrossRef]
90. Baumann, M.; Leineweber, K.; Tewiele, M.; Wu, K.; Türk, T.R.; Su, S.; Gössl, M.; Buck, T.; Wilde, B.; Heemann, U.; et al. Imatinib ameliorates fibrosis in uraemic cardiac disease in BALB/c without improving cardiac function. *Nephrol. Dial. Transplant.* **2010**, *25*, 1817–1824. [CrossRef]
91. Kennedy, D.J.; Elkareh, J.; Shidyak, A.; Shapiro, A.P.; Smaili, S.; Mutgi, K.; Gupta, S.; Tian, J.; Morgan, E.; Khouri, S.; et al. Partial nephrectomy as a model for uremic cardiomyopathy in the mouse. *Am. J. Physiol. Renal Physiol.* **2008**, *294*, F450–F454. [CrossRef] [PubMed]
92. Ham, O.; Jin, W.; Lei, L.; Huang, H.H.; Tsuji, K.; Huang, M.; Roh, J.; Rosenzweig, A.; Lu, H.A.J. Pathological cardiac remodeling occurs early in CKD mice from unilateral urinary obstruction, and is attenuated by Enalapril. *Sci. Rep.* **2018**, *8*, 16087. [CrossRef] [PubMed]
93. Shi, M.; McMillan, K.L.; Wu, J.; Gillings, N.; Flores, B.; Moe, O.W.; Hu, M.C. Cisplatin nephrotoxicity as a model of chronic kidney disease. *Lab. Investig.* **2018**, *98*, 1105–1121. [CrossRef] [PubMed]
94. Neuburg, S.; Dussold, C.; Gerber, C.; Wang, X.; Francis, C.; Qi, L.; David, V.; Wolf, M.; Martin, A. Genetic background influences cardiac phenotype in murine chronic kidney disease. *Nephrol. Dial. Transplant.* **2018**, *33*, 1129–1137. [CrossRef] [PubMed]
95. Rizzi, E.; Guimaraes, D.A.; Ceron, C.S.; Prado, C.M.; Pinheiro, L.C.; Martins-Oliveira, A.; Gerlach, R.F.; Tanus-Santos, J.E. β1-Adrenergic blockers exert antioxidant effects, reduce matrix metalloproteinase activity, and improve renovascular hypertension-induced cardiac hypertrophy. *Free Radic. Biol. Med.* **2014**, *73*, 308–317. [CrossRef]

96. Fuellen, G.; Nacken, W.; Sorg, C.; Kerkhoff, C. Computational Searches for Missing Orthologs: The Case of S100A12 in Mice. *OMICS A J. Integr. Biol.* **2004**, *8*, 334–340. [CrossRef]
97. Kieswich, J.E.; Chen, J.; Alliouachene, S.; Caton, P.W.; McCafferty, K.; Thiemermann, C.; Yaqoob, M.M. A novel model of reno-cardiac syndrome in the C57BL/6 mouse strain. *BMC Nephrol.* **2018**, *19*, 346. [CrossRef]
98. Schneider, M.P.; Scheppach, J.B.; Raff, U.; Toncar, S.; Ritter, C.; Klink, T.; Störk, S.; Wanner, C.; Schlieper, G.; Saritas, T.; et al. Left Ventricular Structure in Patients With Mild-to-Moderate CKD-a Magnetic Resonance Imaging Study. *Kidney Int. Rep.* **2019**, *4*, 267–274. [CrossRef]
99. Thadhani, R.; Appelbaum, E.; Pritchett, Y.; Chang, Y.; Wenger, J.; Tamez, H.; Bhan, I.; Agarwal, R.; Zoccali, C.; Wanner, C.; et al. Vitamin D therapy and cardiac structure and function in patients with chronic kidney disease: The PRIMO randomized controlled trial. *JAMA* **2012**, *307*, 674–684. [CrossRef]
100. J-DAVID Investigators; Shoji, T.; Inaba, M.; Fukagawa, M.; Ando, R.; Emoto, M.; Fujii, H.; Fujimori, A.; Fukui, M.; Hase, H.; et al. Effect of Oral Alfacalcidol on Clinical Outcomes in Patients Without Secondary Hyperparathyroidism Receiving Maintenance Hemodialysis: The J-DAVID Randomized Clinical Trial. *JAMA* **2018**, *320*, 2325–2334.
101. Vera, M.; Torramade-Moix, S.; Martin-Rodriguez, S.; Cases, A.; Cruzado, J.M.; Rivera, J.; Escolar, G.; Palomo, M.; Diaz-Ricart, M. Antioxidant and Anti-Inflammatory Strategies Based on the Potentiation of Glutathione Peroxidase Activity Prevent Endothelial Dysfunction in Chronic Kidney Disease. *Cell. Physiol. Biochem.* **2018**, *51*, 1287–1300. [CrossRef] [PubMed]
102. Haller, S.T.; Yan, Y.; Drummond, C.A.; Xie, J.; Tian, J.; Kennedy, D.J.; Shilova, V.Y.; Xie, Z.; Liu, J.; Cooper, C.J.; et al. Rapamycin Attenuates Cardiac Fibrosis in Experimental Uremic Cardiomyopathy by Reducing Marinobufagenin Levels and Inhibiting Downstream Pro-Fibrotic Signaling. *J. Am. Heart Assoc.* **2016**, *5*, e004106. [CrossRef]
103. Zapolski, T.; Furmaga, J.; Wysokiński, A.P.; Wysocka, A.; Rudzki, S.; Jaroszyński, A. The atrial uremic cardiomyopathy regression in patients after kidney transplantation—The prospective echocardiographic study. *BMC Nephrol.* **2019**, *20*, 152. [CrossRef] [PubMed]
104. Nazzal, L.; Roberts, J.; Singh, P.; Jhawar, S.; Matalon, A.; Gao, Z.; Holzman, R.; Liebes, L.; Blaser, M.J.; Lowenstein, J. Microbiome perturbation by oral vancomycin reduces plasma concentration of two gut-derived uremic solutes, indoxyl sulfate and p-cresyl sulfate, in end-stage renal disease. *Nephrol. Dial. Transplant.* **2017**, *32*, 1809–1817. [CrossRef] [PubMed]
105. Shalhoub, V.; Shatzen, E.M.; Ward, S.C.; Davis, J.; Stevens, J.; Bi, V.; Renshaw, L.; Hawkins, N.; Wang, W.; Chen, C.; et al. FGF23 neutralization improves chronic kidney disease-associated hyperparathyroidism yet increases mortality. *J. Clin. Investig.* **2012**, *122*, 2543–2553. [CrossRef]
106. Hu, M.C.; Shi, M.; Gillings, N.; Flores, B.; Takahashi, M.; Kuro, O.M.; Moe, O.W. Recombinant α-Klotho may be prophylactic and therapeutic for acute to chronic kidney disease progression and uremic cardiomyopathy. *Kidney Int.* **2017**, *91*, 1104–1114. [CrossRef]
107. Coyne, D.W.; Goldsmith, D.; Macdougall, I.C. New options for the anemia of chronic kidney disease. *Kidney Int. Suppl.* **2017**, *7*, 157–163. [CrossRef]
108. Calò, L.A.; Vertolli, U.; Pagnin, E.; Ravarotto, V.; Davis, P.A.; Lupia, M.; Naso, E.; Maiolino, G.; Naso, A. Increased rho kinase activity in mononuclear cells of dialysis and stage 3–4 chronic kidney disease patients with left ventricular hypertrophy: Cardiovascular risk implications. *Life Sci.* **2016**, *148*, 80–85. [CrossRef]

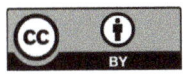

© 2020 by the authors. Licensee MDPI, Basel, Switzerland. This article is an open access article distributed under the terms and conditions of the Creative Commons Attribution (CC BY) license (http://creativecommons.org/licenses/by/4.0/).

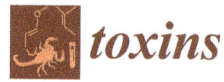

Review

Inflammation and Premature Ageing in Chronic Kidney Disease

Thomas Ebert [1,*,†], Sven-Christian Pawelzik [2,3,†], Anna Witasp [1], Samsul Arefin [1], Sam Hobson [1], Karolina Kublickiene [1], Paul G. Shiels [4], Magnus Bäck [2,3,‡] and Peter Stenvinkel [1,*,‡]

1. Karolinska Institutet, Department of Clinical Science, Intervention and Technology, Division of Renal Medicine, SE-141 86 Stockholm, Sweden; anna.witasp@ki.se (A.W.); samsul.arefin@ki.se (S.A.); sam.hobson@ki.se (S.H.); karolina.kublickiene@ki.se (K.K.)
2. Karolinska Institutet, Department of Medicine Solna, Cardiovascular Medicine Unit, SE-171 76 Stockholm, Sweden; sven-christian.pawelzik@ki.se (S.-C.P.); magnus.back@ki.se (M.B.)
3. Karolinska University Hospital, Theme Heart and Vessels, Division of Valvular and Coronary Disease, SE-171 76 Stockholm, Sweden
4. University of Glasgow, Wolfson Wohl Cancer Research Centre, College of Medical, Veterinary & Life Sciences, Institute of Cancer Sciences, Glasgow G61 1QH, UK; Paul.Shiels@glasgow.ac.uk
* Correspondence: thomas.ebert@ki.se (T.E.); peter.stenvinkel@ki.se (P.S.)
† These authors equally contributed to this work.
‡ These authors equally contributed to this work.

Received: 1 February 2020; Accepted: 29 March 2020; Published: 4 April 2020

Abstract: Persistent low-grade inflammation and premature ageing are hallmarks of the uremic phenotype and contribute to impaired health status, reduced quality of life, and premature mortality in chronic kidney disease (CKD). Because there is a huge global burden of disease due to CKD, treatment strategies targeting inflammation and premature ageing in CKD are of particular interest. Several distinct features of the uremic phenotype may represent potential treatment options to attenuate the risk of progression and poor outcome in CKD. The nuclear factor erythroid 2-related factor 2 (NRF2)–kelch-like erythroid cell-derived protein with CNC homology [ECH]-associated protein 1 (KEAP1) signaling pathway, the endocrine phosphate-fibroblast growth factor-23–klotho axis, increased cellular senescence, and impaired mitochondrial biogenesis are currently the most promising candidates, and different pharmaceutical compounds are already under evaluation. If studies in humans show beneficial effects, carefully phenotyped patients with CKD can benefit from them.

Keywords: ageing; chronic kidney disease; end-stage kidney disease; inflammation; premature ageing; senescence; uremic toxins

Key Contribution: We summarize the current literature on uremic inflammation and premature ageing in Chronic Kidney Disease and discuss potential treatment strategies.

1. Introduction—CKD, Inflammation, and Premature Ageing

Chronic kidney disease (CKD) is a major global health burden that contributes to increased morbidity and mortality in affected patients [1]. Inflammation is a key risk factor for CKD progression [2], and recent data from the CANTOS trial suggest that anti-inflammatory treatment in patients with CKD reduces major adverse cardiovascular events [3]. Compared to the general population, patients with CKD also have a highly accelerated ageing process that is characterized by vascular disease; a persistent, low-grade inflammatory status; sarcopenia; and other maladies [4]. Both inflammation and ageing (i.e., "inflammageing") are established risk factors for mortality in a cluster of "burden of lifestyle diseases", such as CKD [5], which has been recognized as one of the prototype diseases for premature ageing [6]. Persistent inflammation, premature ageing, and CKD share common regulatory patterns of distinct biological pathways. For instance, the transcription factor nuclear factor erythroid 2-related factor 2 (NRF2) is downregulated in all three conditions [7–9]. Thus, both inflammation and premature ageing are major contributing factors to health status and outcome in patients with CKD.

The aim of this review is to summarize the clinical phenotypes of inflammation and premature ageing in CKD. We also summarize the relationship between these two phenotypes. Furthermore, we provide an overview of novel factors contributing to the uremic phenotype, and we describe potential novel targets for the systemic treatment of these interrelated disorders.

2. Inflammation in CKD

2.1. Uremic Inflammation

An impaired renal function leads to the accumulation of nitrogenous substances in the blood that would normally be excreted in the urine. At progressively increasing concentration, these substances exert toxic effects, which eventually become apparent as symptoms of *uremia*. The altering effects of the uremic milieu on the immune system has been described as *uremic inflammation* [10,11], and include mechanisms of both immunoactivation and immunosuppression. Uremic inflammation resembles the premature ageing phenotype in many ways. On the one hand, it is characterized by an abnormal activation of the innate immune system, especially monocytes [6,12]. This immunoactivation contributes to systemic inflammation via increased synthesis of pro-inflammatory cytokines, such as interleukin (IL)-1, IL-6, and tumor necrosis factor (TNF) [12], and is similar to the chronic low-grade state of systemic inflammation that is associated with an ageing immune system and has been coined "inflammageing" [13]. Furthermore, inflammation is also a major component of other diseases that are independent risk factors for CKD, such as obesity [14]. Importantly, an increased synthesis of pro-inflammatory cytokines and chemokines by senescent cells is one of the main features of cellular senescence [15,16], and has been coined senescence-associated secretory phenotype (SASP). The SASP suggests a further bi-directional link between inflammation and ageing in CKD. On the other hand, a downregulation and reduced function of the adaptive immune system, particularly of T and B lymphocytes, during uremic inflammation parallels "immunosenescence" in the premature ageing phenotype [6,10,12].

The causes of uremic inflammation are multifactorial. Exogenous factors, such as catheterization, exposition to microbial contaminants, or biocompatibility issues during dialysis treatment [10] may play an obvious role in the activation of the immune system and are avoidable using good clinical practice. Possible exposure to bacterial endotoxin, which activates the immune system and contributes to systemic inflammation, can furthermore result from comorbidities, such as gingivitis and periodontitis [17]. Patients with CKD may also show signs of intestinal dysbiosis and increased gut permeability [10], which lead to the presence of bacterial DNA and elevated endotoxin levels, as well as elevated plasma levels of the macrophage-derived cluster of differentiation (CD)14 [10], a co-receptor in the recognition of bacterial endotoxin [18].

Conversely, endogenous factors that provoke uremic inflammation in CKD are linked to metabolic deviations from normal physiology and can be categorized as (i) changes in the mineral metabolism, especially in the levels of phosphate and sodium concentrations; (ii) regulation of oxidative stress; and (iii) increased nonenzymatic glycation. However, these categories are interconnected and may influence each other.

The endocrine fibroblast growth factor-23 (FGF-23)–klotho pathway (Figures 1 and 2) is important for the resorption of phosphate in the kidney and is dysregulated in CKD. Decreased renal clearance produces a relative overload of inorganic phosphate (P_i), which results in hyperphosphatemia and contributes to systemic inflammation and vascular calcification/early vascular ageing (EVA) [19] (Figure 2). Hyperphosphatemia promotes endothelial dysfunction and trans-differentiation of vascular smooth muscle cells (VSMC) into osteoblast-like cells [20]. In bovine aortic smooth muscle cells, high P_i promotes an osteogenic phenotype via an inflammatory mechanism involving nuclear factor kappa-light-chain-enhancer of activated B cells (NF-κB) signaling, which increases the generation of reactive oxygen species (ROS). This phenotype can be prevented with the P_i binder lanthanum carbonate [21]. Similarly, another P_i binder, sevelamer, increases levels of fetuin A, an inhibitor of extracellular matrix mineralization, in patients with CKD [22]. As a negative acute phase protein, low levels of fetuin A indicate systemic inflammation and may shorten telomeres in leukocytes [23]. Furthermore, high P_i induces the expression of the pro-inflammatory transcription factor NF-κB in human aortic VSMC [24].

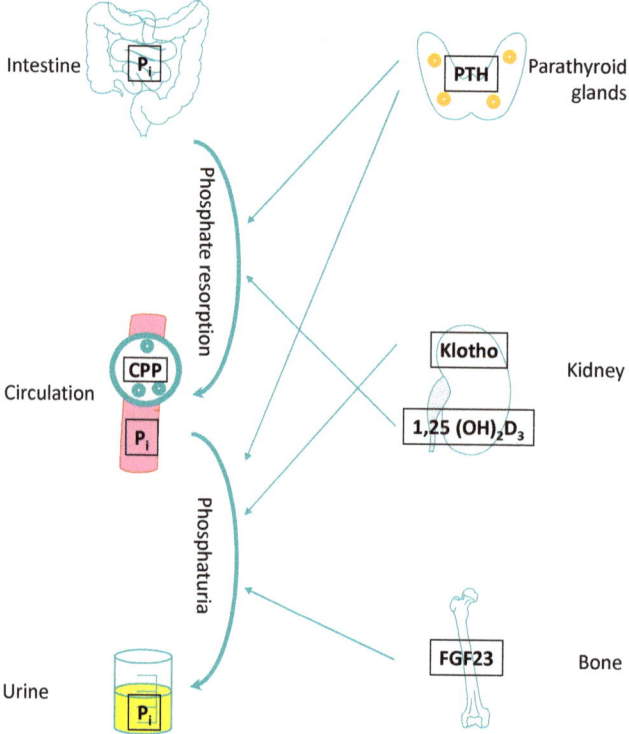

Figure 1

Figure 1. The phosphate-fibroblast growth factor-23 (FGF-23)–klotho endocrine axis. Main effectors of phosphate homeostasis with potential effects on ageing components (simplified overview). Phosphate (P_i) is taken up by the intestine and accumulates in the circulation of patients with advanced chronic kidney disease (CKD). In the circulation, fetuin A (blue circles)-bound calcium P_i in calciprotein particles (CPP) prevents precipitation of calcium P_i in the circulation. Increased P_i is further regulated by parathyroid hormone (PTH) secreted from the four parathyroid glands (orange circles) at the back of thyroid gland by increasing intestinal P_i resorption but also inducing phosphaturia. The 1,25(OH)$_2$ vitamin D$_3$ metabolite is activated in the kidneys and increases intestinal P_i resorption. Furthermore, bone-secreted fibroblast growth factor-23 (FGF-23) also exerts phosphaturic effects through its mandatory co-receptor klotho in the kidneys.

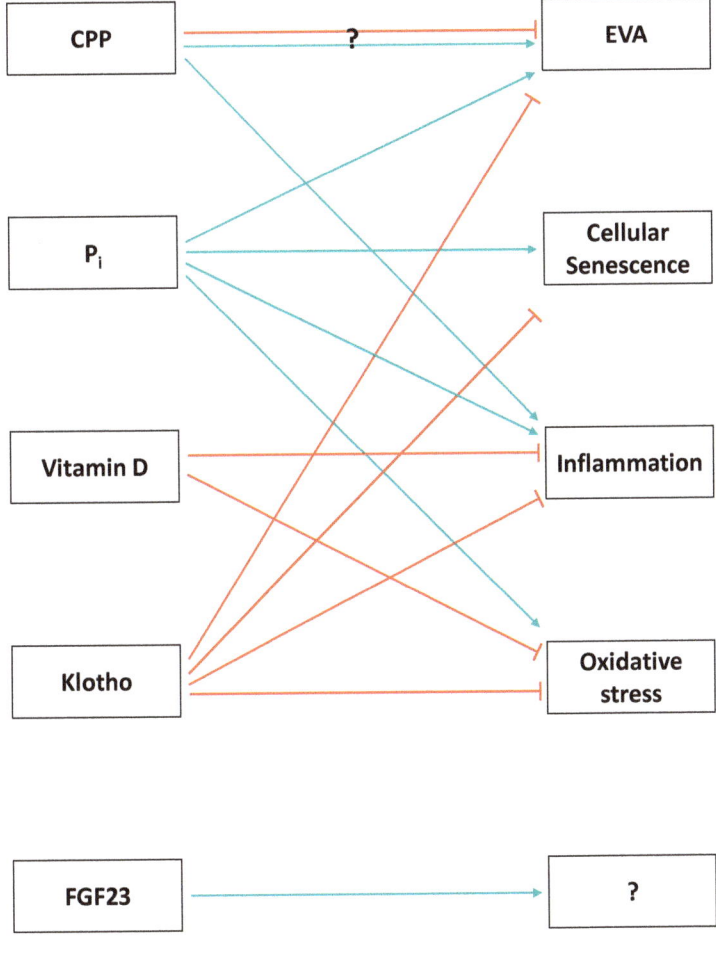

Figure 2

Figure 2. The phosphate-FGF-23–klotho endocrine axis and premature ageing in CKD. Association of the different effectors of the phosphate homeostasis with ageing components (light blue arrows: inducers; red arrows: inhibitors). In advanced CKD, calciprotein particles (CPP) can induce early vascular ageing (EVA) and inflammation. However, contradictory findings also suggest a beneficial role of CPP on EVA. Circulating phosphate (P_i) promotes EVA, cellular senescence, and oxidative stress by different mechanisms. Vitamin D inhibits inflammation and oxidative stress directly or indirectly. The anti-ageing-associated klotho counteracts EVA, cellular senescence, inflammation, and oxidative stress. Data for fibroblast growth factor-23 (FGF-23) are limited and further studies need to investigate whether FGF-23 directly induces different ageing components or whether the clinical associations to ageing are mediated by other factors, such as P_i.

Although P_i levels increase in the circulation of CKD patients, sodium accumulates in the tissue under uremic conditions and may lead to chronic systemic inflammation via activation of the p38 mitogen-activated protein kinase (MAPK) pathway and induction of IL-17-producing $CD4^+$ T helper cells [6,25].

The transcription factor NRF2 plays an important and ancient role in the anti-oxidant response. Following oxidative stress, NRF2 dissociates from its repressor kelch-like erythroid cell-derived protein with CNC homology [ECH]-associated protein 1 (KEAP1) in the cytosol and subsequently translocates to the nucleus, where it binds to the anti-oxidant response element of numerous promoter regions of over 300 genes encoding anti-oxidant and detoxifying molecules [26]. In peripheral blood mononuclear cells from CKD patients, NRF2 is down-regulated, whereas NF-κB is in turn up-regulated [27]. NF-κB plays a key role in regulating the inflammatory response and is stimulated by ROS [10]. This suggests that uremia induces an impaired NRF2 system in CKD and hemodialysis (HD) patients, which contributes to the pathogenesis of oxidative stress and inflammation [27]. Importantly, increased oxidative stress and its sequalae are major contributors to premature atherosclerosis and calcification [28], resulting in increased cardiovascular (CV) morbidity and mortality in CKD [29,30]. Retained uremic toxins may further both become substrates for oxidative injury and increase the burden of oxidative stress [29,30].

Advanced glycation end-products (AGE) are formed from reducing sugars and biomolecules such as proteins, lipids, and nucleic acids by a sequence of nonenzymatic glycation reactions, collectively known as the Maillard reaction [26,31]. Exogenous sources of AGE originate from diet [32] and tobacco smoking [33]. Endogenously, AGE formation is promoted by hyperglycemia, but also by high levels of oxidative stress [26]. In fact, oxidative stress and AGE formation mutually stimulate each other [34]. AGE increase the levels of ROS via activation of Nicotinamide adenine dinucleotide phosphate (NADPH) oxidase through interaction with the advanced glycation end product-specific receptor (RAGE), as well as through receptor-independent pathways, whereas ROS decrease the levels of glyoxalase I (Glo-1), an enzyme that detoxifies AGE precursor molecules [26]. In CKD, AGE accumulate as a result from both a decreased renal clearance and increased formation [26]. AGE–RAGE interaction activates the NF-κB pathway and thus perpetuates uremic inflammation via release of pro-inflammatory cytokines, such as IL-1, IL-6, and TNF [35].

2.2. Consequences of Inflammation on Premature Ageing in CKD

Persistent uremic inflammation directly promotes premature ageing and further increases inflammatory effects through a vicious circle. For instance, NF-κB promotes cellular senescence and accelerated ageing but it is also activated in senescent cells [36–38]. In more detail, senescent cells promote inflammation through the transcription factor GATA4, which increases NF-κB to initiate the SASP [39]. Furthermore, cell replication is amplified in acute and chronic inflammation, resulting in increased telomere attrition, which is directly linked to cellular ageing [40]. Importantly, the association between telomere length and inflammation also seems to be reciprocally. Thus, mice deficient in the telomerase genes telomerase RNA component (*TERC*) and telomerase reverse transcriptase (*TERT*) show a higher amount of mRNA expression of various pro-inflammatory cytokines [41]. In a cross-sectional study, the negative association of leukocyte telomere length with circulating inflammatory markers was also confirmed in prevalent HD patients [23]. Moreover, increased oxidative stress in CKD and adverse lifestyle factors (e.g., smoking and diet), as well as psychological stress, may further promote telomere shortening through inflammation [40].

3. Premature Ageing in CKD

Because the kidneys are involved in the regulation of many systemic processes, patients with CKD are at a high risk to develop multiple systemic complications, including rheologic, metabolic, immunologic, CV, and other disturbances [42]. Importantly, several of these complications show similarities with the ageing process, such as CV diseases (CVD), sarcopenia, bone disease, as well as frailty [43,44], cognitive dysfunction [44], immune deficiency [12], and finally mortality [1]. Thus, patients with CKD appear to have a highly accelerated ageing process as compared to healthy subjects or non-CKD patients. We present possible causes for the premature ageing process in CKD, focusing on uremic toxins including AGE, the endocrine phosphate-FGF-23–klotho axis, as well as

NRF2 as a master regulator of mitochondrial dysfunction/oxidative stress. Importantly, all pathways are linked to hallmarks of the ageing process [45].

3.1. Uremic Toxins and Premature Ageing in CKD

When renal function declines during the progression of CKD, distinct organic compounds accumulate [46], and signs and symptoms of *uremia* occur. The European Uremic Toxins (EUTox) Work Group has provided a comprehensive overview of circulating solutes in CKD [47] describing a large number of uremic toxins with significantly differing circulating levels in end stage kidney disease (ESKD), which can be sorted into three groups: (1) free water-soluble low-molecular-weight solutes, (2) protein-bound solutes, and (3) middle molecules [47]. For a variety of these uremic toxins, associations with the ageing process have been described. Thus, the protein-bound uremic toxins indoxyl sulfate and p-cresyl sulfate induce oxidative stress by different mechanisms [48]. Using an in vitro approach, indoxyl sulfate attenuates mitochondrial activity in human renal proximal tubule epithelial cells [49] and human umbilical vein endothelial cells [50], thereby affecting the cellular metabolic capacity. Furthermore, indoxyl sulfate induces markers of senescence, including senescence-associated beta-galactosidase (SA-β-gal), through oxidative stress [51]. Indoxyl sulfate and p-cresyl sulfate also increased mitochondrial autophagy ("mitophagy") [52]. Although autophagy in general has been suggested as a compensatory and pro-survival mechanism [53], it could also have adverse effects when mitochondrial mass decreased at a level beyond cellular compensation [52]. Thus, mitochondrial dysfunction is one of the key mechanisms linking uremic toxins with hallmarks of the ageing process [45] through increased oxidative stress [54]. It should be noted that indoxyl sulfate dose-dependently decreases protein levels of klotho in human aortic VSMC in vitro by inducing DNA methylation of the klotho-coding *Kl* gene [55]. In accordance, patients with ESKD have increased promoter hypermethylation of the *Kl* gene [55]. Conversely, the inhibition of uremic toxins should have beneficial effects on ageing markers. As an example drug, the oral sorbent AST-120 adsorbs uremic toxins and their precursors within the gastrointestinal tract [56]. AST-120 dose-dependently decreases circulating indoxyl sulfate [56] and was, therefore, tested in several clinical trials [56]. Results of these trials were heterogenous depending on the prespecified primary endpoints, follow-up period, as well as baseline characteristics of the included subjects. In conclusion, there was no effect of adding AST-120 to standard therapy in patients with moderate to severe CKD on a primary composite renal end point in the EPPIC trials [57]. It should be noted, however, that on the basis of the results of a subgroup analysis in the EPPIC trials, AST-120 delayed the time of reaching the primary renal end point in patients from the United States [58].

AGE are another group of uremic toxins that accumulate in CKD [26]. Besides the well-known associations of AGE levels and CVD (mostly investigated in patients with diabetes mellitus) [59,60], AGE and AGE-detoxifying enzymes including Glo-1 also have direct effects on ageing processes. Thus, the AGE–RAGE axis induces renal cytosolic oxidative stress and mitochondrial dysfunction, as well as inflammation [26,61]. The AGE–RAGE axis further promotes premature senescence in proximal tubular epithelial cells via endoplasmatic reticulum stress and p21 activation in an in vivo and in vitro approach [62]. Moreover, AGE-induced endoplasmatic reticulum stress also increases p16 protein expression in tubular epithelial cells in vitro in a dose- and time-dependent manner through the activating transcription factor 4 [63]. Conversely, reduced renal senescence in tubule iss observed in rodents with a transgenic overexpression of the AGE-detoxifying enzyme Glo-1 in vivo and in vitro [54]. More recently, AGE have been shown to induce renal senescence in mesangial cells via the RAGE/Signal transducer and activator of transcription 5 (STAT5) pathway and inhibiting autophagy [64].

Taken together, uremic toxins, including AGE, have distinct and adverse effects on the pro- and anti-oxidative milieu, mitochondrial function, inflammation, and finally cellular senescence; all of which are hallmarks of the ageing process [45] (Figure 3).

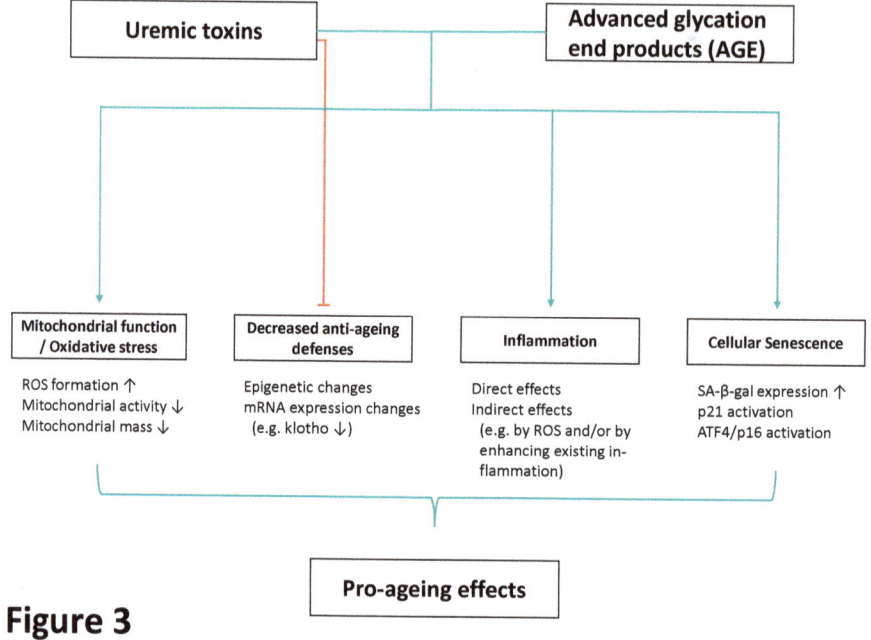

Figure 3. Mechanisms by which uremic toxins and advanced glycation end products (AGE) induce pro-ageing effects. Both uremic toxins and AGE have adverse effects on mitochondrial function including formation of reactive oxygen species (ROS) but also structural disturbances. They impair anti-ageing defenses of the organism, and induce inflammation, as well as cellular senescence. All effects result in an adverse, pro-ageing milieu caused by uremic toxins and AGE. Light blue arrows: inducers; red arrows: inhibitors. ATF4: activating transcription factor 4, ROS: reactive oxygen species, SA-β-gal: senescence-associated beta-galactosidase.

3.2. The Endocrine Phosphate-FGF-23–Klotho Axis and Premature Ageing in CKD

A clear negative association of serum P_i levels with life span has been reported in mammals [8]. Phosphate homeostasis is regulated by a distinct endocrine network involving vitamin D, parathyroid hormone (PTH), klotho, and FGF-23 (Figure 1). In more detail, P_i originating from dietary intake is absorbed by the small intestine by an active transcellular transport or a paracellular pathway [65]. In hypophosphatemia, either normal or increased levels of the active metabolite 1,25(OH)$_2$ vitamin D$_3$ are observed in humans [66], and 1,25(OH)$_2$ vitamin D$_3$ increases the rate of intestinal P_i resorption [67]. Furthermore, the parathyroid glands are affected by elevated serum P_i levels and release PTH, which enhances urinary P_i excretion by PTH-induced removal of the renal sodium P_i cotransporters from the apical membrane [68]. Bone-derived FGF-23 limits hyperphosphatemia by inducing phosphaturia and suppressing vitamin D secretion [69]. FGF-23 signals through endocrine FGF receptor complexes [70] and also associates with distinct metabolic components [71]. FGF-23 requires klotho protein as a co-receptor [70]. The full length klotho protein, which is predominantly expressed in the proximal and distal tubules of the kidneys [72], is cleaved and circulates as a soluble klotho fragment serving as a surrogate marker of renal klotho expression [70]. In the circulation, calciprotein particles (CPP) "capture" calcium (Ca) and P_i with the help of the adipokine fetuin A and prevent the precipitation of Ca-P_i [70,73].

Phosphate induces EVA via different mechanisms, and higher serum P_i concentrations, even if they are within the normal range, have been found to be associated with microvascular dysfunction in a Dutch, population-based cohort study [74] (Figure 2). In human aortic VSMC, P_i treatment arrests the cell cycle [75], mediating cellular senescence. In vitro, P_i further induces vascular calcification and production of ROS [76]. Mediated by Ca-P_i crystals and a disturbed microRNA homeostasis, P_i has additional indirect and negative effects on EVA [77]. Importantly, these in vitro data on EVA are supported by a Scottish general population study showing that P_i is linked to markers of biological age, that is, reduced telomere length, DNA methylation content, and chronological age [78].

Adverse effects of P_i on EVA are at least in part mediated by the Wnt/beta-catenin pathway [79,80]. Thus, high P_i activates the Wnt/beta-catenin pathway in VSMC in vitro, promoting VSMC calcification and osteogenic transition [79]. Conversely, shRNA-mediated knockdown of beta-catenin in CKD rats on a high-phosphate diet reduced vascular calcification [79]. Interestingly, klotho is an inhibitor of the Wnt/beta-catenin pathway [70], ameliorating high P_i-induced VSMC calcification [81], as well as inhibiting osteogenic transition of these cells [82,83]. Taken together, P_i induces EVA at least in part by the Wnt/beta-catenin pathway, and different treatment approaches potentially mitigate the adverse effects of P_i on EVA, including klotho.

Besides preventing the precipitation of Ca-P_i (Figure 2), CPP can induce pro-inflammatory effects in VSMC in vitro [84], further linking inflammation and EVA in CKD. Furthermore, CPP differ between healthy subjects and patients with ESKD and can, therefore, promote widespread calcification in CKD [85].

Because of the above-mentioned evidence of a direct association between P_i and premature ageing in CKD, non-pharmaceutical prevention strategies could potentially reduce the burden of disease, including changes in lifestyle. However, there is a lack of studies linking diets that lower P_i levels to a beneficial clinical outcome [86,87]. Furthermore, whereas low-P_i diets can reduce FGF-23 levels in CKD [88], there was no dose-dependent effect of P_i lowering on FGF-23 reduction when low- and very low phosphate diets were compared in a recent short-term, randomized, crossover trial in 35 ESKD patients [89]. Therefore, non-pharmacological lifestyle-changing prevention strategies might provide a benefit on components of the ageing process, but randomized controlled trials are needed to prove these associations.

Vitamin D has also been linked to distinct components of the ageing process (Figure 2). The negative acute phase reactant vitamin D [90] mitigates oxidative stress at least in part through increased expression of anti-oxidant regulators, including NRF2 and klotho [91–93]. Thus, calcitriol increased renal and circulating klotho expression, whereas it reduced markers of oxidative stress in uninephrectomized, spontaneously hypertensive rats [94]. These data have been confirmed in a recent randomized controlled trial showing increased circulating klotho and total antioxidant capacity after 12 weeks of cholecalciferol treatment compared to the placebo group [95]. Human ex vivo studies indicate that vitamin D exerts anti-inflammatory effects on uremic lymphocytes under renal replacement therapy (RRT) [96]. Meta-analyses demonstrating reduced circulating markers of inflammation in mostly non-CKD subjects on vitamin D supplementation [97,98], further supporting a significant role of vitamin D on the hallmarks of ageing. However, these associations were not seen in CKD patients on vitamin D supplementation [99]. Furthermore, two systematic reviews and meta-analyses did not find strong evidence for a beneficial effect of vitamin D supplementation on arterial stiffness [100] and endothelial function [101], two major components of EVA. Thus, future studies need to validate whether vitamin D has direct effects on premature ageing in CKD or whether its effects are mediated by NRF2, klotho, and others.

FGF-23 has been associated with an adverse outcome in CKD in large studies [102]. However, only a few experimental studies have investigated causal effects of FGF-23 on inflammation and premature ageing as hallmarks in the pathogenesis of CKD and its complications. Thus, FGF-23 induces hepatic inflammation in CKD [103]. Furthermore, some [104,105] but not all [106] studies suggest that FGF-23 might induce EVA. Taken together, data for direct FGF-23 effects on *renal* inflammation and premature ageing in CKD are limited (Figure 2).

Simic et al. [107] recently showed that kidney-derived glycerol-3-phosphate in the renal vein correlated with circulating FGF-23 levels, and they further demonstrated a novel kidney–bone axis by which renal glycerol-3-phosphate increases bone-secreted FGF-23. Future studies need to investigate whether renal glycerol-3-phosphate could also be a potential target for preventing premature ageing.

With respect to premature ageing, klotho (Figure 2) is clearly the most interesting member of this endocrine axis, as Kuro-o et al. [70] described a syndrome that resembles human ageing in mice that have a defect in the klotho-coding *kl* gene. When renal function declines, klotho levels decrease in humans and in rodents with CKD [70]. Klotho-overexpressing mice with CKD have an increased phosphaturia, as well as an improved renal function and EVA phenotype [72]. In mice with an ICR-derived glomerulonephritis, overexpression of the *kl* gene reduces blood urea nitrogen levels, proteinuria, renal SA-β-gal activity, and the development of glomerular and tubulointerstitial changes [108]. Mechanistically, klotho-overexpressing mice show an improved mitochondrial function, as well as a reduced mitochondrial DNA damage and oxidative stress, in the kidneys [108].

Interestingly, both high P_i and inflammation decrease renal *Kl* mRNA expression in vitro [109]. Thus, 5/6 nephrectomized rats on a 0.4% phosphorus diet showed reduced renal klotho protein expression compared to sham-operated animals [109]. Lipopolysaccharide-induced inflammation further reduced klotho expression in all groups [109]. In vivo and ex vivo pharmacological inhibition of NF-κB and Wnt recovered reduced klotho expression after lipopolysaccharide treatment [109] further suggesting that inflammation and the Wnt/beta-catenin pathway are crucially involved in the downregulation of renal klotho in CKD. The pro-fibrotic transforming growth factor (TGF)-β, which is upregulated in CKD, is another mediator of reduced renal klotho in CKD, facilitating adverse Wnt/beta-catenin activation in the kidney [110].

Besides these in vivo data in renal tissue, klotho exerts beneficial effects on the endothelium including attenuation of inflammatory and adhesion molecules, as well as augmented NO production and vasorelaxation [111]. Moreover, klotho-deficient mice show increased vascular calcification [112,113], further supporting a beneficial role of klotho on EVA. In addition, the above-described role of uremic toxins in reducing klotho expression further strengthens these effects in CKD. Finally and most importantly, because overexpression of klotho in mice extends their lifespan [70], klotho is one of the most promising anti-ageing targets in CKD.

3.3. Mitochondrial Dysfunction/Oxidative Stress and Premature Ageing in CKD

Patients with CKD show increased oxidative stress on the basis of an over-production of ROS, as well as decreased anti-oxidant defenses [29,114]. In general, ROS are generated from the reduction of oxygen and can induce oxidation of important macromolecules, including proteins, lipids, carbohydrates, and DNA [29,114], thereby exerting toxic effects on mitochondria [115]. Thus, sufficient anti-oxidative mechanisms are necessary to counteract the excessive ROS formation in cells. One of the most interesting anti-oxidative targets interfering with ageing is the transcription factor NRF2, which is a key regulator of anti-oxidative enzymes. When oxidative stress occurs, NRF2 translocates to the nucleus and activates >300 distinct genes that have an anti-oxidant response element in their promoter regions [26,116]. Mitochondrial dysfunction in CKD is associated with low NRF2 expression in human skeletal muscle [117]. NRF2 is also negatively associated with different other age-related lifestyle diseases [9] and rare progeroid syndromes [7]. Thus, patients with Hutchinson–Gilford progeria syndrome (HGPS) show an impaired activity of the NRF2 pathway, and reactivation of NRF2 in ex vivo cells of patients with HGPS can reverse ageing defects [118]. Mechanistically, NRF2 knockdown in wildtype fibroblasts increases oxidative stress and recapitulates cellular senescence defects of HGPS [118]. Furthermore, caveolin-induced NRF2 inhibition induces senescence in murine adipocytes in vitro and, conversely, less inhibition of NRF2-dependent anti-oxidant signaling results in decreased senescence, as assessed by SA-β-gal and $p21^{Waf1/Cip1}$ [119]. Molecular markers of vascular senescence, that is, $p16^{INK4a}$ and $p21^{Waf1/Cip1}$, as well as cytokines of the SASP, are increased in NRF2-deficient mice compared to control mice [120]. Klotho also exerts some of its beneficial effects on EVA by activating the NRF2 pathway [121]. Furthermore, because testosterone ameliorates age-related renal fibrosis in mice via activation of NRF2 signaling [122], the effects of sex hormones and their supplementation in CKD also need attention. In ESKD, reduced NRF2 expression in peripheral blood mononuclear cells has been reported in addition to an up-regulation of pro-inflammatory NF-κB [27]. Furthermore, uremic toxins correlate positively with NF-κB expression and negatively with NRF2 expression in peripheral blood mononuclear cells [123]. Accordingly, rats undergoing 5/6 nephrectomy also show an impaired activation of NRF2 in the kidneys [124]. Conversely, the NRF2 agonist bardoxolone reduces tubular cell mitochondrial damage and improves redox balance and mitochondrial function in a CKD mouse model [125]. Taken together, mitochondrial dysfunction and oxidative stress promote premature ageing. Because the protective NRF2 pathway is attenuated in CKD and other burden of lifestyle diseases associated with ageing, this offers the potential for future NRF2 agonist-based treatment.

4. Secondary Premature Ageing by CKD-Causing Diseases and CKD Treatment

As described above, many facets of CKD contribute to premature ageing. However, distinct causes of CKD contribute to premature ageing, irrespective of renal function, and are summarized below.

4.1. Glomerular Diseases Excluding Diabetic Kidney Disease (DKD)

In contrast to other CKD causes, the incidence of IgA nephropathy (IgAN) does not increase with age and is, therefore, higher in children and young adults as compared to elderly subjects [126,127]. In Asian cohorts of IgAN, renal biopsies show higher expressions of $p16^{INK4}$ [128], p21 [129], and reduced klotho [128] compared to controls. Furthermore, $p16^{INK4}$, as well as klotho, correlated with IgAN-related renal fibrosis [128]. Because other glomerular diseases, including focal segmental glomerulosclerosis and minimal change disease, are also associated with an increased renal expression of the senescence marker $p16^{INK4A}$ [127], glomerular diseases seem to have direct relations to premature ageing. Patients with Fabry disease have shorter leukocyte telomere length compared to controls [130]. Thus, this rare renal disease could also serve as a model of premature ageing [131].

4.2. Polycystic Kidney Disease as a Model of Adverse Anti-Senescence

Patients with autosomal dominant polycystic kidney disease (ADPKD) often progress to CKD and ESKD [132]. Interestingly and in contrast to most other underlying CKD causes, the senescence marker $p21^{Waf1/Cip1}$ is decreased in both human and rodent ADPKD, suggesting that an anti-senescent milieu promotes cyst formation [127]. In accordance with this hypothesis, the cyclin-dependent kinase inhibitor roscovitine reduces cyst formation in mice with PKD [127]. In contrast, nephronophthisis, another cystic kidney disease, is characterized by cellular senescence [133]. Furthermore, senolytic treatment in mice with nephronophthisis type 7 improves cystic area, inflammation, and renal fibrosis [134]. These contradictory findings indicate that senescence must be viewed as disease-specific and in the context of a spectrum ranging from beneficial to adverse effects.

4.3. Obesity, Diabetes Mellitus, and DKD

Obesity is a major predictor contributing to type 2 diabetes (T2D), CKD, CVD, and increased mortality [135,136]. Besides being risk factors for CKD, obesity and T2D also contribute to cellular senescence per se [137,138]. Furthermore, the adverse effects of an increased fat mass are at least partly related to the secretion of proteins from adipocytes into the circulation, that is, adipocytokines. Indeed, adipocytokines associate with adverse metabolic status and the SASP [71,139]. Interestingly, treatment of obese mice with the senolytic agents dasatinib and quercetin improves glucose tolerance, enhances insulin sensitivity, lowers circulating inflammatory mediators, and increases levels of the beneficial adipocytokine adiponectin [140]. Furthermore, distinct adipocytokines can also contribute to attenuated vascular calcification in CKD, such as chemerin [141].

With respect to DKD, both humans and mice with DKD have an increased expression of senescence markers, including SA-β-gal, $p16^{INK4A}$, and $p21^{Waf1/Cip1}$, in different renal cell types, and diabetic, p21-deficient mice are protected from DKD compared to diabetic wildtype mice [127]. However, future studies need to validate whether hyperglycemia rather than DKD itself might cause this pro-senescent phenotype.

4.4. CKD-/ESKD Treatment-Associated Ageing (Dialysis, Transplantation)

As the uremic milieu associates with premature ageing and senescence, one could speculate that RRT (dialysis and renal transplantation [Rtx]) improves a prematurely aged phenotype. However, the dialysis procedure itself exerts pro-inflammatory and pro-oxidative effects due to multiple factors, such as bio-incompatibility of dialysis membranes or fluids, contaminated/polluted dialysis water, intravenous iron treatment, activation of the renin–angiotensin–aldosterone system (RAAS), and depletion of anti-oxidants [6] potentially resulting in adverse effects on ageing processes in RRT. Ageing-associated phenotypes are also observed after Rtx. Thus, patients undergoing Rtx have an increased risk for complications, including ischemia-reperfusion injury (IRI) and allograft rejection during and after Rtx. These complications can result in an accelerated senescence as assessed by $p21^{Waf1/Cip1}$ and $p16^{Ink4a}$, as well as telomere shortening [127]. Furthermore, transplant biopsies show strong $p16^{INK4a}$ staining beyond the amount predicted by chronological age [142]. Conversely, short-term inhibition of the senescence promoter p53 reduces IRI-induced senescence and improves kidney outcome in mice [143]. Immunosuppressive treatment of the recipients can further result in therapy-induced senescent cells that remain in the transplanted kidney and mediate adverse pro-ageing signals [144]. Thus, patients receiving mycophenolate mofetil after Rtx have an increased telomere attrition compared to azathioprine-treated patients, supporting a direct effect of immunosuppressive treatment on ageing [145]. Taken together, RRT by either dialysis or Rtx does not arrest ageing processes, and RRT might even accelerate the ageing phenotype.

5. Approaches for Handling of Inflammation and Premature Ageing in CKD

Inflammation and premature ageing are hallmarks in the pathogenesis of CKD and its many complications, having highly detrimental effects on health status, quality of life, and mortality. However, current treatment recommendations indicate that each single risk factor for CKD progression and its complications must be treated separately and, at the final stage, RRT has to be provided [42]. This approach led to substantial improvements in reducing example, in patients with T1D, the use of novel insulins, new glucose monitoring devices, and the widespread usage of RAAS blockers has improved the outcome [146,147]. However, because the global burden of disease due to CKD is increasing [148], systemic approaches for the treatment of CKD and its complications are warranted to target the underlying hallmarks of CKD, that is, inflammation and premature ageing. Some of these are summarized below.

5.1. NRF2–KEAP1 Signaling Pathway

Several groups have independently shown beneficial associations and effects of the NRF2 system as a key regulator of anti-oxidative enzymes in CKD, and promote NRF2 as a multiorgan protector.

Concluding the findings discussed above, treatment of the repressed NRF2 system in CKD can improve oxidative stress and mitochondrial function [125,149], inflammation [27,123,149], as well as premature ageing [122], in particular EVA [120,121].

NRF2-inducing treatment options include nutritional components, exercise [150], and pharmaceutical compounds targeting NRF2 or inhibiting the binding of NRF2 to KEAP1 [116]. Although the above-mentioned beneficial effects of NRF2 have drawn interest to this molecular "health promoter", potential caveats should be acknowledged. Firstly, NRF2 has dual roles in its association with carcinogenesis, as well as cancer progression and therapy. Thus, NRF2 activation in normal cells can prevent cancer initiation [151]. In contrast, prolonged NRF2 activation is involved in cancer promotion, progression, and treatment resistance [151]. Consequently, each NRF2-based approach must carefully investigate oncogenic risk as a potential side effect. Secondly, despite promising initial results, previous treatment approaches for patients with DKD using the NRF2 agonist bardoxolone have been stopped due to an excess of heart failure hospitalizations among those assigned to bardoxolone [7]. However, because patients with risk factors for heart failure could be identified and excluded, bardoxolone is currently being re-investigated in different clinical trials comprising patients with CKD and underlying pathologies [116]. When patients in these studies are carefully selected, the NRF2 agonist might have beneficial effects on several hallmarks of the uremic phenotype, such as inflammation, oxidative stress, as well as on premature ageing. Thus, NRF2 is currently a promising and the clinically most advanced signaling pathway for the treatment of both inflammation and premature ageing in CKD. It should be kept in mind that it is also possible to target NRF2 by nutraceuticals, such as sulforaphane [7].

5.2. Klotho Pathway

Kidney-derived klotho is of particular interest as a potential treatment for inflammation and premature ageing in CKD, because klotho-deficient mice and patients with CKD have similar phenotypes, such as EVA and a pro-inflammatory status, and klotho is related to ageing in both humans and mice [70,72]. Similar to the NRF2 system, klotho is repressed in CKD, and stimulation of klotho can ameliorate oxidative stress and mitochondrial function [108], renal fibrosis [152], inflammation [72], as well as premature ageing [108], including EVA [55,81–83,111–113].

Importantly, and possibly in contrast to the NRF2–KEAP1 signaling pathway, klotho is down-regulated in several cancers and is also recognized as a potential anti-tumor therapy [153].

Therapeutic approaches to stimulate klotho expression can aim for the reactivation of endogenous klotho or the administration of exogenous klotho [72]. Several drugs increase endogenous klotho [72]. For instance, the thiazolidinedione pioglitazone protects against renal injury in ageing by an increased expression of klotho [72]. Furthermore, the vitamin D analog paricalcitol induces the tissue-dependent expression of klotho in the kidneys and increases serum and urinary klotho levels in rodent CKD models [72]. In vitro data using murine internal medulla collecting duct epithelial cells further suggest that statins induce *klotho* mRNA expression [72]. Moreover, because angiotensin II and aldosterone decrease *klotho* mRNA expression in vitro and in vivo [70], RAAS blockers potentially reverse the decrease in *klotho* expression in rodents [70]. Recently, testosterone was positively correlated with circulating klotho levels in both men and women, and the association sustained significance after adjustment for cortisol and markers of renal function but not chronological age [154]. However, and in contrast to this study, a randomized controlled trial of transdermal testosterone does not find changes in soluble klotho levels between the verum and placebo group [155]. Finally, direct administration of exogenous, soluble klotho has also been proven effective for increasing circulating klotho levels, as well as protecting against acute kidney injury and CKD [72,156]. It has to be pointed out that, except for direct klotho administration, each of the mentioned pharmacological compounds is already approved for the use in CKD, and for some but not all of these, positive renal outcome data in humans with CKD are available [157]. However, the relative contribution of increased klotho on the outcome of these human studies has not been analyzed thus far. Hence, the direct effect of klotho on uremic inflammation and premature ageing needs to be addressed. However, preliminary safety data appear to be more attractive compared to targeting the NRF2–KEAP1 signaling pathway.

6. Conclusions

Persistent low-grade inflammation and premature ageing are hallmarks of the uremic phenotype and contribute to impaired health status, reduced quality of life, and premature mortality. Several potential treatment options targeting distinct features of the uremic phenotype may attenuate the risk of progression and poor outcome. Because the burden of disease due to CKD is huge, systemic treatment approaches targeting the underlying hallmarks of CKD, that is, inflammation and premature ageing, are currently being investigated. The NRF2–KEAP1 signaling pathway, the endocrine klotho axis, increased cellular senescence, and impaired mitochondrial biogenesis are currently the most promising candidates, and different pharmacological compounds are already in evaluation. If randomized controlled trials show beneficial effects, patients with distinct CKD phenotypes can benefit from them.

Author Contributions: T.E. and S.-C.P. wrote the manuscript and researched the literature. M.B., P.S., A.W., S.A., S.H., K.K., and P.G.S. contributed to the discussion and reviewed/edited the manuscript. All authors have read and agreed to the published version of the manuscript.

Funding: T.E. was supported by a Novo Nordisk postdoctoral fellowship run in partnership with Karolinska Institutet, Stockholm, Sweden. This work was further supported by the Swedish Heart and Lung Foundation (no. 20180571 and 20160384), King Gustaf V and Queen Victoria Freemason Foundation, Professor Nanna Svartz Foundation, the Stockholm County Council (20170365), Njurfonden (Swedish Kidney Foundation), as well as the Strategic Research Programme in Diabetes at Karolinska Institutet (Swedish Research Council grant no. 2009-1068) and other grants from the Swedish Research Council (no. 2018–00932).

Conflicts of Interest: Peter Stenvinkel serves on scientific advisory boards of Baxter, Reata, and Astra Zeneca. The other authors of this manuscript have nothing to declare.

References

1. Bikbov, B.; Purcell, C.A.; Levey, A.S.; Smith, M.; Abdoli, A.; Abebe, M.; Adebayo, O.M.; Afarideh, M.; Agarwal, S.K.; Agudelo-Botero, M.; et al. Global, regional, and national burden of chronic kidney disease, 1990–2017: A systematic analysis for the global burden of disease study 2017. *Lancet* **2020**, *395*, 709–733. [CrossRef]
2. Ruiz-Ortega, M.; Rayego-Mateos, S.; Lamas, S.; Ortiz, A.; Rodrigues-Diez, R.R. Targeting the progression of chronic kidney disease. *Nat. Rev. Nephrol.* **2020**, 1–20. [CrossRef] [PubMed]
3. Ridker, P.M.; MacFadyen, J.G.; Glynn, R.J.; Koenig, W.; Libby, P.; Everett, B.M.; Lefkowitz, M.; Thuren, T.; Cornel, J.H. Inhibition of interleukin-1β by canakinumab and cardiovascular outcomes in patients with chronic kidney disease. *J. Am. Coll. Cardiol.* **2018**, *71*, 2405–2414. [CrossRef] [PubMed]
4. Dai, L.; Qureshi, A.R.; Witasp, A.; Lindholm, B.; Stenvinkel, P. Early vascular ageing and cellular senescence in chronic kidney disease. *Comput. Struct. Biotechnol. J.* **2019**, *17*, 721–729. [CrossRef] [PubMed]
5. Hobson, S.; Arefin, S.; Kublickiene, K.; Shiels, P.G.; Stenvinkel, P. Senescent cells in early vascular ageing and bone disease of chronic kidney disease—A novel target for treatment. *Toxins* **2019**, *11*, 82. [CrossRef] [PubMed]
6. Kooman, J.P.; Kotanko, P.; Schols, A.M.W.J.; Shiels, P.G.; Stenvinkel, P. Chronic kidney disease and premature ageing. *Nat. Rev. Nephrol.* **2014**, *10*, 732–742. [CrossRef] [PubMed]
7. Stenvinkel, P.; Meyer, C.J.; Block, G.A.; Chertow, G.M.; Shiels, P.G. Understanding the role of the cytoprotective transcription factor nuclear factor erythroid 2–related factor 2—Lessons from evolution, the animal kingdom and rare progeroid syndromes. *Nephrol. Dial. Transplant.* **2019**. [CrossRef]
8. Stenvinkel, P.; Painer, J.; Kuro-o, M.; Lanaspa, M.; Arnold, W.; Ruf, T.; Shiels, P.G.; Johnson, R.J. Novel treatment strategies for chronic kidney disease: Insights from the animal kingdom. *Nat. Rev. Nephrol.* **2018**, *14*, 265–284. [CrossRef]
9. Cuadrado, A.; Manda, G.; Hassan, A.; Alcaraz, M.J.; Barbas, C.; Daiber, A.; Ghezzi, P.; León, R.; López, M.G.; Oliva, B.; et al. Transcription factor NRF2 as a therapeutic target for chronic diseases: A systems medicine approach. *Pharmacol. Rev.* **2018**, *70*, 348–383. [CrossRef]
10. Kooman, J.P.; Dekker, M.J.; Usvyat, L.A.; Kotanko, P.; van der Sande, F.M.; Schalkwijk, C.G.; Shiels, P.G.; Stenvinkel, P. Inflammation and premature aging in advanced chronic kidney disease. *Am. J. Physiol. Ren. Physiol.* **2017**, *313*, F938–F950. [CrossRef]
11. Cobo, G.; Lindholm, B.; Stenvinkel, P. Chronic inflammation in end-stage renal disease and dialysis. *Nephrol. Dial. Transplant.* **2018**, *33*, iii35–iii40. [CrossRef] [PubMed]
12. Sato, Y.; Yanagita, M. Immunology of the ageing kidney. *Nat. Rev. Nephrol.* **2019**, *15*, 625–640. [CrossRef] [PubMed]
13. Franceschi, C.; Garagnani, P.; Parini, P.; Giuliani, C.; Santoro, A. Inflammaging: A new immune—Metabolic viewpoint for age-related diseases. *Nat. Rev. Endocrinol.* **2018**, *14*, 576–590. [CrossRef] [PubMed]
14. Pawelzik, S.-C.; Avignon, A.; Idborg, H.; Boegner, C.; Stanke-Labesque, F.; Jakobsson, P.-J.; Sultan, A.; Bäck, M. Urinary prostaglandin D2 and E2 metabolites associate with abdominal obesity, glucose metabolism, and triglycerides in obese subjects. *Prostaglandins Other Lipid Mediat.* **2019**, *145*, 106361. [CrossRef]
15. Ferenbach, D.A.; Bonventre, J.V. Mechanisms of maladaptive repair after AKI leading to accelerated kidney ageing and CKD. *Nat. Rev. Nephrol.* **2015**, *11*, 264–276. [CrossRef]
16. Kirkland, J.L.; Tchkonia, T. Cellular senescence: A translational perspective. *EBioMedicine* **2017**, *21*, 21–28. [CrossRef]

17. Hickey, N.A.; Shalamanova, L.; Whitehead, K.A.; Dempsey-Hibbert, N.; van der Gast, C.; Taylor, R.L. Exploring the putative interactions between chronic kidney disease and chronic periodontitis. *Crit. Rev. Microbiol.* **2020**, *12*, 1–17. [CrossRef]
18. Van Maldeghem, I.; Nusman, C.M.; Visser, D.H. Soluble CD14 subtype (sCD14-ST) as biomarker in neonatal early-onset sepsis and late-onset sepsis: A systematic review and meta-analysis. *BMC Immunol.* **2019**, *20*, 17. [CrossRef]
19. Carracedo, M.; Artiach, G.; Witasp, A.; Clària, J.; Carlström, M.; Laguna-Fernandez, A.; Stenvinkel, P.; Bäck, M. The G-protein coupled receptor ChemR23 determines smooth muscle cell phenotypic switching to enhance high phosphate-induced vascular calcification. *Cardiovasc. Res.* **2019**, *115*, 1557–1566. [CrossRef]
20. Abbasian, N.; Burton, J.O.; Herbert, K.E.; Tregunna, B.-E.; Brown, J.R.; Ghaderi-Najafabadi, M.; Brunskill, N.J.; Goodall, A.H.; Bevington, A. Hyperphosphatemia, phosphoprotein phosphatases, and microparticle release in vascular endothelial cells. *J. Am. Soc. Nephrol.* **2015**, *26*, 2152–2162. [CrossRef]
21. Zhao, W.-H.; Gou, B.-D.; Zhang, T.-L.; Wang, K. Lanthanum chloride bidirectionally influences calcification in bovine vascular smooth muscle cells. *J. Cell. Biochem.* **2012**, *113*, 1776–1786. [CrossRef] [PubMed]
22. Zhou, Z.; Ji, Y.; Ju, H.; Chen, H.; Sun, M. Circulating fetuin-A and risk of all-cause mortality in patients with chronic kidney disease: A systematic review and meta-analysis. *Front. Physiol.* **2019**, *10*, 966. [CrossRef] [PubMed]
23. Carrero, J.J.; Stenvinkel, P.; Fellström, B.; Qureshi, A.R.; Lamb, K.; Heimbürger, O.; Bárány, P.; Radhakrishnan, K.; Lindholm, B.; Soveri, I.; et al. Telomere attrition is associated with inflammation, low fetuin-A levels and high mortality in prevalent haemodialysis patients. *J. Intern. Med.* **2008**, *263*, 302–312. [CrossRef] [PubMed]
24. Voelkl, J.; Tuffaha, R.; Luong, T.T.D.; Zickler, D.; Masyout, J.; Feger, M.; Verheyen, N.; Blaschke, F.; Kuro-o, M.; Tomaschitz, A.; et al. Zinc inhibits phosphate-induced vascular calcification through TNFAIP3-Mediated suppression of NF-κB. *J. Am. Soc. Nephrol.* **2018**, *29*, 1636–1648. [CrossRef]
25. Mikolajczyk, T.P.; Guzik, T.J. Adaptive immunity in hypertension. *Curr. Hypertens. Rep.* **2019**, *21*, 68. [CrossRef]
26. Stinghen, A.E.M.; Massy, Z.A.; Vlassara, H.; Striker, G.E.; Boullier, A. Uremic toxicity of advanced glycation end products in CKD. *J. Am. Soc. Nephrol.* **2016**, *27*, 354–370. [CrossRef]
27. Pedruzzi, L.M.; Cardozo, L.F.M.F.; Daleprane, J.B.; Stockler-Pinto, M.B.; Monteiro, E.B.; Leite, M.; Vaziri, N.D.; Mafra, D. Systemic inflammation and oxidative stress in hemodialysis patients are associated with down-regulation of Nrf2. *J. Nephrol.* **2015**, *28*, 495–501. [CrossRef]
28. Mercier, N.; Pawelzik, S.-C.; Pirault, J.; Carracedo, M.; Persson, O.; Wollensack, B.; Franco-Cereceda, A.; Bäck, M. Semicarbazide-Sensitive Amine Oxidase Increases in Calcific Aortic Valve Stenosis and Contributes to Valvular Interstitial Cell Calcification. *Oxid. Med. Cell. Longev.* **2020**, 5197376. [CrossRef]
29. Daenen, K.; Andries, A.; Mekahli, D.; Van Schepdael, A.; Jouret, F.; Bammens, B. Oxidative stress in chronic kidney disease. *Pediatr. Nephrol.* **2019**, *34*, 975–991. [CrossRef]
30. Huang, M.; Zheng, L.; Xu, H.; Tang, D.; Lin, L.; Zhang, J.; Li, C.; Wang, W.; Yuan, Q.; Tao, L.; et al. Oxidative stress contributes to vascular calcification in patients with chronic kidney disease. *J. Mol. Cell. Cardiol.* **2020**, *138*, 256–268. [CrossRef]
31. Rabbani, N.; Thornalley, P.J. Advanced glycation end products in the pathogenesis of chronic kidney disease. *Kidney Int.* **2018**, *93*, 803–813. [CrossRef] [PubMed]
32. Snelson, M.; Coughlan, M.T. Dietary advanced glycation end products: Digestion, metabolism and modulation of gut microbial ecology. *Nutrients* **2019**, *11*, 215. [CrossRef] [PubMed]
33. Chapman, S.; Mick, M.; Hall, P.; Mejia, C.; Sue, S.; Wase, B.A.; Nguyen, M.A.; Whisenant, E.C.; Wilcox, S.H.; Winden, D.; et al. Cigarette smoke extract induces oral squamous cell carcinoma cell invasion in a receptor for advanced glycation end-products-dependent manner. *Eur. J. Oral Sci.* **2018**, *126*, 33–40. [CrossRef] [PubMed]
34. Nowotny, K.; Jung, T.; Höhn, A.; Weber, D.; Grune, T. Advanced glycation end products and oxidative stress in type 2 diabetes mellitus. *Biomolecules* **2015**, *5*, 194–222. [CrossRef] [PubMed]
35. Sanajou, D.; Ghorbani Haghjo, A.; Argani, H.; Aslani, S. Age-Rage axis blockade in diabetic nephropathy: Current status and future directions. *Eur. J. Pharmacol.* **2018**, *833*, 158–164. [CrossRef] [PubMed]
36. Taniguchi, K.; Karin, M. NF-κB, inflammation, immunity and cancer: Coming of age. *Nat. Rev. Immunol.* **2018**, *18*, 309–324. [CrossRef]
37. Osorio, F.G.; Soria-Valles, C.; Santiago-Fernández, O.; Freije, J.M.P.; López-Otín, C. Chapter Four—NF-κB signaling as a driver of ageing. In *International Review of Cell and Molecular Biology*; Jeon, K.W., Galluzzi, L., Eds.; Academic Press: Cambridge, MA, USA, 2016; Volume 326, pp. 133–174.

38. Costantino, S.; Paneni, F.; Cosentino, F. Ageing, metabolism and cardiovascular disease. *J. Physiol.* **2016**, *594*, 2061–2073. [CrossRef]
39. Kang, C.; Xu, Q.; Martin, T.D.; Li, M.Z.; Demaria, M.; Aron, L.; Lu, T.; Yankner, B.A.; Campisi, J.; Elledge, S.J. The DNA damage response induces inflammation and senescence by inhibiting autophagy of GATA4. *Science* **2015**, *349*, aaa5612. [CrossRef]
40. Zhang, J.; Rane, G.; Dai, X.; Shanmugam, M.K.; Arfuso, F.; Samy, R.P.; Lai, M.K.P.; Kappei, D.; Kumar, A.P.; Sethi, G. Ageing and the telomere connection: An intimate relationship with inflammation. *Ageing Res. Rev.* **2016**, *25*, 55–69. [CrossRef]
41. Chen, R.; Zhang, K.; Chen, H.; Zhao, X.; Wang, J.; Li, L.; Cong, Y.; Ju, Z.; Xu, D.; Williams, B.R.G.; et al. Telomerase deficiency causes alveolar stem cell senescence-associated low-grade inflammation in lungs. *J. Biol. Chem.* **2015**, *290*, 30813–30829. [CrossRef]
42. Romagnani, P.; Remuzzi, G.; Glassock, R.; Levin, A.; Jager, K.J.; Tonelli, M.; Massy, Z.; Wanner, C.; Anders, H.-J. Chronic kidney disease. *Nat. Rev. Dis. Primer* **2017**, *3*, 17088. [CrossRef] [PubMed]
43. Chowdhury, R.; Peel, N.M.; Krosch, M.; Hubbard, R.E. Frailty and chronic kidney disease: A systematic review. *Arch. Gerontol. Geriatr.* **2017**, *68*, 135–142. [CrossRef] [PubMed]
44. Drew, D.A.; Weiner, D.E.; Sarnak, M.J. Cognitive impairment in CKD: Pathophysiology, management, and prevention. *Am. J. Kidney Dis.* **2019**, *74*, 782–790. [CrossRef]
45. López-Otín, C.; Blasco, M.A.; Partridge, L.; Serrano, M.; Kroemer, G. The hallmarks of aging. *Cell* **2013**, *153*, 1194–1217. [CrossRef] [PubMed]
46. Underwood, C.F.; Hildreth, C.M.; Wyse, B.F.; Boyd, R.; Goodchild, A.K.; Phillips, J.K. Uraemia: An unrecognized driver of central neurohumoral dysfunction in chronic kidney disease? *Acta Physiol.* **2017**, *219*, 305–323. [CrossRef] [PubMed]
47. Duranton, F.; Cohen, G.; Smet, R.D.; Rodriguez, M.; Jankowski, J.; Vanholder, R.; Argiles, A.; European Uremic Toxin Work Group. Normal and pathologic concentrations of uremic toxins. *J. Am. Soc. Nephrol.* **2012**, *23*, 1258–1270. [CrossRef]
48. Fujii, H.; Goto, S.; Fukagawa, M. Role of uremic toxins for kidney, cardiovascular, and bone dysfunction. *Toxins* **2018**, *10*, 202. [CrossRef]
49. Mutsaers, H.A.M.; Wilmer, M.J.G.; Reijnders, D.; Jansen, J.; van den Broek, P.H.H.; Forkink, M.; Schepers, E.; Glorieux, G.; Vanholder, R.; van den Heuvel, L.P.; et al. Uremic toxins inhibit renal metabolic capacity through interference with glucuronidation and mitochondrial respiration. *Biochim. Biophys. Acta BBA Mol. Basis Dis.* **2013**, *1832*, 142–150. [CrossRef]
50. Lee, W.-C.; Li, L.-C.; Chen, J.-B.; Chang, H.-W. Indoxyl sulfate-induced oxidative stress, mitochondrial dysfunction, and impaired biogenesis are partly protected by vitamin C and N-Acetylcysteine. *Sci. World J.* **2015**, *2015*, 1–6. [CrossRef]
51. Muteliefu, G.; Shimizu, H.; Enomoto, A.; Nishijima, F.; Takahashi, M.; Niwa, T. Indoxyl sulfate promotes vascular smooth muscle cell senescence with upregulation of p53, p21, and prelamin A through oxidative stress. *Am. J. Physiol. Cell Physiol.* **2012**, *303*, C126–C134.
52. Sun, C.-Y.; Cheng, M.-L.; Pan, H.-C.; Lee, J.-H.; Lee, C.-C. Protein-bound uremic toxins impaired mitochondrial dynamics and functions. *Oncotarget* **2017**, *8*, 77722–77733. [CrossRef] [PubMed]
53. Carracedo, M.; Persson, O.; Saliba-Gustafsson, P.; Artiach, G.; Ehrenborg, E.; Eriksson, P.; Franco-Cereceda, A.; Bäck, M. Upregulated autophagy in calcific aortic valve stenosis confers protection of valvular interstitial cells. *Int. J. Mol. Sci.* **2019**, *20*, 1486. [CrossRef] [PubMed]
54. Hirakawa, Y.; Jao, T.-M.; Inagi, R. Pathophysiology and therapeutics of premature ageing in chronic kidney disease, with a focus on glycative stress. *Clin. Exp. Pharmacol. Physiol.* **2017**, *44*, 70–77. [CrossRef]
55. Chen, J.; Zhang, X.; Zhang, H.; Liu, T.; Zhang, H.; Teng, J.; Ji, J.; Ding, X. Indoxyl sulfate enhance the hypermethylation of klotho and promote the process of vascular calcification in chronic kidney disease. *Int. J. Biol. Sci.* **2016**, *12*, 1236–1246. [CrossRef] [PubMed]
56. Asai, M.; Kumakura, S.; Kikuchi, M. Review of the efficacy of AST-120 (KREMEZIN®) on renal function in chronic kidney disease patients. *Ren. Fail.* **2019**, *41*, 47–56. [CrossRef]
57. Schulman, G.; Berl, T.; Beck, G.J.; Remuzzi, G.; Ritz, E.; Arita, K.; Kato, A.; Shimizu, M. Randomized placebo-controlled EPPIC trials of AST-120 in CKD. *J. Am. Soc. Nephrol.* **2015**, *26*, 1732–1746. [CrossRef] [PubMed]

58. Schulman, G.; Berl, T.; Beck, G.J.; Remuzzi, G.; Ritz, E.; Shimizu, M.; Shobu, Y.; Kikuchi, M. The effects of AST-120 on chronic kidney disease progression in the United States of America: A post hoc subgroup analysis of randomized controlled trials. *BMC Nephrol.* **2016**, *17*, 141. [CrossRef]
59. Koska, J.; Saremi, A.; Howell, S.; Bahn, G.; Courten, B.D.; Ginsberg, H.; Beisswenger, P.J.; Reaven, P.D. Advanced glycation end products, oxidation products, and incident cardiovascular events in patients with type 2 diabetes. *Diabetes Care* **2018**, *41*, 570–576. [CrossRef]
60. De Vos, L.C.; Lefrandt, J.D.; Dullaart, R.P.F.; Zeebregts, C.J.; Smit, A.J. Advanced glycation end products: An emerging biomarker for adverse outcome in patients with peripheral artery disease. *Atherosclerosis* **2016**, *254*, 291–299. [CrossRef]
61. Chaudhuri, J.; Bains, Y.; Guha, S.; Kahn, A.; Hall, D.; Bose, N.; Gugliucci, A.; Kapahi, P. The role of advanced glycation end products in aging and metabolic diseases: Bridging association and causality. *Cell Metab.* **2018**, *28*, 337–352. [CrossRef]
62. Liu, J.; Huang, K.; Cai, G.-Y.; Chen, X.-M.; Yang, J.-R.; Lin, L.-R.; Yang, J.; Huo, B.-G.; Zhan, J.; He, Y.-N. Receptor for advanced glycation end-products promotes premature senescence of proximal tubular epithelial cells via activation of endoplasmic reticulum stress-dependent p21 signaling. *Cell Signal.* **2014**, *26*, 110–121. [CrossRef] [PubMed]
63. Liu, J.; Yang, J.-R.; Chen, X.-M.; Cai, G.-Y.; Lin, L.-R.; He, Y.-N. Impact of ER stress-regulated ATF4/p16 signaling on the premature senescence of renal tubular epithelial cells in diabetic nephropathy. *Am. J. Physiol. Cell Physiol.* **2015**, *308*, C621–C630. [CrossRef] [PubMed]
64. Shi, M.; Yang, S.; Zhu, X.; Sun, D.; Sun, D.; Jiang, X.; Zhang, C.; Wang, L. The RAGE/STAT5/autophagy axis regulates senescence in mesangial cells. *Cell Signal.* **2019**, *62*, 109334. [CrossRef] [PubMed]
65. Knöpfel, T.; Himmerkus, N.; Günzel, D.; Bleich, M.; Hernando, N.; Wagner, C.A. Paracellular transport of phosphate along the intestine. *Am. J. Physiol. Gastrointest. Liver Physiol.* **2019**, *317*, G233–G241. [CrossRef] [PubMed]
66. Florenzano, P.; Cipriani, C.; Roszko, K.L.; Fukumoto, S.; Collins, M.T.; Minisola, S.; Pepe, J. Approach to patients with hypophosphataemia. *Lancet Diabetes Endocrinol.* **2020**, *8*, 163–174. [CrossRef]
67. Hernando, N.; Wagner, C.A. Mechanisms and regulation of intestinal phosphate absorption. *Compr. Physiol.* **2018**, *8*, 1065–1090.
68. Jacquillet, G.; Unwin, R.J. Physiological regulation of phosphate by vitamin D, parathyroid hormone (PTH) and phosphate (Pi). *Pflügers Arch. Eur. J. Physiol.* **2019**, *471*, 83–98. [CrossRef]
69. Vervloet, M. Renal and extrarenal effects of fibroblast growth factor 23. *Nat. Rev. Nephrol.* **2019**, *15*, 109–120. [CrossRef]
70. Kuro-o, M. The klotho proteins in health and disease. *Nat. Rev. Nephrol.* **2019**, *15*, 27–44. [CrossRef]
71. Ebert, T.; Gebhardt, C.; Scholz, M.; Wohland, T.; Schleinitz, D.; Fasshauer, M.; Blüher, M.; Stumvoll, M.; Kovacs, P.; Tönjes, A. Relationship between 12 adipocytokines and distinct components of the metabolic syndrome. *J. Clin. Endocrinol. Metab.* **2018**, *103*, 1015–1023. [CrossRef]
72. Zou, D.; Wu, W.; He, Y.; Ma, S.; Gao, J. The role of klotho in chronic kidney disease. *BMC Nephrol.* **2018**, *19*, 285. [CrossRef] [PubMed]
73. Bäck, M.; Aranyi, T.; Cancela, M.L.; Carracedo, M.; Conceição, N.; Leftheriotis, G.; Macrae, V.; Martin, L.; Nitschke, Y.; Pasch, A.; et al. Endogenous calcification inhibitors in the prevention of vascular calcification: A consensus statement from the COST action EuroSoftCalcNet. *Front. Cardiovasc. Med.* **2019**, *5*, 196. [CrossRef] [PubMed]
74. Ginsberg, C.; Houben, A.J.H.M.; Malhotra, R.; Berendschot, T.T.J.M.; Dagnelie, P.C.; Kooman, J.P.; Webers, C.A.; Stehouwer, C.D.A.; Ix, J.H. Serum phosphate and microvascular function in a population-based cohort. *Clin. J. Am. Soc. Nephrol.* **2019**, *14*, 1626–1633. [CrossRef] [PubMed]
75. Rahabi-Layachi, H.; Ourouda, R.; Boullier, A.; Massy, Z.A.; Amant, C. Distinct effects of inorganic phosphate on cell cycle and apoptosis in human vascular smooth muscle cells. *J. Cell. Physiol.* **2015**, *230*, 347–355. [CrossRef]
76. Zhao, M.-M.; Xu, M.-J.; Cai, Y.; Zhao, G.; Guan, Y.; Kong, W.; Tang, C.; Wang, X. Mitochondrial reactive oxygen species promote p65 nuclear translocation mediating high-phosphate-induced vascular calcification in vitro and in vivo. *Kidney Int.* **2011**, *79*, 1071–1079. [CrossRef]
77. Vervloet, M.G.; Sezer, S.; Massy, Z.A.; Johansson, L.; Cozzolino, M.; Fouque, D.; ERA–EDTA Working Group on Chronic Kidney Disease–Mineral and Bone Disorders and the European Renal Nutrition Working Group. The role of phosphate in kidney disease. *Nat. Rev. Nephrol.* **2017**, *13*, 27–38. [CrossRef]

78. McClelland, R.; Christensen, K.; Mohammed, S.; McGuinness, D.; Cooney, J.; Bakshi, A.; Demou, E.; MacDonald, E.; Caslake, M.; Stenvinkel, P.; et al. Accelerated ageing and renal dysfunction links lower socioeconomic status and dietary phosphate intake. *Aging* **2017**, *8*, 1135–1149. [CrossRef]
79. Yao, L.; Sun, Y.; Sun, W.; Xu, T.; Ren, C.; Fan, X.; Sun, L.; Liu, L.; Feng, J.; Ma, J.; et al. High phosphorus level leads to aortic calcification via β-catenin in chronic kidney disease. *Am. J. Nephrol.* **2015**, *41*, 28–36. [CrossRef]
80. Cai, T.; Sun, D.; Duan, Y.; Wen, P.; Dai, C.; Yang, J.; He, W. WNT/β-catenin signaling promotes VSMCs to osteogenic transdifferentiation and calcification through directly modulating Runx2 gene expression. *Exp. Cell Res.* **2016**, *345*, 206–217. [CrossRef]
81. Chen, Y.-X.; Huang, C.; Duan, Z.-B.; Xu, C.-Y.; Chen, Y. Klotho/FGF23 axis mediates high phosphate-induced vascular calcification in vascular smooth muscle cells via Wnt7b/β-catenin pathway. *Kaohsiung J. Med. Sci.* **2019**, *35*, 393–400. [CrossRef]
82. Chen, T.; Mao, H.; Chen, C.; Wu, L.; Wang, N.; Zhao, X.; Qian, J.; Xing, C. The Role and Mechanism of α-Klotho in the Calcification of Rat Aortic Vascular Smooth Muscle Cells. Available online: https://www.hindawi.com/journals/bmri/2015/194362/ (accessed on 28 February 2020).
83. Mencke, R.; Hillebrands, J.-L. The role of the anti-ageing protein Klotho in vascular physiology and pathophysiology. *Ageing Res. Rev.* **2017**, *35*, 124–146. [CrossRef] [PubMed]
84. Aghagolzadeh, P.; Bachtler, M.; Bijarnia, R.; Jackson, C.; Smith, E.R.; Odermatt, A.; Radpour, R.; Pasch, A. Calcification of vascular smooth muscle cells is induced by secondary calciprotein particles and enhanced by tumor necrosis factor-α. *Atherosclerosis* **2016**, *251*, 404–414. [CrossRef] [PubMed]
85. Viegas, C.S.B.; Santos, L.; Macedo, A.L.; Matos, A.A.; Silva, A.P.; Neves, P.L.; Staes, A.; Gevaert, K.; Morais, R.; Vermeer, C.; et al. Chronic kidney disease circulating calciprotein particles and extracellular vesicles promote vascular calcification. *Arterioscler. Thromb. Vasc. Biol.* **2018**, *38*, 575–587. [CrossRef] [PubMed]
86. Barreto, F.C.; Barreto, D.V.; Massy, Z.A.; Drüeke, T.B. Strategies for phosphate control in patients with CKD. *Kidney Int. Rep.* **2019**, *4*, 1043–1056. [CrossRef] [PubMed]
87. Elder, G.J.; Malik, A.; Lambert, K. Role of dietary phosphate restriction in chronic kidney disease. *Nephrology* **2018**, *23*, 1107–1115. [CrossRef] [PubMed]
88. Tsai, W.-C.; Wu, H.-Y.; Peng, Y.-S.; Hsu, S.-P.; Chiu, Y.-L.; Chen, H.-Y.; Yang, J.-Y.; Ko, M.-J.; Pai, M.-F.; Tu, Y.-K.; et al. Effects of lower versus higher phosphate diets on fibroblast growth factor-23 levels in patients with chronic kidney disease: A systematic review and meta-analysis. *Nephrol. Dial. Transplant.* **2018**, *33*, 1977–1983. [CrossRef]
89. Tsai, W.-C.; Wu, H.-Y.; Peng, Y.-S.; Hsu, S.-P.; Chiu, Y.-L.; Yang, J.-Y.; Chen, H.-Y.; Pai, M.-F.; Lin, W.-Y.; Hung, K.-Y.; et al. Short-term effects of very-low-phosphate and low-phosphate diets on fibroblast growth factor 23 in hemodialysis patients: A randomized crossover trial. *Clin. J. Am. Soc. Nephrol.* **2019**, *14*, 1475–1483. [CrossRef]
90. Czarnik, T.; Czarnik, A.; Gawda, R.; Gawor, M.; Piwoda, M.; Marszalski, M.; Maj, M.; Chrzan, O.; Said, R.; Rusek-Skora, M.; et al. Vitamin D kinetics in the acute phase of critical illness: A prospective observational study. *J. Crit. Care* **2018**, *43*, 294–299. [CrossRef]
91. Norris, K.C.; Olabisi, O.; Barnett, M.E.; Meng, Y.-X.; Martins, D.; Obialo, C.; Lee, J.E.; Nicholas, S.B. The role of vitamin D and oxidative stress in chronic kidney disease. *Int. J. Environ. Res. Public Health* **2018**, *15*, 2701. [CrossRef]
92. Berridge, M.J. Vitamin D deficiency accelerates ageing and age-related diseases: A novel hypothesis. *J. Physiol.* **2017**, *595*, 6825–6836. [CrossRef]
93. Haussler, M.R.; Whitfield, G.K.; Haussler, C.A.; Sabir, M.S.; Khan, Z.; Sandoval, R.; Jurutka, P.W. Chapter eight–1,25-Dihydroxyvitamin D and Klotho: A tale of two renal hormones coming of age. In *Vitamins & Hormones*; Litwack, G., Ed.; Vitamin D Hormone; Academic Press: Cambridge, MA, USA, 2016; Volume 100, pp. 165–230.
94. Takenaka, T.; Inoue, T.; Ohno, Y.; Miyazaki, T.; Nishiyama, A.; Ishii, N.; Suzuki, H. Calcitriol supplementation improves endothelium-dependent vasodilation in rat hypertensive renal injury. *Kidney Blood Press. Res.* **2014**, *39*, 17–27. [CrossRef] [PubMed]
95. Jebreal Azimzadeh, M.; Shidfar, F.; Jazayeri, S.; Hosseini, A.F.; Ranjbaran, F. Effect of vitamin D supplementation on klotho protein, antioxidant status and nitric oxide in the elderly: A randomized, double-blinded, placebo-controlled clinical trial. *Eur. J. Integr. Med.* **2020**, *35*, 101089. [CrossRef]

96. Carvalho, J.T.G.; Schneider, M.; Cuppari, L.; Grabulosa, C.C.; Aoike, D.T.; Redublo, B.M.Q.; Batista, M.C.; Cendoroglo, M.; Moyses, R.M.; Dalboni, M.A. Cholecalciferol decreases inflammation and improves vitamin D regulatory enzymes in lymphocytes in the uremic environment: A randomized controlled pilot trial. *PLoS ONE* **2017**, *12*, e0179540. [CrossRef] [PubMed]
97. Mansournia, M.A.; Ostadmohammadi, V.; Doosti-Irani, A.; Ghayour-Mobarhan, M.; Ferns, G.; Akbari, H.; Ghaderi, A.; Talari, H.R.; Asemi, Z. The effects of vitamin d supplementation on biomarkers of inflammation and oxidative stress in diabetic patients: A systematic review and meta-analysis of randomized controlled trials. *Horm. Metab. Res.* **2018**, *50*, 429–440. [CrossRef]
98. Kruit, A.; Zanen, P. The association between vitamin D and C-reactive protein levels in patients with inflammatory and non-inflammatory diseases. *Clin. Biochem.* **2016**, *49*, 534–537. [CrossRef]
99. Hu, C.; Wu, X. Effect of vitamin D supplementation on vascular function and inflammation in patients with chronic kidney disease: A controversial issue. *Ther. Apher. Dial.* **2019**. [CrossRef]
100. Rodríguez, A.J.; Scott, D.; Srikanth, V.; Ebeling, P. Effect of vitamin D supplementation on measures of arterial stiffness: A systematic review and meta-analysis of randomized controlled trials. *Clin. Endocrinol. (Oxf.)* **2016**, *84*, 645–657. [CrossRef]
101. Hussin, A.M.; Ashor, A.W.; Schoenmakers, I.; Hill, T.; Mathers, J.C.; Siervo, M. Effects of vitamin D supplementation on endothelial function: A systematic review and meta-analysis of randomised clinical trials. *Eur. J. Nutr.* **2017**, *56*, 1095–1104. [CrossRef]
102. Gutiérrez, O.M.; Mannstadt, M.; Isakova, T.; Rauh-Hain, J.A.; Tamez, H.; Shah, A.; Smith, K.; Lee, H.; Thadhani, R.; Jüppner, H.; et al. Fibroblast growth factor 23 and mortality among patients undergoing hemodialysis. *N. Engl. J. Med.* **2008**, *359*, 584–592. [CrossRef]
103. Singh, S.; Grabner, A.; Yanucil, C.; Schramm, K.; Czaya, B.; Krick, S.; Czaja, M.J.; Bartz, R.; Abraham, R.; Di Marco, G.S.; et al. Fibroblast growth factor 23 directly targets hepatocytes to promote inflammation in chronic kidney disease. *Kidney Int.* **2016**, *90*, 985–996. [CrossRef]
104. Silswal, N.; Touchberry, C.D.; Daniel, D.R.; McCarthy, D.L.; Zhang, S.; Andresen, J.; Stubbs, J.R.; Wacker, M.J. FGF23 directly impairs endothelium-dependent vasorelaxation by increasing superoxide levels and reducing nitric oxide bioavailability. *Am. J. Physiol. Endocrinol. Metab.* **2014**, *307*, E426–E436. [CrossRef] [PubMed]
105. Verkaik, M.; Juni, R.P.; van Loon, E.P.M.; van Poelgeest, E.M.; Kwekkeboom, R.F.J.; Gam, Z.; Richards, W.G.; Ter Wee, P.M.; Hoenderop, J.G.; Eringa, E.C.; et al. FGF23 impairs peripheral microvascular function in renal failure. *Am. J. Physiol. Heart Circ. Physiol.* **2018**, *315*, H1414–H1424. [CrossRef] [PubMed]
106. Lindberg, K.; Olauson, H.; Amin, R.; Ponnusamy, A.; Goetz, R.; Taylor, R.F.; Mohammadi, M.; Canfield, A.; Kublickiene, K.; Larsson, T.E. Arterial klotho expression and FGF23 effects on vascular calcification and function. *PLoS ONE* **2013**, *8*, e60658. [CrossRef] [PubMed]
107. Simic, P.; Kim, W.; Zhou, W.; Pierce, K.A.; Chang, W.; Sykes, D.B.; Aziz, N.B.; Elmariah, S.; Ngo, D.; Pajevic, P.D.; et al. Glycerol-3-phosphate is an FGF23 regulator derived from the injured kidney. *J. Clin. Investig.* **2020**, *130*, 1513–1526. [CrossRef]
108. Haruna, Y.; Kashihara, N.; Satoh, M.; Tomita, N.; Namikoshi, T.; Sasaki, T.; Fujimori, T.; Xie, P.; Kanwar, Y.S. Amelioration of progressive renal injury by genetic manipulation of Klotho gene. *Proc. Natl. Acad. Sci. USA* **2007**, *104*, 2331–2336. [CrossRef]
109. Rodríguez-Ortiz, M.E.; Díaz-Tocados, J.M.; Muñoz-Castañeda, J.R.; Herencia, C.; Pineda, C.; Martínez-Moreno, J.M.; Montes de Oca, A.; López-Baltanás, R.; Alcalá-Díaz, J.; Ortiz, A.; et al. Inflammation both increases and causes resistance to FGF23 in normal and uremic rats. *Clin. Sci.* **2020**, *134*, 15–32. [CrossRef]
110. Zhou, L.; Li, Y.; Zhou, D.; Tan, R.J.; Liu, Y. Loss of klotho contributes to kidney injury by derepression of Wnt/β-catenin signaling. *J. Am. Soc. Nephrol.* **2013**, *24*, 771–785. [CrossRef]
111. Vila Cuenca, M.; Hordijk, P.L.; Vervloet, M.G. Most exposed: The endothelium in chronic kidney disease. *Nephrol. Dial. Transplant.* **2019**. [CrossRef]
112. Ter Braake, A.D.; Smit, A.E.; Bos, C.; van Herwaarden, A.E.; Alkema, W.; van Essen, H.W.; Bravenboer, N.; Vervloet, M.G.; Hoenderop, J.G.J.; de Baaij, J.H.F. Magnesium prevents vascular calcification in Klotho deficiency. *Kidney Int.* **2020**, *97*, 487–501. [CrossRef]
113. Leibrock, C.B.; Alesutan, I.; Voelkl, J.; Pakladok, T.; Michael, D.; Schleicher, E.; Kamyabi-Moghaddam, Z.; Quintanilla-Martinez, L.; Kuro-o, M.; Lang, F. NH4Cl treatment prevents tissue calcification in klotho deficiency. *J. Am. Soc. Nephrol.* **2015**, *26*, 2423–2433. [CrossRef]

114. Ravarotto, V.; Simioni, F.; Pagnin, E.; Davis, P.A.; Calò, L.A. Oxidative stress—Chronic kidney disease—Cardiovascular disease: A vicious circle. *Life Sci.* **2018**, *210*, 125–131. [CrossRef] [PubMed]
115. Bhargava, P.; Schnellmann, R.G. Mitochondrial energetics in the kidney. *Nat. Rev. Nephrol.* **2017**, *13*, 629–646. [CrossRef] [PubMed]
116. Cuadrado, A.; Rojo, A.I.; Wells, G.; Hayes, J.D.; Cousin, S.P.; Rumsey, W.L.; Attucks, O.C.; Franklin, S.; Levonen, A.-L.; Kensler, T.W.; et al. Therapeutic targeting of the NRF2 and KEAP1 partnership in chronic diseases. *Nat. Rev. Drug Discov.* **2019**, *18*, 295–317. [CrossRef] [PubMed]
117. Liu, C.; Gidlund, E.; Witasp, A.; Qureshi, A.R.; Söderberg, M.; Thorell, A.; Nader, G.A.; Barany, P.; Stenvinkel, P.; von Walden, F. Reduced skeletal muscle expression of mitochondrial derived peptides humanin and MOTS-C and Nrf2 in chronic kidney disease. *Am. J. Physiol.-Ren. Physiol.* **2019**, *317*, F1122–F1131.
118. Kubben, N.; Zhang, W.; Wang, L.; Voss, T.C.; Yang, J.; Qu, J.; Liu, G.-H.; Misteli, T. Repression of the antioxidant NRF2 pathway in premature aging. *Cell* **2016**, *165*, 1361–1374. [CrossRef]
119. Volonte, D.; Liu, Z.; Musille, P.M.; Stoppani, E.; Wakabayashi, N.; Di, Y.-P.; Lisanti, M.P.; Kensler, T.W.; Galbiati, F. Inhibition of nuclear factor-erythroid 2–related factor (Nrf2) by caveolin-1 promotes stress-induced premature senescence. *Mol. Biol. Cell* **2013**, *24*, 1852–1862. [CrossRef] [PubMed]
120. Fulop, G.A.; Kiss, T.; Tarantini, S.; Balasubramanian, P.; Yabluchanskiy, A.; Farkas, E.; Bari, F.; Ungvari, Z.; Csiszar, A. Nrf2 deficiency in aged mice exacerbates cellular senescence promoting cerebrovascular inflammation. *GeroScience* **2018**, *40*, 513–521. [CrossRef] [PubMed]
121. Romero, A.; Hipólito-Luengo, Á.S.; Villalobos, L.A.; Vallejo, S.; Valencia, I.; Michalska, P.; Pajuelo-Lozano, N.; Sánchez-Pérez, I.; León, R.; Bartha, J.L.; et al. The angiotensin-(1-7)/Mas receptor axis protects from endothelial cell senescence via klotho and Nrf2 activation. *Aging Cell* **2019**, *18*, e12913. [CrossRef]
122. Zhang, G.; Kang, Y.; Zhou, C.; Cui, R.; Jia, M.; Hu, S.; Ji, X.; Yuan, J.; Cui, H.; Shi, G. Amelioratory effects of testosterone propionate on age-related renal fibrosis via suppression of TGF-β1/Smad signaling and activation of Nrf2-ARE signaling. *Sci. Rep.* **2018**, *8*, 1–11. [CrossRef]
123. Stockler-Pinto, M.B.; Soulage, C.O.; Borges, N.A.; Cardozo, L.F.M.F.; Dolenga, C.J.; Nakao, L.S.; Pecoits-Filho, R.; Fouque, D.; Mafra, D. From bench to the hemodialysis clinic: Protein-bound uremic toxins modulate NF-κB/Nrf2 expression. *Int. Urol. Nephrol.* **2018**, *50*, 347–354. [CrossRef]
124. Zhang, H.; Wang, J.; Wang, Y.; Gao, C.; Gu, Y.; Huang, J.; Wang, J.; Zhang, Z. Salvianolic acid a protects the kidney against oxidative stress by activating the Akt/GSK-3 β/Nrf2 signaling pathway and inhibiting the NF-κ B signaling pathway in 5/6 nephrectomized rats. *Oxid. Med. Cell. Longev.* **2019**, *2019*, 1–16. [CrossRef]
125. Nagasu, H.; Sogawa, Y.; Kidokoro, K.; Itano, S.; Yamamoto, T.; Satoh, M.; Sasaki, T.; Suzuki, T.; Yamamoto, M.; Wigley, W.C.; et al. Bardoxolone methyl analog attenuates proteinuria-induced tubular damage by modulating mitochondrial function. *FASEB J.* **2019**, *33*, 12253–12263. [CrossRef] [PubMed]
126. Lai, K.N.; Tang, S.C.W.; Schena, F.P.; Novak, J.; Tomino, Y.; Fogo, A.B.; Glassock, R.J. IgA nephropathy. *Nat. Rev. Dis. Primer* **2016**, *2*, 1–20. [CrossRef] [PubMed]
127. Sturmlechner, I.; Durik, M.; Sieben, C.J.; Baker, D.J.; van Deursen, J.M. Cellular senescence in renal ageing and disease. *Nat. Rev. Nephrol.* **2017**, *13*, 77–89. [CrossRef] [PubMed]
128. Yamada, K.; Doi, S.; Nakashima, A.; Kawaoka, K.; Ueno, T.; Doi, T.; Yokoyama, Y.; Arihiro, K.; Kohno, N.; Masaki, T. Expression of age-related factors during the development of renal damage in patients with IgA nephropathy. *Clin. Exp. Nephrol.* **2015**, *19*, 830–837. [CrossRef] [PubMed]
129. Jiang, H.; Liang, L.; Qin, J.; Lu, Y.; Li, B.; Wang, Y.; Lin, C.; Zhou, Q.; Feng, S.; Yip, S.H.; et al. Functional networks of aging markers in the glomeruli of IgA nephropathy: A new therapeutic opportunity. *Oncotarget* **2016**, *7*, 33616–33626. [CrossRef]
130. Cokan Vujkovac, A.; Novaković, S.; Vujkovac, B.; Števanec, M.; Škerl, P.; Šabovič, M. Aging in fabry disease: Role of telomere length, telomerase activity, and kidney disease. *Nephron* **2020**, *144*, 5–13. [CrossRef]
131. Kooman, J.P.; Stenvinkel, P.; Shiels, P.G. Fabry disease: A new model of premature ageing? *Nephron* **2020**, *144*, 1–4. [CrossRef]
132. Bergmann, C.; Guay-Woodford, L.M.; Harris, P.C.; Horie, S.; Peters, D.J.M.; Torres, V.E. Polycystic kidney disease. *Nat. Rev. Dis. Primer* **2018**, *4*, 1–24. [CrossRef]
133. Lu, D.; Rauhauser, A.; Li, B.; Ren, C.; McEnery, K.; Zhu, J.; Chaki, M.; Vadnagara, K.; Elhadi, S.; Jetten, A.M.; et al. Loss of Glis2/NPHP7 causes kidney epithelial cell senescence and suppresses cyst growth in the Kif3a mouse model of cystic kidney disease. *Kidney Int.* **2016**, *89*, 1307–1323. [CrossRef]

134. Jin, H.; Zhang, Y.; Liu, D.; Wang, S.S.; Ding, Q.; Rastogi, P.; Purvis, M.; Wang, A.; Elhadi, S.; Ren, C.; et al. Innate immune signaling contributes to tubular cell senescence in the Glis2 knockout mouse model of nephronophthisis. *Am. J. Pathol.* **2020**, *190*, 176–189. [CrossRef]
135. Larsson, S.C.; Bäck, M.; Rees, J.M.B.; Mason, A.M.; Burgess, S. Body mass index and body composition in relation to 14 cardiovascular conditions in UK Biobank: A Mendelian randomization study. *Eur. Heart J.* **2020**, *41*, 221–226. [CrossRef]
136. Blüher, M. Obesity: Global epidemiology and pathogenesis. *Nat. Rev. Endocrinol.* **2019**, *15*, 288–298. [CrossRef] [PubMed]
137. Schafer, M.J.; Miller, J.D.; LeBrasseur, N.K. Cellular senescence: Implications for metabolic disease. *Mol. Cell. Endocrinol.* **2017**, *455*, 93–102. [CrossRef] [PubMed]
138. Liu, Z.; Wu, K.K.L.; Jiang, X.; Xu, A.; Cheng, K.K.Y. The role of adipose tissue senescence in obesity- and ageing-related metabolic disorders. *Clin. Sci.* **2020**, *134*, 315–330. [CrossRef] [PubMed]
139. Ebert, T.; Roth, I.; Richter, J.; Tönjes, A.; Kralisch, S.; Lossner, U.; Kratzsch, J.; Blüher, M.; Stumvoll, M.; Fasshauer, M. Different associations of adipokines in lean and healthy adults. *Horm. Metab. Res.* **2014**, *46*, 41–47. [CrossRef] [PubMed]
140. Palmer, A.K.; Xu, M.; Zhu, Y.; Pirtskhalava, T.; Weivoda, M.M.; Hachfeld, C.M.; Prata, L.G.; van Dijk, T.H.; Verkade, E.; Casaclang-Verzosa, G.; et al. Targeting senescent cells alleviates obesity-induced metabolic dysfunction. *Aging Cell* **2019**, *18*, e12950. [CrossRef] [PubMed]
141. Carracedo, M.; Witasp, A.; Qureshi, A.R.; Laguna-Fernandez, A.; Brismar, T.; Stenvinkel, P.; Bäck, M. Chemerin inhibits vascular calcification through ChemR23 and is associated with lower coronary calcium in chronic kidney disease. *J. Intern. Med.* **2019**, *286*, 449–457. [CrossRef] [PubMed]
142. Melk, A.; Schmidt, B.M.W.; Vongwiwatana, A.; Rayner, D.C.; Halloran, P.F. Increased expression of senescence-associated cell cycle inhibitor p16INK4a in deteriorating renal transplants and diseased native kidney. *Am. J. Transplant.* **2005**, *5*, 1375–1382. [CrossRef]
143. Baisantry, A.; Berkenkamp, B.; Rong, S.; Bhayadia, R.; Sörensen-Zender, I.; Schmitt, R.; Melk, A. Time-dependent p53 inhibition determines senescence attenuation and long-term outcome after renal ischemia-reperfusion. *Am. J. Physiol. Ren. Physiol.* **2019**, *316*, F1124–F1132. [CrossRef]
144. Childs, B.G.; Durik, M.; Baker, D.J.; van Deursen, J.M. Cellular senescence in aging and age-related disease: From mechanisms to therapy. *Nat. Med.* **2015**, *21*, 1424–1435. [CrossRef]
145. Luttropp, K.; Nordfors, L.; McGuinness, D.; Wennberg, L.; Curley, H.; Quasim, T.; Genberg, H.; Sandberg, J.; Sönnerborg, I.; Schalling, M.; et al. Increased telomere attrition after renal transplantation—Impact of antimetabolite therapy. *Transplant. Direct* **2016**, *2*, e116. [CrossRef] [PubMed]
146. Toppe, C.; Möllsten, A.; Waernbaum, I.; Schön, S.; Gudbjörnsdottir, S.; Landin-Olsson, M.; Dahlquist, G. Decreasing cumulative incidence of end-stage renal disease in young patients with type 1 diabetes in Sweden: A 38-year prospective nationwide study. *Diabetes Care* **2019**, *42*, 27–31. [CrossRef] [PubMed]
147. Helve, J.; Sund, R.; Arffman, M.; Harjutsalo, V.; Groop, P.-H.; Grönhagen-Riska, C.; Finne, P. Incidence of end-stage renal disease in patients with type 1 diabetes. *Diabetes Care* **2018**, *41*, 434–439. [CrossRef] [PubMed]
148. Thomas, B.; Matsushita, K.; Abate, K.H.; Al-Aly, Z.; Ärnlöv, J.; Asayama, K.; Atkins, R.; Badawi, A.; Ballew, S.H.; Banerjee, A.; et al. Global cardiovascular and renal outcomes of reduced GFR. *J. Am. Soc. Nephrol.* **2017**, *28*, 2167–2179. [CrossRef] [PubMed]
149. Wardyn, J.D.; Ponsford, A.H.; Sanderson, C.M. Dissecting molecular cross-talk between Nrf2 and NF-κB response pathways. *Biochem. Soc. Trans.* **2015**, *43*, 621–626. [CrossRef]
150. Abreu, C.C.; Cardozo, L.F.M.F.; Stockler-Pinto, M.B.; Esgalhado, M.; Barboza, J.E.; Frauches, R.; Mafra, D. Does resistance exercise performed during dialysis modulate Nrf2 and NF-κB in patients with chronic kidney disease? *Life Sci.* **2017**, *188*, 192–197. [CrossRef] [PubMed]
151. Vega, M.R.; de la Chapman, E.; Zhang, D.D. NRF2 and the hallmarks of cancer. *Cancer Cell* **2018**, *34*, 21–43. [CrossRef]
152. Qiao, X.; Rao, P.; Zhang, Y.; Liu, L.; Pang, M.; Wang, H.; Hu, M.; Tian, X.; Zhang, J.; Zhao, Y.; et al. Redirecting TGF-β signaling through the β-Catenin/Foxo complex prevents kidney fibrosis. *J. Am. Soc. Nephrol.* **2018**, *29*, 557–570. [CrossRef]
153. Zhou, X.; Wang, X. Klotho: A novel biomarker for cancer. *J. Cancer Res. Clin. Oncol.* **2015**, *141*, 961–969. [CrossRef]

154. Dote-Montero, M.; Amaro-Gahete, F.J.; De-la-O, A.; Jurado-Fasoli, L.; Gutierrez, A.; Castillo, M.J. Study of the association of DHEAS, testosterone and cortisol with S-Klotho plasma levels in healthy sedentary middle-aged adults. *Exp. Gerontol.* **2019**, *121*, 55–61. [CrossRef]
155. Pedersen, L.; Christensen, L.L.; Pedersen, S.M.; Andersen, M. Reduction of calprotectin and phosphate during testosterone therapy in aging men: A randomized controlled trial. *J. Endocrinol. Investig.* **2017**, *40*, 529–538. [CrossRef] [PubMed]
156. Neyra, J.A.; Hu, M.C. Potential application of klotho in human chronic kidney disease. *Bone* **2017**, *100*, 41–49. [CrossRef] [PubMed]
157. Gregg, L.P.; Hedayati, S.S. Management of traditional cardiovascular risk factors in CKD: What are the data? *Am. J. Kidney Dis.* **2018**, *72*, 728–744. [CrossRef] [PubMed]

© 2020 by the authors. Licensee MDPI, Basel, Switzerland. This article is an open access article distributed under the terms and conditions of the Creative Commons Attribution (CC BY) license (http://creativecommons.org/licenses/by/4.0/).

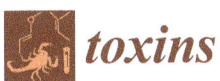

Review

Molecular and Cellular Mechanisms that Induce Arterial Calcification by Indoxyl Sulfate and P-Cresyl Sulfate

Britt Opdebeeck, Patrick C. D'Haese * and Anja Verhulst

Laboratory of Pathophysiology, Department of Biomedical Sciences, University of Antwerp, 2000 Antwerpen, Belgium; britt.opdebeeck2@uantwerpen.be (B.O.); anja.verhulst@uantwerpen.be (A.V.)
* Correspondence: patrick.dhaese@uantwerpen.be; Tel.: +32-3-265-2599

Received: 18 December 2019; Accepted: 17 January 2020; Published: 19 January 2020

Abstract: The protein-bound uremic toxins, indoxyl sulfate (IS) and p-cresyl sulfate (PCS), are considered to be harmful vascular toxins. Arterial media calcification, or the deposition of calcium phosphate crystals in the arteries, contributes significantly to cardiovascular complications, including left ventricular hypertrophy, hypertension, and impaired coronary perfusion in the elderly and patients with chronic kidney disease (CKD) and diabetes. Recently, we reported that both IS and PCS trigger moderate to severe calcification in the aorta and peripheral vessels of CKD rats. This review describes the molecular and cellular mechanisms by which these uremic toxins induce arterial media calcification. A complex interplay between inflammation, coagulation, and lipid metabolism pathways, influenced by epigenetic factors, is crucial in IS/PCS-induced arterial media calcification. High levels of glucose are linked to these events, suggesting that a good balance between glucose and lipid levels might be important. On the cellular level, effects on endothelial cells, which act as the primary sensors of circulating pathological triggers, might be as important as those on vascular smooth muscle cells. Endothelial dysfunction, provoked by IS and PCS triggered oxidative stress, may be considered a key event in the onset and development of arterial media calcification. In this review a number of important outstanding questions such as the role of miRNA's, phenotypic switching of both endothelial and vascular smooth muscle cells and new types of programmed cell death in arterial media calcification related to protein-bound uremic toxins are put forward and discussed.

Keywords: uremic toxins; arterial calcification; lipid metabolism; inflammation; coagulation; endothelial dysfunction; epigenetics

Key Contribution: Indoxyl sulfate and p-cresyl sulfate promote arterial calcification, and this is linked to a complex interplay between inflammation, coagulation, and lipid metabolism pathways.

---

1. Introduction

During chronic kidney disease (CKD), uremic retention solutes accumulate in the bloodstream due to progressive kidney function loss. Three classes of uremic retention solutes exist: (i) low-molecular-weight water-soluble solutes (<500 Da), (ii) middle-molecular-weight solutes (>500 Da), and (iii) protein-bound solutes. This latter class is characterized by a limited dialytic removal due to the high molecular weight of the protein complexes that complicates their movement across the dialysis membrane [1]. Both indoxyl sulfate (IS) and p-cresyl sulfate (PCS) belong to the protein-bound uremic toxins and originate from protein fermentation in the intestine. The intestinal microbiota facilitates the breakdown of tyrosine/phenylalanine and tryptophan into, respectively, p-cresol and indole, which are absorbed and detoxified by oxidation and conjugation with sulfate [2]. In the bloodstream, IS and PCS bind to albumin, which implies that glomerular filtration does not take place and thus requires tubular transporter systems in the kidney to excrete these two protein-bound uremic toxins. Basolateral organic anion transporter 1 (OAT1) and 3 (OAT3), breast cancer resistance protein (BCRP) and multidrug resistance protein 4 (MRP4) belong to the IS and PCS tubular transport system [3]. Due to progressive kidney function loss, the concentration of IS and PCS increases with CKD stage in humans, as shown in Table 1 (adapted from Lin et al., *J. Food Drug Anal.*, 2019 [4]), ending up with levels of around 20-fold CKD stage 1. Moreover, free IS and PCS levels are 100-fold higher in pretreatment hemodialysis patients as compared to normal subjects [5]. There is, however, a high inter-individual variability, reflected by high standard deviations, which is also observed in other studies [6–8]. An explanation might be (i) alterations in colon microbiome attributed in part to dietary restrictions in CKD patients [9], (ii) modulation of IS and PCS transporters [10] and (iii) residual kidney function [11]. This inter-patient variability might influence the interpretation on the association between of IS and PCS concentrations and clinical outcomes. However, unbound PCS serum levels are suggested to hold a substantial predictive value for the survival in CKD patients [8]. Moreover, IS and PCS serum levels are also associated with cardiovascular disease and mortality [12,13]. Furthermore, Shafi et al. reported no association between total IS and PCS serum concentrations with cardiac death, sudden cardiac death, and first cardiovascular event [14]. These conflicting clinical associations demand for experimental study designs to unravel the role of IS and PCS in cardiovascular disease, which is crucial, as cardiovascular defects account for 50% of all deaths in CKD patients [15], having high serum IS and PCS levels.

Table 1. Serum levels of albumin bound (total) and unbound (free) IS and PCS.

CKD	Stage 1	Stage 2	Stage 3	Stage 4	Stage 5
N	29	49	64	40	22
Total IS (mg/L)	1.03 ± 0.85	1.54 ± 1.11	2.22 ± 1.79	4.74 ± 4.34	18.21 ± 15.06
Total PCS (mg/L)	2.69 ± 4.34	4.42 ± 4.47	6.45 ± 7.12	16.10 ± 13.98	27.00 ± 17.66
Free IS (mg/L)	0.08 ± 0.06	0.11 ± 0.09	0.17 ± 0.13	0.49 ± 0.72	2.36 ± 2.64
Free PCS (mg/L)	0.15 ± 0.20	0.24 ± 0.29	0.36 ± 0.37	1.36 ± 2.58	2.38 ± 2.03

Data represent the mean ± standard deviation.

2. Molecular Mechanisms by Which IS and PCS Induce Vascular Calcification

Arterial media calcification is a life-threatening disease that manifests in elderly and patients with chronic kidney disease (CKD) and diabetes mellitus. The disease phenotype is characterized by a passive and active deposition of calcium phosphate crystals in the media layer of the arterial wall that leads to arterial stiffness, which in turn induces hypertension, left ventricular hypertrophy, and impaired coronary perfusion. Arterial media calcification occurs already in the early stages of CKD, and more than half of the CKD patients on dialysis suffer from it [16,17]. Moreover, calcifications in the arterial wall are also present in children with CKD [18]. Moreover, CKD patients who also suffer from diabetes mellitus have a higher incidence of arterial calcification compared to nondiabetic hemodialysis patients [19]. Poor control of glucose levels is a predictor of arterial calcification in humans [19,20]. Our laboratory recently reported that both IS and PCS are important harmful vascular toxins, as they trigger moderate to severe arterial media calcification in CKD rats, which goes along with the activation of inflammation (i.e., acute phase response signaling pathway) and coagulation (i.e., intrinsic/extrinsic prothrombin activation pathway) pathways linked with increased circulating glucose levels and insulin resistance. These changes were even observed after four days of IS or PCS exposure, i.e., before arterial media calcifications had developed, indicating that the IS/PCS mediated upregulation of inflammation and coagulation precedes the vascular calcification process [21]. Additionally, in this study, escape from uremic-toxin-induced calcification was linked with liver X receptor and farnesoid X/liver X receptor signaling pathways, discussed more in detail below. This review focuses on these signaling pathways, as well as on the connection with endothelial dysfunction and the effects on microRNAs.

2.1. Inflammation and Coagulation Signaling Pathways

The inflammatory acute phase response signaling pathway is a physiological host-defense mechanism to injury, including trauma, acute infection, and myocardial infarction [22]. In addition, a low-grade chronic acute phase response exists and is characterized by chronically elevated levels of acute phase proteins in response to metabolically triggered inflammation [23]. During CKD, the human body undergoes a permanent status of low-grade inflammation. The uremic retention solutes IS and PCS regulate inflammation in multiple cell types, including adipocytes, endothelial cells, macrophages, proximal tubular cells, and glial cells [24–28]. Inflammatory responses are associated with the development of arterial calcification [29]. Moreover, a recent study in 112 chronic hemodialysis patients correlated acute-phase proteins (i.e., C-reactive protein, ferritin, hepcidin, and albumin) with the development of abdominal aortic calcification [30]. In addition, the acute-phase proteins serum amyloid A and C-reactive protein have been reported not to be solely produced by hepatocytes, but also in the arterial wall, by vascular smooth muscle cells (VSMCs). Both proteins stimulate the phenotypic switch of VSMCs into bone-like cells through activation of the p38 MAPK pathway and oxidative stress pathways [31,32]. As mentioned above, our study also revealed that, after proteomic analysis of aortic tissue from either IS or PCS exposed CKD rats, coagulation pathways (intrinsic/extrinsic prothrombin activation pathways) play a central role in the arterial calcification process [21]. A close link between coagulation and inflammation exists as coagulation factors, such as fibrinogens and prothrombin, also belong to the acute phase proteins [22]. A recent study showed that IS induces platelet hyperactivity, with an elevated response to collagen and thrombin, through activation of the p38 MAPK and oxidative stress pathways [33]. Moreover, other studies reported an association between increased serum IS levels and thrombotic complications in CKD patients [33,34]. Then again, the thrombin–antithrombin complex level, used as a marker for thrombin formation in vivo, correlates with the presence and severity of coronary artery calcification [35,36]. An in vitro study of Kapustin et al. showed that Gla-containing coagulation factors (i.e., prothrombin and protein C and S) inhibit the vascular calcification process [37]. This might mean that the calcification-inducing effects of warfarin [38,39] can also be ascribed to its anti-coagulant actions, next to the fact that it prevents the production of the active form of matrix Gla protein, an important endogenous calcification inhibitor (warfarin inhibits carboxylation of Gla-proteins by inhibiting vitamin K recycling). All of these data suggest that coagulation and vascular calcification are interconnected and that the uremic toxins IS and PCS could play an important role herein. However, a recent multicenter randomized controlled trial showed that withdrawal of vitamin K antagonists in hemodialysis patients did not influence progression of arterial calcification progression after 18 months [40]. These conflicting data again indicate that the arterial calcification process is the result of a complex interplay between different pathological pathways.

Interestingly, in our experimental study, a minority (3 out of 15) of CKD rats exposed to either IS or PCS did not develop arterial media calcification. This escape from uremic toxin-induced arterial calcification was related to liver X receptor and farnesoid X/liver X receptor signaling pathways, an important pathway in lipid metabolism. Activation of the liver X receptor (LXR) by the agonist GW3965 leads to anti-inflammatory actions in endothelial cells and macrophages by attenuation of the NF-kB pathway and IL-8 production [41,42]. Moreover, LXR activation inhibits cardiomyocyte apoptosis by restored mitochondrial membrane potential level and thus decreased reactive oxygen species (ROS) production [43]. These studies suggest that IS- and PCS-induced vascular calcification could be counteracted by preventing inflammation and oxidative stress events through the LXR pathway. This is further strengthened by results from our study in which, next to upregulation of acute phase response (inflammation), also oxidative stress pathways, i.e., Glutathione Mediated Detoxification and Glutathione Redox Reactions I, were observed in calcified aortic tissue of rats exposed to either IS or PCS for 7 weeks [21]. Furthermore, epigenetic involvement, often influenced by inflammation and oxidative stress, adds to the complexity by which uremic toxins trigger cardiovascular complications in CKD patients. IS has been associated with the regulating mammalian methyltransferase Set7/9, an epigenetic inducer of inflammatory genes, in VSMCs [44]. Moreover, data from an experimental rat study showed that IS exposure induces arterial thrombosis via decreased aortic levels of sirtuin 1, a class III histone deacetylase involved in oxidative stress [45]. We conducted a curated chemical and genomic/proteomic perturbagen matching analysis to predict upstream regulators that could be responsible for the observed changes in the arterial proteins linked to inflammation and coagulation signaling pathways. This analysis revealed a major role for altered energy and glucose metabolism, including elevated glucose levels and insulin receptor dysfunction [21]. This is interesting in view of the fact that diabetes increases the risk for vascular calcification in CKD patients [19]. Koppe et al. showed that chronic PCS exposure promoted insulin resistance and hyperglycemia in CKD mice [46]. Taken together, our study [21] suggests that IS and PCS stimulate the aortic media calcification via alterations in glucose metabolism, which in turn may stimulate inflammation, coagulation, and oxidative stress pathways in the aorta. It is worth noting that other studies have reported that the aryl hydrocarbon receptor, activated by IS, also regulates coagulation in VSMCs [47] and endothelial cells [48]. Interestingly, transient hyperglycemia also triggers Set7/9-mediated epigenetic changes in the promoter of NF-kB subunit p65, favoring overexpression of inflammatory genes [49]. Moreover, hyperglycemia favors the downregulation of sirtuin 1 in endothelial cells, and, by this, it upregulates vascular p66Shc gene transcription, which is implicated in mitochondrial ROS production and induction of apoptotic cell death. Moreover, metformin, an antidiabetic drug, has been reported to stimulate sirtuin 1 activation, which suppressed the increase of poly (ADP-ribose) polymerase (PARP) mediated mitochondrial ROS and thereby halted oxidative stress and inflammation in the retina of diabetic rats [50]. Remarkably, both metformin [51] and minocycline (PARP-inhibitor) [52] inhibit the development of arterial calcification in rats, pointing to the importance of oxidative stress and cell death events in the process of vascular calcification. Figure 1 gives a schematic overview of the interplay between inflammation, coagulation, and lipid metabolism and the role of epigenetics in IS and PCS-induced arterial calcification.

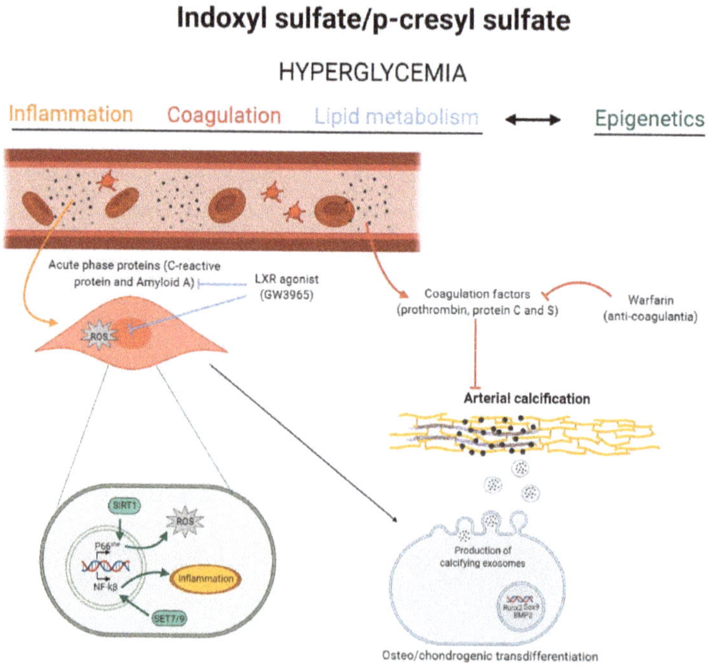

Figure 1. The role of inflammation, coagulation, lipid metabolism, and epigenetics in indoxyl sulfate and p-cresyl sulfate induced arterial calcification. High levels of indoxyl sulfate (IS) and p-cresyl sulfate

(PCS) induce a state of hyperglycemia, which activates inflammation, coagulation, lipid, and epigenetic pathways in the vascular cell. Inflammation (yellow): acute-phase response proteins induce reactive oxygen species (ROS) production in the vascular smooth muscle cell, stimulating the phenotypic switch into osteo-/chondrogenic cells. Coagulation (red): circulating coagulation factors inhibit arterial media calcification, while the anti-coagulant warfarin stimulates the calcification process. Lipid metabolism (blue): the liver-X-receptor (LXR) agonist blocks the inflammation mediated ROS production and, by this, inhibits arterial media calcification. Epigenetics (green): IS and PCS induced hyperglycemia might trigger sirtuin 1 (SIRT1)- and Set7/9-mediated epigenetic changes in the promoter of, respectively, p66She gene and NF-kB subunit p65, favoring, respectively, mitochondrial ROS production and inflammation in the cell. Figure was created with BioRender.com.

2.2. MicroRNAs, Upcoming Important Epigenetic Regulators in Uremic Toxins-Induced Vascular Calcification

MicroRNAs, small noncoding RNAs, are approximately 18–25 nucleotides long and regulate the protein expression of the target mRNA without affecting the gene sequence [53]. It has been well established that microRNAs play an important role in the vascular calcification process [54]. Protein-bound uremic toxins stimulate the expression of microRNA miR-92a in endothelial cells and, by this, suppress the gene expression of sirtuin 1, Krüppel-like factors 2 and 4, and endothelial nitric oxide synthase (eNOS) [55]. Interestingly, nitric oxide (NO) may be protective against arterial calcification, as in vitro NO inhibits murine VSMCs calcification and osteochondrogenic transdifferentiation via inhibition of TGFβ-induced phosphorylation of SMAD2/3 [56] and metformin halts arterial calcification through restoration of NO bioavailability (via the AMPK-eNOS-NO pathway) in rats [51,57]. As already mentioned above, metformin also increases the expression of sirtuin 1 [50] and thus might be able to counteract the IS/PCS-miR-92a triggered suppression of sirtuin 1 and, by this, decrease oxidative stress and inflammation events.

Another microRNA, miR-29b, has been reported to influence the development of arterial calcification in VSMC cell cultures and 5/6th nephrectomized rats [58]. Moreover, a recent study showed that miR-29b was downregulated in human aortic smooth muscle cells in which IS induced calcification, and by this increased Wnt7b/β catenin signaling [59]. IS also promotes renal fibrosis by DNA hypermethylation of sFRP5, leading to activation of the Wnt/β catenin signaling pathway [60]. Interestingly, our laboratory found that sclerostin, a Wnt/β catenin inhibitor, might be linked to prevention of vascular calcification development [39]. Furthermore, uremic toxins also correlate with elevated serum levels of miR-126, miR-143, miR-145, and miR-223 [61]. This latter microRNA, when overexpressed, triggers the uptake of glucose via the glucose transporter GLUT4 in cardiomyocytes [62] and stimulates the arterial calcification process by acting on the VSMC phenotypic switch [63], which is further discussed in the next paragraph. For this reason, miR-223 might have played a role in the hyperglycemia seen in our previous study concomitantly with the development of IS/PCS induced aortic media calcification. This, in turn, could have stimulated inflammation, coagulation, and oxidative stress pathways in the aorta. Again, this points to an important role of hyperglycemia in the toxic effects of IS and PCS on the vasculature.

2.3. Novel Research Fields to be Explored

2.3.1. Protein-Bound Uremic Toxins Influence Phenotypic Switch of Multiple Cell Types

The phenotypic transition of VSMCs into osteo/chondrogenic cells is a hallmark of the arterial calcification process [64]. Studies have shown that both IS and PCS are able to induce osteo/chondrogenic transdifferentiation of VSMCs by downregulation of smooth muscle genes (i.e., smooth muscle 22α, α-smooth muscle actin) and upregulation of bone-like genes (i.e., runx2, alkaline phosphatase, and osteopontin) [65,66]. This genotypic switching stimulates the VSMCs to produce calcifying exosomes, in which calcium phosphate crystals aggregate and, by this, mineralize the extracellular matrix [64]. Interestingly, IS and PCS also induce the transdifferentiation of other cell types, such as proximal renal tubular cells. When these cells are exposed to either IS or PCS, an epithelial to mesenchymal transition (EMT) occurs. During EMT, proximal renal tubular cells lose their adhesive characteristics with downregulation of E-cadherin in favor of mesenchymal fibroblast-like characteristics with upregulation of α-smooth muscle actin, fibronectin, N-cadherin, and vimentin. Several studies have shown that exposure to IS or PCS induces these phenotypic alterations, leading to glomerular sclerosis and interstitial fibrosis, with further stimulation of the progression of CKD [67–69]. Moreover, AST120, an oral spherical carbonaceous adsorbent, absorbs the precursors of IS and PCS and ameliorates the EMT process in renal tubular cells, and this is correlated with a decrease of serum IS levels [70]. Both TGFβ/Smad signaling and β-catenin signaling have been reported to act as main regulators of the uremic-toxin-induced EMT process in renal tubular cells [69,71]. In addition to EMT, endothelial to mesenchymal transition (EndMT), a subtype of EMT, involves the transdifferentiation of endothelial cells into mesenchymal stem-like cells which can differentiate further into multiple cell lineages: fibroblasts/myofibroblasts, osteoblasts/osteocytes, chondrocytes, and/or adipocytes [72]. Various studies have linked EndMT to the development of arterial calcification [73–75]. Its specific role in the calcification process, however, is not yet completely understood. It would be interesting to investigate whether IS and PCS are involved in the EndMT process, as (i) IS and PCS are known to promote arterial media calcification, and (ii) IS and PCS stimulate the EMT process in proximal tubular cells. Moreover, research so far predominantly focused on the transdifferentiation of VSMCs into bone-like cells, whilst the phenotypic transition of endothelial cells (EndMT) is often neglected and might be more important than generally thought [76]. Subsequently, in vitro experiments have demonstrated that both IS and PCS induce endothelial dysfunction, underlining even more that the endothelium plays a crucial role during uremic-toxin-induced arterial media calcification.

2.3.2. The Endothelium, an Overlooked Structure in the Process of Uremic Toxin Induced Vascular Calcification

IS and PCS induce deleterious effects in the endothelium, including the inhibition of cell proliferation and wound healing, and the increase in oxidative stress responses, cell senescence, and the release of endothelial microparticles [77–80]. A prospective observational study in 41 CKD patients revealed that AST-120 treatment decreased serum IS levels, as well as the oxidized/reduced glutathione ratio [79]. Interestingly, a depletion of glutathione triggers ferroptotic events [81], a novel type of iron-mediated programmed cell death characterized by the accumulation of lipid peroxides. Moreover, IS-generated oxidative stress in human umbilical vein endothelial cells induces endothelial senescence [79,82]. Additionally, in other cell types, including proximal renal tubular cells and VSMCs, IS has been reported to accelerate the process of cell senescence, as evidenced by the upregulation of p53 activity [83,84]. Activation of this tumor-suppressor protein p53 in the cell initiates apoptosis, senescence, and ferroptosis [85]. Which of these cell fates eventually occurs depends on yet unknown mechanisms that direct allow p53 to selectively activate downstream targets. The involvement of cell senescence and apoptosis in arterial calcification has been reported [86,87]. To which extent ferroptosis is involved in the calcification process remains unknown and, therefore, could be a new research field that is worth being explored, in order to further unravel the mechanisms underlying the effects of IS and PCS, as well as other toxins on the development of vascular calcification.

An additional challenging approach would consist in a further in-depth investigation at which extent the IS-induced release of microparticles derived from the endothelial cell membranes plays a role in the development of arterial calcification [88]. These endothelial microparticles (EMPs) have pro-inflammatory and pro-coagulant characteristics by interacting with monocytes. Moreover, EMPs accumulate different substances which influence the behavior of recipient cells. Buendia et al. reported that endothelial dysfunction favors the release of EMPs with a high content of calcium and bone morphogenetic protein-2, two important stimulators of the osteo/chondrogenic transdifferentiation of VSMCs [89]. In addition, microRNAs can be released via EMPs and influence endothelial function, i.e., through modulation of eNOS bioavailability, as mentioned above. Figure 2 gives an overview of the IS- and PCS-induced effects on VSMCs and endothelial cells.

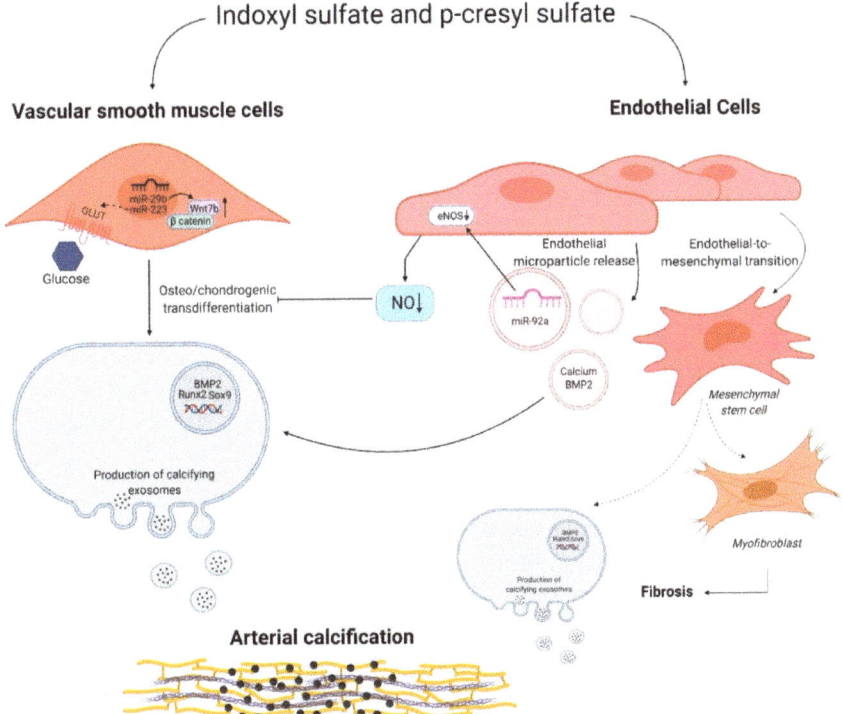

Figure 2. Indoxyl sulfate and p-cresyl sulfate induced molecular mechanisms in vascular smooth muscle cells and endothelial cells. Indoxyl sulfate (IS) and p-cresyl sulfate (PCS) influence the behavior of vascular smooth muscle cells (VSMCs) and endothelial cells. Right side: microRNA miR-29b and miR-223 favor the osteo/chondrogenic switch of VSMCs by promoting the expression of Wnt7b/β catenin signaling and potentially increasing the uptake of glucose via a glucose transporter (GLUT), respectively. Left side: IS and PCS stimulate endothelial microparticle release. These microparticles secrete microRNA miR-92a, calcium, and bone morphogenic protein 2 (BMP2), which in turn induce a phenotypic switch of VSMCs into osteo/chondrogenic cells directly or indirectly through influencing endothelial nitric oxide synthase (eNOS) and thus decreasing nitric oxide (NO) bioavailability. Moreover, IS and PCS could trigger the endothelial to mesenchymal transition of endothelial cells into osteo/chondrogenic cells and myofibroblast, stimulating arterial calcification and fibrosis. Figure was created with BioRender.com.

3. Concluding Remarks

In conclusion, the protein-bound uremic toxins IS and PCS are considered to be harmful vascular toxins. Their vascular toxicity is associated with the upregulation of inflammation, coagulation, and oxidative stress pathways. Moreover, hyperglycemia seems to be an important player in these events. On the other hand, escape from IS/PCS-induced arterial media calcification was linked to activation of lipid metabolism. This suggests that the balance in glucose versus lipid metabolism could be crucial in uremic-toxin-induced vascular calcification.

Author Contributions: Drafted and revised the manuscript, B.O.; Revised the manuscript, P.C.D. and A.V. All authors have read and agreed to the published version of the manuscript.

Funding: This research was funded by the Fund of Scientific Research-Flanders (FWO) grant number 1S22217N. The APC was funded by Laboratory of Pathophysiology.

Conflicts of Interest: The authors declare no conflicts of interest.

References

1. Vanholder, R.; De Smet, R.; Glorieux, G.; Argiles, A.; Baurmeister, U.; Brunet, P.; Clark, W.; Cohen, G.; De Deyn, P.P.; Deppisch, R.; et al. Review on uremic toxins: classification, concentration, and interindividual variability. *Kidney Int.* **2003**, *63*, 1934–1943. [CrossRef]
2. Evenepoel, P.; Meijers, B.K.; Bammens, B.R.; Verbeke, K. Uremic toxins originating from colonic microbial metabolism. *Kidney Int. Suppl.* **2009**, *76*, S12–S19. [CrossRef] [PubMed]
3. Mutsaers, H.A.; van den Heuvel, L.P.; Ringens, L.H.; Dankers, A.C.; Russel, F.G.; Wetzels, J.F.; Hoenderop, J.G.; Masereeuw, R. Uremic toxins inhibit transport by breast cancer resistance protein and multidrug resistance protein 4 at clinically relevant concentrations. *PLoS ONE* **2011**, *6*, e18438. [CrossRef] [PubMed]
4. Lin, C.N.; Wu, I.W.; Huang, Y.F.; Peng, S.Y.; Huang, Y.C.; Ning, H.C. Measuring serum total and free indoxyl sulfate and p-cresyl sulfate in chronic kidney disease using UPLC-MS/MS. *J. Food Drug Anal.* **2019**, *27*, 502–509. [CrossRef] [PubMed]
5. Sirich, T.L.; Funk, B.A.; Plummer, N.S.; Hostetter, T.H.; Meyer, T.W. Prominent accumulation in hemodialysis patients of solutes normally cleared by tubular secretion. *J. Am. Soc. Nephrol.* **2014**, *25*, 615–622. [CrossRef] [PubMed]
6. Barreto, F.C.; Barreto, D.V.; Liabeuf, S.; Meert, N.; Glorieux, G.; Temmar, M.; Choukroun, G.; Vanholder, R.; Massy, Z.A. Serum indoxyl sulfate is associated with vascular disease and mortality in chronic kidney disease patients. *Clin. J. Am. Soc. Nephro.* **2009**, *4*, 1551–1558. [CrossRef]
7. Eloot, S.; Van Biesen, W.; Roels, S.; Delrue, W.; Schepers, E.; Dhondt, A.; Vanholder, R.; Glorieux, G. Spontaneous variability of pre-dialysis concentrations of uremic toxins over time in stable hemodialysis patients. *PLoS ONE* **2017**, *12*, e0186010. [CrossRef]
8. Liabeuf, S.; Barreto, D.V.; Barreto, F.C.; Meert, N.; Glorieux, G.; Schepers, E.; Temmar, M.; Choukroun, G.; Vanholder, R.; Massy, Z.A.; et al. Free p-cresylsulphate is a predictor of mortality in patients at different stages of chronic kidney disease. *Nephrol. Dial. Transpl.* **2010**, *25*, 1183–1191. [CrossRef]
9. Poesen, R.; Windey, K.; Neven, E.; Kuypers, D.; De Preter, V.; Augustijns, P.; D'Haese, P.; Evenepoel, P.; Verbeke, K.; Meijers, B.; et al. The Influence of CKD on Colonic Microbial Metabolism. *J. Am. Soc. Nephrol.* **2016**, *27*, 1389–1399. [CrossRef]
10. Hsueh, C.H.; Yoshida, K.; Zhao, P.; Meyer, T.W.; Zhang, L.; Huang, S.M.; Giacomini, K.M. Identification and Quantitative Assessment of Uremic Solutes as Inhibitors of Renal Organic Anion Transporters, OAT1 and OAT3. *Mol. Pharm.* **2016**, *13*, 3130–3140. [CrossRef]
11. Toth-Manikowski, S.M.; Sirich, T.L.; Meyer, T.W.; Hostetter, T.H.; Hwang, S.; Plummer, N.S.; Hai, X.; Coresh, J.; Powe, N.R.; Shafi, T.; et al. Contribution of 'clinically negligible' residual kidney function to clearance of uremic solutes. *Nephrol. Dial. Transpl.* **2019**. [CrossRef] [PubMed]
12. Kaminski, T.W.; Pawlak, K.; Karbowska, M.; Mysliwiec, M.; Pawlak, D. Indoxyl sulfate - the uremic toxin linking hemostatic system disturbances with the prevalence of cardiovascular disease in patients with chronic kidney disease. *BMC Nephrol.* **2017**, *18*, 35. [CrossRef] [PubMed]
13. Lin, C.J.; Wu, V.; Wu, P.C.; Wu, C.J. Meta-Analysis of the Associations of p-Cresyl Sulfate (PCS) and Indoxyl Sulfate (IS) with Cardiovascular Events and All-Cause Mortality in Patients with Chronic Renal Failure. *PLoS ONE* **2015**, *10*, e0132589. [CrossRef] [PubMed]
14. Shafi, T.; Sirich, T.L.; Meyer, T.W.; Hostetter, T.H.; Plummer, N.S.; Hwang, S.; Melamed, M.L.; Banerjee, T.; Coresh, J.; Powe, N.R.; et al. Results of the HEMO Study suggest that p-cresol sulfate and indoxyl sulfate are not associated with cardiovascular outcomes. *Kidney Int.* **2017**, *92*, 1484–1492. [CrossRef] [PubMed]
15. Cozzolino, M.; Mangano, M.; Stucchi, A.; Ciceri, P.; Conte, F.; Galassi, A. Cardiovascular disease in dialysis patients. *Nephrol. Dial. Transpl.* **2018**, *33*, iii28–iii34. [CrossRef] [PubMed]
16. Russo, D.; Palmiero, G.; De Blasio, A.P.; Balletta, M.M.; Andreucci, V.E. Coronary artery calcification in patients with CRF not undergoing dialysis. *Am. J. Kidney. Dis.* **2004**, *44*, 1024–1030. [CrossRef]

17. Sigrist, M.K.; Taal, M.W.; Bungay, P.; McIntyre, C.W. Progressive vascular calcification over 2 years is associated with arterial stiffening and increased mortality in patients with stages 4 and 5 chronic kidney disease. *Clin. J. Am. Soc. Nephrol.* **2007**, *2*, 1241–1248. [CrossRef]
18. Wilson, A.C.; Mitsnefes, M.M. Cardiovascular disease in CKD in children: update on risk factors, risk assessment, and management. *Am. J. Kidney. Dis.* **2009**, *54*, 345–360. [CrossRef]
19. Ishimura, E.; Okuno, S.; Kitatani, K.; Kim, M.; Shoji, T.; Nakatani, T.; Inaba, M.; Nishizawa, Y. Different risk factors for peripheral vascular calcification between diabetic and non-diabetic haemodialysis patients–importance of glycaemic control. *Diabetologia* **2002**, *45*, 1446–1448. [CrossRef]
20. Katz, R.; Budoff, M.J.; O'Brien, K.D.; Wong, N.D.; Nasir, K. The metabolic syndrome and diabetes mellitus as predictors of thoracic aortic calcification as detected by non-contrast computed tomography in the Multi-Ethnic Study of Atherosclerosis. *Diabetic Med.* **2016**, *33*, 912–919. [CrossRef]
21. Opdebeeck, B.; Maudsley, S.; Azmi, A.; De Mare, A.; De Leger, W.; Meijers, B.; Verhulst, A.; Evenepoel, P.; D'Haese, P.C.; Neven, E.; et al. Indoxyl Sulfate and p-Cresyl Sulfate Promote Vascular Calcification and Associate with Glucose Intolerance. *J. Am. Soc. Nephrol.* **2019**, *30*, 751–766. [CrossRef]
22. Gruys, E.; Toussaint, M.J.; Niewold, T.A.; Koopmans, S.J. Acute phase reaction and acute phase proteins. *J. Zhejiang Univ. Sci. B* **2005**, *6*, 1045–1056. [CrossRef]
23. Venteclef, N.; Jakobsson, T.; Steffensen, K.R.; Treuter, E. Metabolic nuclear receptor signaling and the inflammatory acute phase response. *Trends Endocrin. Met.* **2011**, *22*, 333–343. [CrossRef]
24. Adesso, S.; Magnus, T.; Cuzzocrea, S.; Campolo, M.; Rissiek, B.; Paciello, O.; Autore, G.; Pinto, A.; Marzocco, S. Indoxyl Sulfate Affects Glial Function Increasing Oxidative Stress and Neuroinflammation in Chronic Kidney Disease: Interaction between Astrocytes and Microglia. *Front. Pharmacol.* **2017**, *8*, 370. [CrossRef]
25. Ito, S.; Osaka, M.; Edamatsu, T.; Itoh, Y.; Yoshida, M. Crucial Role of the Aryl Hydrocarbon Receptor (AhR) in Indoxyl Sulfate-Induced Vascular Inflammation. *J. Atheroscler. Thromb.* **2016**, *23*, 960–975. [CrossRef]
26. Nakano, T.; Katsuki, S.; Chen, M.; Decano, J.L.; Halu, A.; Lee, L.H.; Pestana, D.V.S.; Kum, A.S.T.; Kuromoto, R.K.; Golden, W.S.; et al. Uremic Toxin Indoxyl Sulfate Promotes Proinflammatory Macrophage Activation Via the Interplay of OATP2B1 and Dll4-Notch Signaling. *Circulation* **2019**, *139*, 78–96. [CrossRef]
27. Stockler-Pinto, M.B.; Saldanha, J.F.; Yi, D.; Mafra, D.; Fouque, D.; Soulage, C.O. The uremic toxin indoxyl sulfate exacerbates reactive oxygen species production and inflammation in 3T3-L1 adipose cells. *Free Radical Res.* **2016**, *50*, 337–344. [CrossRef]
28. Watanabe, H.; Miyamoto, Y.; Honda, D.; Tanaka, H.; Wu, Q.; Endo, M.; Noguchi, T.; Kadowaki, D.; Ishima, Y.; Kotani, S.; et al. p-Cresyl sulfate causes renal tubular cell damage by inducing oxidative stress by activation of NADPH oxidase. *Kidney Int.* **2013**, *83*, 582–592. [CrossRef]
29. Bessueille, L.; Magne, D. Inflammation: a culprit for vascular calcification in atherosclerosis and diabetes. *Cell. Mol. Life Sci.* **2015**, *72*, 2475–2489. [CrossRef]
30. Avramovski, P.; Avramovska, M.; Sotiroski, K.; Sikole, A. Acute-phase proteins as promoters of abdominal aortic calcification in chronic dialysis patients. *Saudi J. Kidney Dis. Transpl.* **2019**, *30*, 376–386. [CrossRef]
31. Henze, L.A.; Luong, T.T.D.; Boehme, B.; Masyout, J.; Schneider, M.P.; Brachs, S.; Lang, F.; Pieske, B.; Pasch, A.; Eckardt, K.U.; et al. Impact of C-reactive protein on osteo-/chondrogenic transdifferentiation and calcification of vascular smooth muscle cells. *Aging* **2019**, *11*, 5445–5462. [CrossRef]
32. Zhang, X.; Chen, J.; Wang, S. Serum Amyloid a Induces a Vascular Smooth Muscle Cell Phenotype Switch through the p38 MAPK Signaling Pathway. *Biomed Res. Int.* **2017**, *2017*, 4941379. [CrossRef]
33. Yang, K.; Du, C.; Wang, X.; Li, F.; Xu, Y.; Wang, S.; Chen, S.; Chen, F.; Shen, M.; Chen, M.; et al. Indoxyl sulfate induces platelet hyperactivity and contributes to chronic kidney disease-associated thrombosis in mice. *Blood* **2017**, *129*, 2667–2679. [CrossRef]
34. Wu, C.C.; Hsieh, M.Y.; Hung, S.C.; Kuo, K.L.; Tsai, T.H.; Lai, C.L.; Chen, J.W.; Lin, S.J.; Huang, P.H.; Tarng, D.C.; et al. Serum Indoxyl Sulfate Associates with Postangioplasty Thrombosis of Dialysis Grafts. *J. Am. Soc. Nephrol.* **2016**, *27*, 1254–1264. [CrossRef]
35. Borissoff, J.I.; Joosen, I.A.; Versteylen, M.O.; Spronk, H.M.; ten Cate, H.; Hofstra, L. Accelerated in vivo thrombin formation independently predicts the presence and severity of CT angiographic coronary atherosclerosis. *JACC Cardiovasc. Imag.* **2012**, *5*, 1201–1210. [CrossRef]
36. Horn, P.; Erkilet, G.; Veulemans, V.; Kropil, P.; Schurgers, L.; Zeus, T.; Heiss, C.; Kelm, M.; Westenfeld, R. Microparticle-Induced Coagulation Relates to Coronary Artery Atherosclerosis in Severe Aortic Valve Stenosis. *PLoS ONE* **2016**, *11*, e0151499. [CrossRef]

37. Kapustin, A.N.; Schoppet, M.; Schurgers, L.J.; Reynolds, J.L.; McNair, R.; Heiss, A.; Jahnen-Dechent, W.; Hackeng, T.M.; Schlieper, G.; Harrison, P.; et al. Prothrombin Loading of Vascular Smooth Muscle Cell-Derived Exosomes Regulates Coagulation and Calcification. *Arter. Thromb. Vasc. Biol.* **2017**, *37*, e22–e32. [CrossRef]
38. Wuyts, J.; Dhondt, A. The role of vitamin K in vascular calcification of patients with chronic kidney disease. *Acta Clin. Belg.* **2016**, *71*, 462–467. [CrossRef]
39. De Mare, A.; Maudsley, S.; Azmi, A.; Hendrickx, J.O.; Opdebeeck, B.; Neven, E.; D'Haese, P.C.; Verhulst, A. Sclerostin as Regulatory Molecule in Vascular Media Calcification and the Bone-Vascular Axis. *Toxins* **2019**, *11*, 428. [CrossRef]
40. De Vriese, A.S.; Caluwe, R.; Pyfferoen, L.; De Bacquer, D.; De Boeck, K.; Delanote, J.; De Surgeloose, D.; Van Hoenacker, P.; Van Vlem, B.; Verbeke, F.; et al. Multicenter Randomized Controlled Trial of Vitamin K Antagonist Replacement by Rivaroxaban with or without Vitamin K2 in Hemodialysis Patients with Atrial Fibrillation: the Valkyrie Study. *J. Am. Soc. Nephrol.* **2020**, *31*, 186–196. [CrossRef]
41. Bi, X.; Song, J.; Gao, J.; Zhao, J.; Wang, M.; Scipione, C.A.; Koschinsky, M.L.; Wang, Z.V.; Xu, S.; Fu, G.; et al. Activation of liver X receptor attenuates lysophosphatidylcholine-induced IL-8 expression in endothelial cells via the NF-kappaB pathway and SUMOylation. *J. Cell. Mol. Med.* **2016**, *20*, 2249–2258. [CrossRef]
42. Zhang, X.Q.; Even-Or, O.; Xu, X.; van Rosmalen, M.; Lim, L.; Gadde, S.; Farokhzad, O.C.; Fisher, E.A. Nanoparticles containing a liver X receptor agonist inhibit inflammation and atherosclerosis. *Adv. Healthc. Mater.* **2015**, *4*, 228–236. [CrossRef]
43. Cheng, Y.; Zhang, D.; Zhu, M.; Wang, Y.; Guo, S.; Xu, B.; Hou, G.; Feng, Y.; Liu, G. Liver X receptor alpha is targeted by microRNA-1 to inhibit cardiomyocyte apoptosis through a ROS-mediated mitochondrial pathway. *Biochem. Cell. Biol.* **2018**, *96*, 11–18. [CrossRef]
44. Chen, J.; Gu, Y.; Zhang, H.; Ning, Y.; Song, N.; Hu, J.; Cai, J.; Shi, Y.; Ding, X.; Zhang, X.; et al. Amelioration of Uremic Toxin Indoxyl Sulfate-Induced Osteoblastic Calcification by SET Domain Containing Lysine Methyltransferase 7/9 Protein. *Nephron* **2019**, *141*, 287–294. [CrossRef]
45. Karbowska, M.; Kaminski, T.W.; Znorko, B.; Domaniewski, T.; Misztal, T.; Rusak, T.; Pryczynicz, A.; Guzinska-Ustymowicz, K.; Pawlak, K.; Pawlak, D.; et al. Indoxyl Sulfate Promotes Arterial Thrombosis in Rat Model via Increased Levels of Complex TF/VII, PAI-1, Platelet Activation as Well as Decreased Contents of SIRT1 and SIRT3. *Front. Physiol.* **2018**, *9*, 1623. [CrossRef]
46. Koppe, L.; Pillon, N.J.; Vella, R.E.; Croze, M.L.; Pelletier, C.C.; Chambert, S.; Massy, Z.; Glorieux, G.; Vanholder, R.; Dugenet, Y.; et al. p-Cresyl sulfate promotes insulin resistance associated with CKD. *J. Am. Soc. Nephrol.* **2013**, *24*, 88–99. [CrossRef]
47. Shivanna, S.; Kolandaivelu, K.; Shashar, M.; Belghasim, M.; Al-Rabadi, L.; Balcells, M.; Zhang, A.; Weinberg, J.; Francis, J.; Pollastri, M.P.; et al. The Aryl Hydrocarbon Receptor is a Critical Regulator of Tissue Factor Stability and an Antithrombotic Target in Uremia. *J. Am. Soc. Nephrol.* **2016**, *27*, 189–201. [CrossRef]
48. Gondouin, B.; Cerini, C.; Dou, L.; Sallee, M.; Duval-Sabatier, A.; Pletinck, A.; Calaf, R.; Lacroix, R.; Jourde-Chiche, N.; Poitevin, S.; et al. Indolic uremic solutes increase tissue factor production in endothelial cells by the aryl hydrocarbon receptor pathway. *Kidney Int.* **2013**, *84*, 733–744. [CrossRef]
49. El-Osta, A.; Brasacchio, D.; Yao, D.; Pocai, A.; Jones, P.L.; Roeder, R.G.; Cooper, M.E.; Brownlee, M. Transient high glucose causes persistent epigenetic changes and altered gene expression during subsequent normoglycemia. *J. Exp. Med.* **2008**, *205*, 2409–2417. [CrossRef]
50. Zheng, Z.; Chen, H.; Li, J.; Li, T.; Zheng, B.; Zheng, Y.; Jin, H.; He, Y.; Gu, Q.; Xu, X.; et al. Sirtuin 1-mediated cellular metabolic memory of high glucose via the LKB1/AMPK/ROS pathway and therapeutic effects of metformin. *Diabetes* **2012**, *61*, 217–228. [CrossRef]
51. Zhang, X.; Xiao, J.; Li, R.; Qin, X.; Wang, F.; Mao, Y.; Liang, W.; Sheng, X.; Guo, M.; Song, Y.; et al. Metformin alleviates vascular calcification induced by vitamin D3 plus nicotine in rats via the AMPK pathway. *Vasc. Pharmacol.* **2016**, *81*, 83–90. [CrossRef] [PubMed]
52. Muller, K.H.; Hayward, R.; Rajan, R.; Whitehead, M.; Cobb, A.M.; Ahmad, S.; Sun, M.; Goldberga, I.; Li, R.; Bashtanova, U.; et al. Poly(ADP-Ribose) Links the DNA Damage Response and Biomineralization. *Cell Rep.* **2019**, *27*, 3124–3138.e3113. [CrossRef]
53. Yao, Q.; Chen, Y.; Zhou, X. The roles of microRNAs in epigenetic regulation. *Curr. Opin. Chem. Biol.* **2019**, *51*, 11–17. [CrossRef] [PubMed]
54. Paloian, N.J.; Giachelli, C.M. A current understanding of vascular calcification in CKD. *Am. J. Physiol.-Renal. 2014*, *307*, F891–F900. [CrossRef] [PubMed]

55. Shang, F.; Wang, S.C.; Hsu, C.Y.; Miao, Y.; Martin, M.; Yin, Y.; Wu, C.C.; Wang, Y.T.; Wu, G.; Chien, S.; et al. MicroRNA-92a Mediates Endothelial Dysfunction in CKD. *J. Am. Soc. Nephrol.* **2017**, *28*, 3251–3261. [CrossRef]
56. Kanno, Y.; Into, T.; Lowenstein, C.J.; Matsushita, K. Nitric oxide regulates vascular calcification by interfering with TGF- signalling. *Cardiovasc. Res.* **2008**, *77*, 221–230. [CrossRef]
57. Sambe, T.; Mason, R.P.; Dawoud, H.; Bhatt, D.L.; Malinski, T. Metformin treatment decreases nitroxidative stress, restores nitric oxide bioavailability and endothelial function beyond glucose control. *Biomed. Pharmacother.* **2018**, *98*, 149–156. [CrossRef]
58. Du, Y.; Gao, C.; Liu, Z.; Wang, L.; Liu, B.; He, F.; Zhang, T.; Wang, Y.; Wang, X.; Xu, M.; et al. Upregulation of a disintegrin and metalloproteinase with thrombospondin motifs-7 by miR-29 repression mediates vascular smooth muscle calcification. *Arterioscler. Thromb. Vasc. Biol.* **2012**, *32*, 2580–2588. [CrossRef]
59. Zhang, H.; Chen, J.; Shen, Z.; Gu, Y.; Xu, L.; Hu, J.; Zhang, X.; Ding, X. Indoxyl sulfate accelerates vascular smooth muscle cell calcification via microRNA-29b dependent regulation of Wnt/beta-catenin signaling. *Toxicol. Lett.* **2018**, *284*, 29–36. [CrossRef]
60. Yu, Y.; Guan, X.; Nie, L.; Liu, Y.; He, T.; Xiong, J.; Xu, X.; Li, Y.; Yang, K.; Wang, Y.; et al. DNA hypermethylation of sFRP5 contributes to indoxyl sulfate-induced renal fibrosis. *J. Mol. Med.* **2017**, *95*, 601–613. [CrossRef]
61. Massy, Z.A.; Metzinger-Le Meuth, V.; Metzinger, L. MicroRNAs Are Associated with Uremic Toxicity, Cardiovascular Calcification, and Disease. *Contrib. Nephrol.* **2017**, *189*, 160–168. [CrossRef]
62. Lu, H.; Buchan, R.J.; Cook, S.A. MicroRNA-223 regulates Glut4 expression and cardiomyocyte glucose metabolism. *Cardiovasc. Res.* **2010**, *86*, 410–420. [CrossRef]
63. Rangrez, A.Y.; M'Baya-Moutoula, E.; Metzinger-Le Meuth, V.; Henaut, L.; Djelouat, M.S.; Benchitrit, J.; Massy, Z.A.; Metzinger, L. Inorganic phosphate accelerates the migration of vascular smooth muscle cells: evidence for the involvement of miR-223. *PLoS ONE* **2012**, *7*, e47807. [CrossRef] [PubMed]
64. Neven, E.; De Schutter, T.M.; De Broe, M.E.; D'Haese, P.C. Cell biological and physicochemical aspects of arterial calcification. *Kidney Int.* **2011**, *79*, 1166–1177. [CrossRef] [PubMed]
65. Adijiang, A.; Goto, S.; Uramoto, S.; Nishijima, F.; Niwa, T. Indoxyl sulphate promotes aortic calcification with expression of osteoblast-specific proteins in hypertensive rats. *Nephrol. Dial. Transpl.* **2008**, *23*, 1892–1901. [CrossRef]
66. Muteliefu, G.; Enomoto, A.; Jiang, P.; Takahashi, M.; Niwa, T. Indoxyl sulphate induces oxidative stress and the expression of osteoblast-specific proteins in vascular smooth muscle cells. *Nephrol. Dial. Transpl.* **2009**, *24*, 2051–2058. [CrossRef]
67. Kim, S.H.; Yu, M.A.; Ryu, E.S.; Jang, Y.H.; Kang, D.H. Indoxyl sulfate-induced epithelial-to-mesenchymal transition and apoptosis of renal tubular cells as novel mechanisms of progression of renal disease. *Lab. Invest.* **2012**, *92*, 488–498. [CrossRef]
68. Sun, C.Y.; Chang, S.C.; Wu, M.S. Uremic toxins induce kidney fibrosis by activating intrarenal renin-angiotensin-aldosterone system associated epithelial-to-mesenchymal transition. *PLoS ONE* **2012**, *7*, e34026. [CrossRef]
69. Bolati, D.; Shimizu, H.; Higashiyama, Y.; Nishijima, F.; Niwa, T. Indoxyl sulfate induces epithelial-to-mesenchymal transition in rat kidneys and human proximal tubular cells. *Am. J. Nephrol.* **2011**, *34*, 318–323. [CrossRef]
70. Bolati, D.; Shimizu, H.; Niwa, T. AST-120 ameliorates epithelial-to-mesenchymal transition and interstitial fibrosis in the kidneys of chronic kidney disease rats. *J. Renal. Nutr.* **2012**, *22*, 176–180. [CrossRef]
71. Chang, L.C.; Sun, H.L.; Tsai, C.H.; Kuo, C.W.; Liu, K.L.; Lii, C.K.; Huang, C.S.; Li, C.C. 1,25(OH)2 D3 attenuates indoxyl sulfate-induced epithelial-to-mesenchymal cell transition via inactivation of PI3K/Akt/beta-catenin signaling in renal tubular epithelial cells. *Nutrition* **2019**, *69*, 110554. [CrossRef] [PubMed]
72. Medici, D.; Kalluri, R. Endothelial-mesenchymal transition and its contribution to the emergence of stem cell phenotype. *Semin. Cancer Biol.* **2012**, *22*, 379–384. [CrossRef] [PubMed]
73. Medici, D.; Olsen, B.R. The role of endothelial-mesenchymal transition in heterotopic ossification. *J. Bone Miner. Res.* **2012**, *27*, 1619–1622. [CrossRef]
74. Yao, J.; Guihard, P.J.; Blazquez-Medela, A.M.; Guo, Y.; Moon, J.H.; Jumabay, M.; Bostrom, K.I.; Yao, Y. Serine Protease Activation Essential for Endothelial-Mesenchymal Transition in Vascular Calcification. *Circ. Res.* **2015**, *117*, 758–769. [CrossRef]

75. Yao, Y.; Jumabay, M.; Ly, A.; Radparvar, M.; Cubberly, M.R.; Bostrom, K.I. A role for the endothelium in vascular calcification. *Circ. Res.* **2013**, *113*, 495–504. [CrossRef]
76. Van den Bergh, G.; Opdebeeck, B.; D'Haese, P.C.; Verhulst, A. The Vicious Cycle of Arterial Stiffness and Arterial Media Calcification. *Trends Mol. Med.* **2019**. [CrossRef]
77. Dou, L.; Bertrand, E.; Cerini, C.; Faure, V.; Sampol, J.; Vanholder, R.; Berland, Y.; Brunet, P. The uremic solutes p-cresol and indoxyl sulfate inhibit endothelial proliferation and wound repair. *Kidney Int.* **2004**, *65*, 442–451. [CrossRef]
78. Faure, V.; Dou, L.; Sabatier, F.; Cerini, C.; Sampol, J.; Berland, Y.; Brunet, P.; Dignat-George, F. Elevation of circulating endothelial microparticles in patients with chronic renal failure. *J. Thromb. Haemost.* **2006**, *4*, 566–573. [CrossRef]
79. Yu, M.; Kim, Y.J.; Kang, D.H. Indoxyl sulfate-induced endothelial dysfunction in patients with chronic kidney disease via an induction of oxidative stress. *Clin. J. Am. Soc. Nephro.* **2011**, *6*, 30–39. [CrossRef]
80. Guo, J.; Lu, L.; Hua, Y.; Huang, K.; Wang, I.; Huang, L.; Fu, Q.; Chen, A.; Chan, P.; Fan, H.; et al. Vasculopathy in the setting of cardiorenal syndrome: roles of protein-bound uremic toxins. *Am. J. Physiol. Heart Circ. Physiol.* **2017**, *313*, H1–H13. [CrossRef]
81. Sun, Y.; Zheng, Y.; Wang, C.; Liu, Y. Glutathione depletion induces ferroptosis, autophagy, and premature cell senescence in retinal pigment epithelial cells. *Cell Death Dis.* **2018**, *9*, 753. [CrossRef] [PubMed]
82. Itoh, Y.; Ezawa, A.; Kikuchi, K.; Tsuruta, Y.; Niwa, T. Protein-bound uremic toxins in hemodialysis patients measured by liquid chromatography/tandem mass spectrometry and their effects on endothelial ROS production. *Anal. Bioanal. Chem.* **2012**, *403*, 1841–1850. [CrossRef] [PubMed]
83. Muteliefu, G.; Shimizu, H.; Enomoto, A.; Nishijima, F.; Takahashi, M.; Niwa, T. Indoxyl sulfate promotes vascular smooth muscle cell senescence with upregulation of p53, p21, and prelamin A through oxidative stress. *Am. J. Physiol.-Cell Physiol.* **2012**, *303*, C126–134. [CrossRef] [PubMed]
84. Shimizu, H.; Bolati, D.; Adijiang, A.; Enomoto, A.; Nishijima, F.; Dateki, M.; Niwa, T. Senescence and dysfunction of proximal tubular cells are associated with activated p53 expression by indoxyl sulfate. *Am. J. Physiol.-Cell Physiol.* **2010**, *299*, C1110–C1117. [CrossRef] [PubMed]
85. Gnanapradeepan, K.; Basu, S.; Barnoud, T.; Budina-Kolomets, A.; Kung, C.P.; Murphy, M.E. The p53 Tumor Suppressor in the Control of Metabolism and Ferroptosis. *Front. Endocrinol.* **2018**, *9*, 124. [CrossRef]
86. Liu, Y.; Drozdov, I.; Shroff, R.; Beltran, L.E.; Shanahan, C.M. Prelamin A accelerates vascular calcification via activation of the DNA damage response and senescence-associated secretory phenotype in vascular smooth muscle cells. *Circ. Res.* **2013**, *112*, e99–e109. [CrossRef]
87. Proudfoot, D.; Skepper, J.N.; Hegyi, L.; Bennett, M.R.; Shanahan, C.M.; Weissberg, P.L. Apoptosis regulates human vascular calcification in vitro: evidence for initiation of vascular calcification by apoptotic bodies. *Circ. Res.* **2000**, *87*, 1055–1062. [CrossRef]
88. Carmona, A.; Guerrero, F.; Buendia, P.; Obrero, T.; Aljama, P.; Carracedo, J. Microvesicles Derived from Indoxyl Sulfate Treated Endothelial Cells Induce Endothelial Progenitor Cells Dysfunction. *Front. Physiol.* **2017**, *8*, 666. [CrossRef]
89. Buendia, P.; Montes de Oca, A.; Madueno, J.A.; Merino, A.; Martin-Malo, A.; Aljama, P.; Ramirez, R.; Rodriguez, M.; Carracedo, J. Endothelial microparticles mediate inflammation-induced vascular calcification. *FASEB J.* **2015**, *29*, 173–181. [CrossRef]

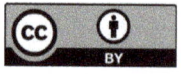

© 2020 by the authors. Licensee MDPI, Basel, Switzerland. This article is an open access article distributed under the terms and conditions of the Creative Commons Attribution (CC BY) license (http://creativecommons.org/licenses/by/4.0/).

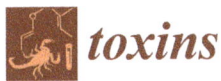

Article

Serum *P*-Cresyl Sulfate Is a Predictor of Central Arterial Stiffness in Patients on Maintenance Hemodialysis

Yu-Hsien Lai [1,2], Chih-Hsien Wang [1,2], Chiu-Huang Kuo [1,2], Yu-Li Lin [1,2], Jen-Pi Tsai [1,3,*] and Bang-Gee Hsu [1,2,*]

1. School of Medicine, Tzu Chi University, Hualien 97004, Taiwan; hsienhsien@gmail.com (Y.-H.L.); wangch33@gmail.com (C.-H.W.); hermit.kuo@gmail.com (C.-H.K.); nomo8931126@gmail.com (Y.-L.L.)
2. Division of Nephrology, Hualien Tzu Chi Hospital, Buddhist Tzu Chi Medical Foundation, Hualien 97004, Taiwan
3. Division of Nephrology, Department of Internal Medicine, Dalin Tzu Chi Hospital, Buddhist Tzu Chi Medical Foundation, Chiayi 62247, Taiwan
* Correspondence: tsaininimd1491@gmail.com (J.-P.T.); gee.lily@msa.hinet.net (B.-G.H.)

Received: 30 October 2019; Accepted: 19 December 2019; Published: 21 December 2019

Abstract: Arterial stiffness (AS) has an important impact on the outcomes of patients on hemodialysis (HD), and *p*-cresyl sulfate (PC) can mediate the process of vascular damage. We aimed to investigate the relationship between carotid–femoral pulse wave velocity (cfPWV) and the level of PCs in HD patients. Serum PCs were quantified using liquid chromatography mass spectrometry. Patients who were on standard HD for more than 3 months were enrolled and categorized according to the cfPWV into the high AS (>10 m/s) and control (≤10 m/s) groups. Forty-nine (41.5%) patients belonged to the high AS group and had a higher incidence of diabetes mellitus (DM) and increased systolic blood pressure, serum C-reactive protein, and PC levels but had lower creatinine, compared with those in the control group. In HD patients, the risk for developing high AS increased in the presence of DM (OR 4.147, 95% confidence interval (CI) 1.497–11.491) and high PCs (OR 1.067, 95% CI 1.002–1.136). Having DM (r = 0.446) and high PC level (r = 0.174) were positively associated with cfPWV. The most optimal cutoff value of PC for predicting AS was 18.99 mg/L (area under the curve 0.661, 95% CI 0.568–0.746). We concluded that DM and PCs were promising predictors of high AS in patients on maintenance HD.

Keywords: arterial stiffness; carotid–femoral pulse wave velocity; hemodialysis; *p*-cresyl sulfate

Key Contribution: Serum PC level was positively associated with cfPWV and was a risk factor for developing AS in HD patients.

1. Introduction

Arterial stiffness (AS), which is a risk factor for cardiovascular (CV) disease (CVD), has long been recognized as the main cause of mortality in patients with chronic kidney disease (CKD) [1–3]. Along with the other traditional risk factors, such as age, hypertension (HTN), diabetes mellitus (DM), and uremia-related factors, including inflammation and abnormal bone and mineral metabolism, vascular calcification has been well known to be associated with CVD [4]. Increasing evidence has shown that the process of vascular damage is mediated by proteins, such as alkaline phosphatase, fetuin A, and parathyroid hormone; abnormal calcium and phosphate homeostasis; and protein-bound uremic toxins [5,6]. Pulse wave velocity (PWV) is a noninvasive method to measure vascular function and has been regarded as a strong predictor of CV events and mortality in patients with end-stage renal disease (ESRD), independent of the classical CV risk factors [2,3]. In the Chronic Renal Insufficiency Cohort (CRIC) study, CKD patients with high PWV were shown to be more likely to develop adverse renal outcomes, including decrease in renal function by half, ESRD, or death [7].

P-cresyl sulfate (PC), which is a 188-kDa gut-derived and protein-bound uremic toxin, was shown to progressively accumulate as renal function worsened [8] and has been regarded as a detrimental factor for renal fibrosis by enhancing the production of reactive oxygen species and by activating transforming growth factor β and the renal–angiotensin–aldosterone system [9,10]. Furthermore, PC has been linked with endothelial dysfunction in vitro [11,12], AS, vascular calcification [13], CV events, and even all-cause mortality in patients with CKD and on hemodialysis (HD) [13–15].

Given the aforementioned data, PWV could predict CV morbidity and mortality and PCs could play a role in AS and lead to adverse outcomes. However, the relationship between PCs and carotid–femoral PWV (cfPWV) in a CKD population is unknown. We conducted this study to noninvasively measure vascular function using cfPWV and to examine the possible risk factors, especially serum PC levels, for developing AS in patients on HD.

2. Results

Of all the HD patients, 59 (50%) were women, the mean age was 63.05 ± 13.28 years, and the median duration of receiving HD was 56.02 months (interquartile range (IQR) 24.6–111.45 months); 55 (46.6%) and 66 (55.9%) patients had DM and HTN, respectively. As measures of adequacy of dialysis, the mean Kt/V was 1.35 ± 0.17, and the mean urea reduction ratio was 0.74 ± 0.04. The mean total PC level of all HD patients was 16.57 ± 9.07 mg/L (Table 1).

Table 1. Clinical variables of the 118 hemodialysis patients with high and low arterial stiffness.

Characteristics	All Patients (n = 118)	Control Group (n = 69)	High Arterial Stiffness Group (n = 49)	p
Carotid–femoral PWV (m/s)	9.63 ± 2.55	7.83 ± 1.30	12.16 ± 1.48	<0.001 *
Age (years)	63.05 ± 13.28	61.32 ± 13.74	65.49 ± 12.34	0.093
Female, n (%)	59 (50.0)	36 (52.2)	23 (46.9)	0.575
Body mass index (kg/m^2)	24.92 ± 5.13	24.92 ± 5.45	24.92 ± 4.69	0.994
Hemodialysis duration (months)	56.02 (24.60–111.45)	80.40 (22.38–133.80)	45.72 (26.22–74.50)	0.069
Diabetes mellitus, n (%)	55 (46.6)	19 (27.5)	36 (73.5)	<0.001 *
Hypertension, n (%)	66 (55.9)	34 (49.3)	32 (65.3)	0.084
Systolic blood pressure (mmHg)	142.13 ± 25.64	138.07 ± 26.99	147.84 ± 22.38	0.021 *
Diastolic blood pressure (mmHg)	76.02 ± 15.61	76.17 ± 16.29	75.29 ± 15.17	0.765
Heart rate (beats per minute)	75.37 ± 12.79	76 ± 13.17	74.49 ± 12.32	0.629
Blood urea nitrogen (mg/dL)	60.36 ± 14.75	59.77 ± 13.64	61.20 ± 16.31	0.604
Creatinine (mg/dL)	9.17 ± 1.99	9.47 ± 1.98	8.73 ± 1.94	0.047 *
Urea reduction rate	0.74 ± 0.04	0.74 ± 0.05	0.73 ± 0.04	0.501
Kt/V (Gotch)	1.35 ± 0.17	1.36 ± 0.19	1.33 ± 0.16	0.396
Total cholesterol (mg/dL)	143.19 ± 35.25	146.35 ± 38.11	138.73 ± 30.60	0.244
Triglyceride (mg/dL)	113.00 (86.75–178.75)	109.00 (86.50–199.00)	121.00 (85.00–174.50)	0.785
Glucose (mg/dL)	136.50 (113.75–177.00)	132.00 (110.50–162.00)	143.00 (119.50–206.00)	0.042 *
Total calcium (mg/dL)	8.96 ± 0.75	8.94 ± 0.76	8.99 ± 0.75	0.732
Phosphorus (mg/dL)	4.65 ± 1.32	4.69 ± 1.35	4.61 ± 1.31	0.746
Intact parathyroid hormone (pg/mL)	186.50 (66.60–353.35)	211.70 (101.10–413.15)	136.80 (44.40–281.75)	0.098
C-reactive protein (mg/dL)	0.34 (0.09–0.95)	0.24 (0.08–0.86)	0.57 (0.13–1.09)	0.029 *
Total p-cresyl sulfate (mg/L)	16.57 ± 9.07	13.95 ± 5.93	20.26 ± 11.27	<0.001 *
Angiotensin receptor blocker, n (%)	35 (29.7)	19 (27.)	16 (32.7)	0.549
β-blocker, n (%)	39 (33.1)	22 (31.9)	17 (34.7)	0.749
Calcium channel blocker, n (%)	46 (39.0)	29 (42.0)	17 (34.7)	0.421
Statin, n (%)	19 (16.1)	8 (11.6)	11(22.4)	0.114
Fibrate, n (%)	13 (11.0)	9 (13.0)	4 (8.2)	0.404

Values for continuous variables are shown as mean ± standard deviation or as median and interquartile range, after analysis by Student's t-test or Mann–Whitney U test and according to the normality of distribution. Values that are presented as number (%) were analyzed by the chi-square test. * $p < 0.05$.

Forty-nine patients (41.5%) were diagnosed as high central AS. Compared with the control group, the high central AS group had higher percentage of DM (73.5% vs. 27.5%, $p < 0.001$); higher systolic blood pressure (SBP; 147.84 ± 23.38 mmHg vs. 138.07 ± 26.99 mmHg, $p = 0.021$); higher serum levels of glucose (143.00 (IQR 119.50–206.00) mg/dL vs. 132.00 (IQR 110.50–162.00) mg/dL, $p = 0.042$); higher C-reactive protein (CRP; 0.57 (IQR 0.13–1.09) vs. 0.24 (IQR 0.08–0.86) mg/dL, $p = 0.029$); and higher total PC levels (20.26 ± 11.27 mg/dL vs. 13.95 ± 5.93 mg/dL, $p = 0.047$) but had lower levels of creatinine (8.73 ± 1.94 mg/L vs. 9.47 ± 1.98 mg/L, $p < 0.001$) (Table 1). There were no significant differences in HTN prevalence, HD duration, body composition, HD adequacy, lipid profiles, and the other clinical characteristics or medications between these two groups.

After adjusting for various factors, including overall age, sex, HD duration, PC levels, DM, SBP, heart rate, CRP, glucose, and creatinine, multivariate logistic regression analysis showed that total PC levels (adjusted odds ratio (aOR) 1.072, 95% confidence interval (CI) 1.002–1.147, $p = 0.043$) and DM (aOR 4.095, 95% CI 1.429–11.739, $p = 0.009$) were the significant independent risk factors for developing high AS (Table 2).

Table 2. Multivariate logistic regression analysis of the factors that correlated with arterial stiffness in 118 hemodialysis patients.

Variables	Odds Ratio	95% Confidence Interval	p
Presence of diabetes mellitus	4.095	1.429–11.739	0.009 *
Total p-cresyl sulfate, 1 mg/L	1.072	1.002–1.147	0.043 *
Age, 1 year	1.026	0.987–1.066	0.191
Sex (female)	0.610	0.223–1.690	0.336
C-reactive protein, 0.1 mg/dL	1.822	0.831–3.997	0.134
Glucose, 1 mg/dL	1.004	0.997–1.011	0.286
Creatinine, 1 mg/dL	0.945	0.710–1.259	0.700
Systolic blood pressure, 1 mmHg	1.002	0.983–1.022	0.838
Heart rate, 1 beat per minute	0.991	0.954–1.030	0.657
Hemodialysis duration, 1 month	0.997	0.988–1.005	0.433

Data analysis was done using the multivariate logistic regression analysis, which was adjusted for the following factors: age, sex, diabetes mellitus, systolic blood pressure, heart rate, hemodialysis duration, C-reactive protein, glucose, creatinine, and total p-cresyl sulfate. * $p < 0.05$.

Simple linear regression analysis showed that the value of cfPWV was significantly positively correlated with DM, SBP, logarithmically transformed glucose, and total PC levels, but was negatively correlated with the logarithmically transformed HD duration (Table 3). On multivariate stepwise linear regression analysis, DM ($r = 0.446$, $p < 0.001$) and PC levels ($r = 0.174$, $p = 0.018$) had significant positive correlations with cfPWV.

Table 3. Correlation between central PWV levels and the clinical variables among 118 HD patients.

Variables	Central PWV (m/s)				
	Simple Regression		Multivariate Regression		
	r	p	Beta	Adjusted R^2 Change	p
Age (years)	0.078	0.402	-	-	-
Female sex	−0.085	0.357	-	-	-
Body mass index (kg/m^2)	0.056	0.545	-	-	-
Log-HD duration (months)	−0.255	0.005 *	-	-	-
Diabetes mellitus	0.538	<0.001 *	0.446	0.283	<0.001 *
Hypertension	0.081	0.381	-	-	-
Systolic blood pressure (mmHg)	0.263	0.004 *	-	-	-

Table 3. Cont.

Variables	Central PWV (m/s)				
	Simple Regression		Multivariate Regression		
	r	p	Beta	Adjusted R^2 Change	p
Diastolic blood pressure (mmHg)	0.055	0.551	-	-	-
Heart rate (beats per minute)	−0.112	0.228	-	-	-
Blood urea nitrogen (mg/dL)	0.016	0.867	-	-	-
Creatinine (mg/dL)	−0.094	0.313	-	-	-
Urea reduction rate	−0.099	0.285	-	-	-
Kt/V (Gotch)	−0.104	0.264	-	-	-
Total cholesterol (mg/dL)	−0.068	0.462	-	-	-
Log-triglyceride (mg/dL)	−0.015	0.872	-	-	-
Log-glucose (mg/dL)	0.198	0.031 *	-	-	-
Total calcium (mg/dL)	0.028	0.763	-	-	-
Phosphorus (mg/dL)	0.065	0.487	-	-	-
Log-iPTH (pg/mL)	−0.088	0.341	-	-	-
Log-CRP (mg/dL)	0.135	0.144	-	-	-
Total p-cresyl sulfate (mg/L)	0.382	<0.001 *	0.174	0.028	0.018 *

Data on HD duration, triglyceride, glucose, iPTH, and CRP levels showed skewed distributions and, therefore, were log-transformed before analysis. Data analysis was done using univariate linear regression analyses or multivariate stepwise linear regression analysis adjusted for the following factors: diabetes mellitus, log-HD duration, systolic blood pressure, log-glucose, and total p-cresyl sulfate. * $p < 0.05$.

Receiver-operating characteristic (ROC) curve analysis (Figure 1) showed that the best cutoff serum level of PC to predict high AS in HD patients was 18.99 mg/L with area under the curve (AUC) of 0.661 (95% CI 0.568–0.746, $p = 0.002$), sensitivity of 48.98% (95% CI 34.4% to 63.7%), and specificity of 84.06% (95% CI 73.3% to 91.8%).

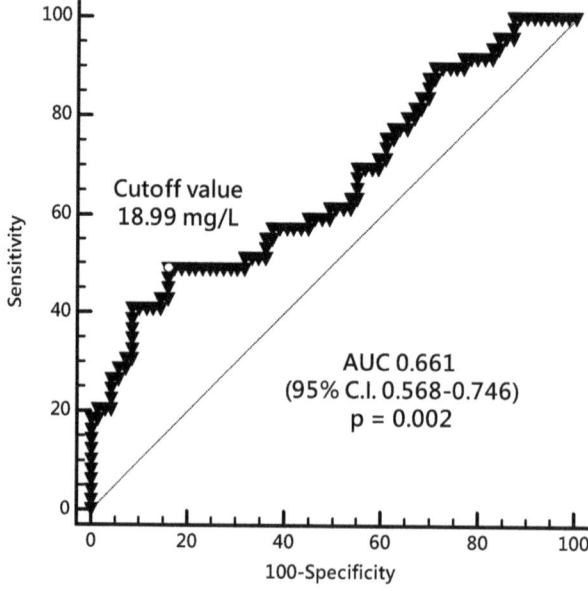

Figure 1. Receiver-operating characteristic curve and the p-cresyl sulfate cutoff level that predicts arterial stiffness in HD patients. AUC, area under the curve; CI, confidence interval; HD, hemodialysis.

3. Discussion

This study showed that DM and high serum PC levels were associated with high cfPWV and could be predictors of high AS in patients on HD. In patients with decline in renal function, AS has been well known to cross-talk with CV events and could lead to poor long-term outcomes in CKD and ESRD patients [2,3,16]. AS that is caused by vascular calcification, which is secondary to an imbalance between the inhibitors and promoters of vascular osteogenesis, and by the traditional and CKD-related risk factors has been reported to progressively increase as renal function declines [5,17]. Vlachopoulos et al. showed that vascular function, which was noninvasively measured and presented as PWV, had a linear correlation with the pooled relative risks for CV events and mortality [3]. Risk factors, such as DM and HTN, had been shown to be related with AS, as measured by cfPWV [18]. Moreover, evidence has shown that deteriorating glucose tolerance was independently associated with central AS with decreasing arterial compliance, carotid–femoral transit time, and increased aortic augmentation index [19]. Furthermore, Agnoletti et al. demonstrated that longer duration of DM led to a higher cfPWV, independent of the other risk factors for AS [20]. In a healthy population, McEniery et al. showed that aortic PWV was associated with higher computed tomography-proven calcification score and isolated systolic HTN [21]. Together with these studies, Cecelja et al. conducted a systemic review and reported that PWV was associated with old age, BP, and DM [18]. Inflammation has been postulated to be associated with endothelial dysfunction and AS. However, the CRIC study showed that baseline inflammation could not predict the long-term AS changes, although there was a positive correlation between several inflammatory markers and AS; these findings highlighted that there were other factors more important than inflammation that cause AS in patients with CKD [22]. Taken together, we found that HD patients with high AS had higher prevalence of DM, SBP, CRP levels, and degree of cfPWV. Similarly, after adjusting for the confounders, we found that DM was the independently significant predictor for the development of high AS in patients on HD.

Initially being known as a gut-derived and protein-bound uremic toxin, PC levels have been shown to increase and accumulate as renal function declined and led to the progression of renal dysfunction and all-cause mortality in patients with CKD [8]. In one systemic review, PC was found to activate oxidative stress, enhance cytokine and inflammatory genes, and induce renal tubular damage [6]. In addition to being regarded as a detrimental factor for renal fibrosis through enhancement of the production of reactive oxygen species, activating transforming growth factor β and the renal–angiotensin–aldosterone system [9,10], PC levels have been reported by in vitro and human studies to induce endothelial dysfunction by increasing the number of circulating endothelial microparticles [23]. Furthermore, an in vitro study on human umbilical vein endothelial cells revealed that PCs could contribute to endothelial dysfunction through the mechanism of increased endothelial permeability, along with reorganized presentation of endothelial actin and VE cadherin and inhibition of endothelial proliferation and wound repair in a dose-dependent manner [11,12]. In addition to playing a role in the progression of endothelial dysfunction, PCs were found to be correlated with image-proven vascular calcification and cfPWV, together with an inverse relationship with the estimated glomerular filtration rate of CKD patients [13]. Recently, Opdebeeck et al. proved that short- and long-term exposures to PCs promoted aortic inflammation and calcification, respectively, in vivo through the acute-phase response and coagulation signaling pathway [24]. In a cross-sectional study, Rossi et al. reported that serum PC was independently associated with interleukin 6 and PWV, highlighting its role in inflammation and its contribution to CV damages in CKD stages 3–4 [25]. Some cohort studies showed that beyond the traditional risk factors, such as age, DM, CRP, malnutrition, or Framingham risk scores, PC levels and severity of vascular calcification led to higher CV events and mortality in CKD and HD patients [13–15]. In accordance with these studies, we found that PCs correlated positively with cfPWV and could be regarded as a main risk factor for developing AS in patients on HD.

A limitation of this study was its cross-sectional and single-center design and the limited number of HD patients. Therefore, the causal relationship between serum PC levels and central AS in patients on HD should be investigated in longitudinal studies on a larger number of patients.

4. Conclusions

Together with DM, serum PC level of >18.99 mg/L may be a risk factor and a predictor of the development of AS in patients on HD. These findings indicated that the gut-derived uremic toxin PC might mediate the process of AS, but its definite mechanism needs to be further elucidated.

5. Materials and Methods

5.1. Participants

From October 2017 to February 2018, 118 patients on HD at a medical center were enrolled. The inclusion criteria were age older than 20 years and receipt of standard 4-h HD three times per week for at least 3 months using standard bicarbonate dialysate and disposable high flux polysulfone artificial kidney (FX class dialyzer, Fresenius Medical Care, Bad Homburg, Germany). The exclusion criteria were active infection, acute myocardial infarction, stroke, peripheral arterial occlusive disease, pulmonary edema, or refusal to provide informed consent. This study was approved by the Protection of Human Subjects Institutional Review Board of Tzu Chi University and Hospital (IRB 103-136-B and 108-96-B).

5.2. Biochemical and Anthropometic Analyses

After an HD session, the body weight and height were measured to the nearest half kilogram and half centimeter, respectively, with the patients wearing light clothing. Body mass index was calculated as the weight (kg)/height (m)^2.

Before HD, approximately 5 mL of blood was collected from each patient. This blood sample was centrifuged at 3000× g for 10 min, stored at 4 °C, and used for biochemical analyses within 1 h after collection. The serum levels of blood urea nitrogen, creatinine, glucose, total cholesterol, triglyceride, total calcium, and phosphorus were examined by an autoanalyzer (Siemens Advia 1800, Siemens Healthcare GmbH, Henkestr, Germany). The adequacy of HD was calculated as the fractional clearance index for urea (Kt/V) and the urea reduction ratio, using the single compartment dialysis urea kinetic model. The levels of intact parathyroid hormone were measured by a commercially available enzyme-linked immunosorbent assay (Diagnostic Systems Laboratories, Webster, TX, USA).

5.3. Determination of Serum P-Cresyl Sulfate Levels

A Waters e2695 HPLC system that comprised a mass spectrometer (ACQUITY QDa, Waters Corporation, Milford, MA, USA) was used in this study [26]. The analytical column was a Phenomenex Luna® C18 (2) (5 µ, 250 × 4.60 mm, 100 Å) with the following settings: column temperature 40 °C, flow 0.8 mL/min, and 30-µL injection. A binary gradient was applied on the mobile phase: the initial composition (95% (A) water with 0.1% formic acid/5% (B) methanol with 0.1% formic acid) was kept constant for 1 min; solvent B was then increased linearly up to 70% over 12 min and was kept constant for 2 min. For column equilibration, solvent B was reduced to 50% over 1 min and was kept constant for 2 min.

The liquid chromatography–mass spectrometry (LC–MS) gradient condition was modified as the pretreated samples were synchronously assessed in positive- or negative-ion (i.e., PCs) mode electrospray ionization. The instrument settings were as follows: desolvation temperature 600 °C, capillary voltage 0.8 kV, and sample cone 15.0 V. The mass spectrometer was operated in full scan at 50 to 450 m/z for positive-ion mode and 100 to 350 m/z for negative-ion mode. The single ion recording mode was used to monitor the individual masses of each compound (PCs: 187.0 m/z). Empower® 3.0 software (Waters Corporation, Milford, MA, USA) was used for data acquisition and processing. The retention time for PCs was approximately 16.56 min. Endogenous compounds were quantified by measuring and comparing the peak areas with the calibration curve obtained from standard solutions. All the determination coefficients of linearity (r^2) were more than 0.995. LC–MS single ion recording mode was used for single ion analysis.

5.4. Carotid–Femoral PWV Measurements

An applanation tonometer (SphygmoCor system, AtCor Medical, Sydney, Australia) was applied to measure the carotid–femoral pulse wave velocity (cfPWV), as previously reported [27]. After resting in a supine position for at least 10 min, patients underwent cfPWV recordings concurrent with an electrocardiogram as a timing reference for the R wave signal. The carotid-femoral distance was obtained by subtracting the carotid measurement site to sternal notch distance from the sternal notch to femoral measurement site distance. Recordings of the successive pulse waves from the carotid and femoral arteries were measured. Using integral software, which contained indices of quality to assure consistency of data on a beat-to-beat basis, the data on pulse wave and electrocardiogram were used to compute the mean interval between the pulse wave and the R wave within an average of 10 cardiac cycles. The carotid–femoral distance was obtained by subtracting the distance of the carotid measurement site to the sternal notch from the distance of the sternal notch to the femoral measurement site. Thereafter, the elapsed time and the difference in distance between the carotid and femoral arteries were used to calculate cfPWV. On the basis of the European Society of Cardiology and the European Society of Hypertension Guidelines [28], patients were sorted according to the cfPWV into the high central AS (>10 m/s) or control (≤10 m/s) group.

5.5. Statistical Analysis

The Kolmogorov–Smirnov test was used to examine the normality of distribution of continuous variables, which were expressed as mean ± standard deviation or as median with IQR. Comparisons between the high AS and control groups were analyzed by the independent Student's t-test or two-tailed Mann–Whitney U test, as appropriate. Categorical data were represented as number and percentage and were analyzed using the χ^2 test. Continuous variables that did not have a normal distribution were logarithmically transformed for use in the linear regression analysis. Multivariate logistic and linear regression analyses were used to assess the risk factors for high central AS and the relationship between all variables and cfPWV, respectively. The best cutoff PC level to predict high central AS was determined using the ROC curve to calculate the area under the curve (AUC). An analysis was regarded as significant if the *p* value was <0.05. SPSS for Windows (version 19.0; SPSS Inc., Chicago, IL, USA) was used for analyses.

Author Contributions: Conceptualization, Y.-H.L. and B.-G.H.; methodology, Y.-H.L. and B.-G.H.; formal analysis, C.-H.W. and B.-G.H.; investigation, Y.-H.L., C.-H.W., C.-H.K., and Y.-L.L.; data curation, Y.-H.L., C.-H.W., C. H.K., and Y.-L.L.; funding acquisition, Y.-H.L.; writing—original draft preparation, C.-H.W. and J.-P.T.; writing—review and editing, J.-P.T. and B.-G.H.; supervision, B.-G.H. All authors have read and agreed to the published version of the manuscript.

Funding: This study was supported by a grant from Hualien Tzu Chi Hospital, Buddhist Tzu Chi Medical Foundation, Taiwan (TCRD107-56).

Conflicts of Interest: The authors declare no conflict of interest.

References

1. Wen, C.P.; Cheng, T.Y.; Tsai, M.K.; Chang, Y.C.; Chan, H.T.; Tsai, S.P.; Chiang, P.H.; Hsu, C.C.; Sung, P.K.; Hsu, Y.H.; et al. All-cause mortality attributable to chronic kidney disease: A prospective cohort study based on 462 293 adults in Taiwan. *Lancet* **2008**, *371*, 2173–2182. [CrossRef]
2. Blacher, J.; Guerin, A.P.; Pannier, B.; Marchais, S.J.; Safar, M.E.; London, G.M. Impact of aortic stiffness on survival in end-stage renal disease. *Circulation* **1999**, *99*, 2434–2439. [CrossRef] [PubMed]

3. Vlachopoulos, C.; Aznaouridis, K.; Stefanadis, C. Prediction of cardiovascular events and all-cause mortality with arterial stiffness: A systematic review and meta-analysis. *J. Am. Coll. Cardiol.* **2010**, *55*, 1318–1327. [CrossRef] [PubMed]
4. Jono, S.; McKee, M.D.; Murry, C.E.; Shioi, A.; Nishizawa, Y.; Mori, K.; Morii, H.; Giachelli, C.M. Phosphate regulation of vascular smooth muscle cell calcification. *Circ. Res.* **2000**, *87*, E10–E17. [CrossRef]
5. Ossareh, S. Vascular calcification in chronic kidney disease: Mechanisms and clinical implications. *Iran. J. Kidney Dis.* **2011**, *5*, 285–299.
6. Vanholder, R.; Schepers, E.; Pletinck, A.; Nagler, E.V.; Glorieux, G. The uremic toxicity of indoxyl sulfate and p-cresyl sulfate: A systematic review. *J. Am. Soc. Nephrol.* **2014**, *25*, 1897–1907. [CrossRef]
7. Townsend, R.R.; Anderson, A.H.; Chirinos, J.A.; Feldman, H.I.; Grunwald, J.E.; Nessel, L.; Roy, J.; Weir, M.R.; Wright, J.T., Jr.; Bansal, N.; et al. Association of pulse wave velocity with chronic kidney disease progression and mortality: Findings from the cric study (chronic renal insufficiency cohort). *Hypertension* **2018**, *71*, 1101–1107. [CrossRef]
8. Wu, I.W.; Hsu, K.H.; Lee, C.C.; Sun, C.Y.; Hsu, H.J.; Tsai, C.J.; Tzen, C.Y.; Wang, Y.C.; Lin, C.Y.; Wu, M.S. P-cresyl sulphate and indoxyl sulphate predict progression of chronic kidney disease. *Nephrol. Dial. Transplant.* **2011**, *26*, 938–947. [CrossRef]
9. Sun, C.Y.; Chang, S.C.; Wu, M.S. Uremic toxins induce kidney fibrosis by activating intrarenal renin-angiotensin-aldosterone system associated epithelial-to-mesenchymal transition. *PLoS ONE* **2012**, *7*, e34026. [CrossRef]
10. Watanabe, H.; Miyamoto, Y.; Honda, D.; Tanaka, H.; Wu, Q.; Endo, M.; Noguchi, T.; Kadowaki, D.; Ishima, Y.; Kotani, S.; et al. P-cresyl sulfate causes renal tubular cell damage by inducing oxidative stress by activation of nadph oxidase. *Kidney Int.* **2013**, *83*, 582–592. [CrossRef]
11. Cerini, C.; Dou, L.; Anfosso, F.; Sabatier, F.; Moal, V.; Glorieux, G.; De Smet, R.; Vanholder, R.; Dignat-George, F.; Sampol, J.; et al. P-cresol, a uremic retention solute, alters the endothelial barrier function in vitro. *Thromb. Haemost.* **2004**, *92*, 140–150. [PubMed]
12. Dou, L.; Bertrand, E.; Cerini, C.; Faure, V.; Sampol, J.; Vanholder, R.; Berland, Y.; Brunet, P. The uremic solutes p-cresol and indoxyl sulfate inhibit endothelial proliferation and wound repair. *Kidney Int.* **2004**, *65*, 442–451. [CrossRef] [PubMed]
13. Liabeuf, S.; Barreto, D.V.; Barreto, F.C.; Meert, N.; Glorieux, G.; Schepers, E.; Temmar, M.; Choukroun, G.; Vanholder, R.; Massy, Z.A.; et al. Free p-cresylsulphate is a predictor of mortality in patients at different stages of chronic kidney disease. *Nephrol. Dial. Transplant.* **2010**, *25*, 1183–1191. [CrossRef] [PubMed]
14. Bammens, B.; Evenepoel, P.; Keuleers, H.; Verbeke, K.; Vanrenterghem, Y. Free serum concentrations of the protein-bound retention solute p-cresol predict mortality in hemodialysis patients. *Kidney Int.* **2006**, *69*, 1081–1087. [CrossRef] [PubMed]
15. Meijers, B.K.; Claes, K.; Bammens, B.; de Loor, H.; Viaene, L.; Verbeke, K.; Kuypers, D.; Vanrenterghem, Y.; Evenepoel, P. P-cresol and cardiovascular risk in mild-to-moderate kidney disease. *Clin. J. Am. Soc. Nephrol.* **2010**, *5*, 1182–1189. [CrossRef] [PubMed]
16. Karras, A.; Haymann, J.P.; Bozec, E.; Metzger, M.; Jacquot, C.; Maruani, G.; Houillier, P.; Froissart, M.; Stengel, B.; Guardiola, P.; et al. Large artery stiffening and remodeling are independently associated with all-cause mortality and cardiovascular events in chronic kidney disease. *Hypertension* **2012**, *60*, 1451–1457. [CrossRef]
17. Moe, S.M.; Chen, N.X. Mechanisms of vascular calcification in chronic kidney disease. *J. Am. Soc. Nephrol.* **2008**, *19*, 213–216. [CrossRef]
18. Cecelja, M.; Chowienczyk, P. Dissociation of aortic pulse wave velocity with risk factors for cardiovascular disease other than hypertension: A systematic review. *Hypertension* **2009**, *54*, 1328–1336. [CrossRef]
19. Schram, M.T.; Henry, R.M.; van Dijk, R.A.; Kostense, P.J.; Dekker, J.M.; Nijpels, G.; Heine, R.J.; Bouter, L.M.; Westerhof, N.; Stehouwer, C.D. Increased central artery stiffness in impaired glucose metabolism and type 2 diabetes: The hoorn study. *Hypertension* **2004**, *43*, 176–181. [CrossRef]
20. Agnoletti, D.; Mansour, A.S.; Zhang, Y.; Protogerou, A.D.; Ouerdane, S.; Blacher, J.; Safar, M.E. Clinical interaction between diabetes duration and aortic stiffness in type 2 diabetes mellitus. *J. Hum. Hypertens.* **2017**, *31*, 189–194. [CrossRef]

21. McEniery, C.M.; McDonnell, B.J.; So, A.; Aitken, S.; Bolton, C.E.; Munnery, M.; Hickson, S.S.; Yasmin; Maki-Petaja, K.M.; Cockcroft, J.R.; et al. Aortic calcification is associated with aortic stiffness and isolated systolic hypertension in healthy individuals. *Hypertension* **2009**, *53*, 524–531. [CrossRef] [PubMed]
22. Peyster, E.; Chen, J.; Feldman, H.I.; Go, A.S.; Gupta, J.; Mitra, N.; Pan, Q.; Porter, A.; Rahman, M.; Raj, D.; et al. Inflammation and arterial stiffness in chronic kidney disease: Findings from the cric study. *Am. J. Hypertens.* **2017**, *30*, 400–408. [CrossRef] [PubMed]
23. Meijers, B.K.; Van Kerckhoven, S.; Verbeke, K.; Dehaen, W.; Vanrenterghem, Y.; Hoylaerts, M.F.; Evenepoel, P. The uremic retention solute p-cresyl sulfate and markers of endothelial damage. *Am. J. Kidney Dis.* **2009**, *54*, 891–901. [CrossRef] [PubMed]
24. Opdebeeck, B.; Maudsley, S.; Azmi, A.; De Mare, A.; De Leger, W.; Meijers, B.; Verhulst, A.; Evenepoel, P.; D'Haese, P.C.; Neven, E. Indoxyl sulfate and p-cresyl sulfate promote vascular calcification and associate with glucose intolerance. *J. Am. Soc. Nephrol.* **2019**, *30*, 751–766. [CrossRef] [PubMed]
25. Rossi, M.; Campbell, K.L.; Johnson, D.W.; Stanton, T.; Vesey, D.A.; Coombes, J.S.; Weston, K.S.; Hawley, C.M.; McWhinney, B.C.; Ungerer, J.P.; et al. Protein-bound uremic toxins, inflammation and oxidative stress: A cross-sectional study in stage 3–4 chronic kidney disease. *Arch. Med. Res.* **2014**, *45*, 309–317. [CrossRef]
26. Wang, C.H.; Lai, Y.H.; Kuo, C.H.; Lin, Y.L.; Tsai, J.P.; Hsu, B.G. Association between serum indoxyl sulfate levels and endothelial function in non-dialysis chronic kidney disease. *Toxins* **2019**, *11*, 589. [CrossRef]
27. Wang, J.H.; Lee, C.J.; Chen, M.L.; Yang, C.F.; Chen, Y.C.; Hsu, B.G. Association of serum osteoprotegerin levels with carotid-femoral pulse wave velocity in hypertensive patients. *J. Clin. Hypertens.* **2014**, *16*, 301–308. [CrossRef]
28. Williams, B.; Mancia, G.; Spiering, W.; Agabiti Rosei, E.; Azizi, M.; Burnier, M.; Clement, D.L.; Coca, A.; de Simone, G.; Dominiczak, A.; et al. 2018 esc/esh guidelines for the management of arterial hypertension. *Eur. Heart J.* **2018**, *39*, 3021–3104. [CrossRef]

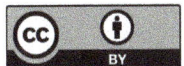

© 2019 by the authors. Licensee MDPI, Basel, Switzerland. This article is an open access article distributed under the terms and conditions of the Creative Commons Attribution (CC BY) license (http://creativecommons.org/licenses/by/4.0/).

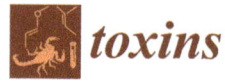

Review

Cardiovascular Calcification in Chronic Kidney Disease—Therapeutic Opportunities

Anika Himmelsbach [†], Carina Ciliox [†] and Claudia Goettsch *

Department of Internal Medicine I, Cardiology, Medical Faculty, RWTH, Aachen University, 52074 Aachen, Germany; ahimmelsbach@ukaachen.de (A.H.); cciliox@ukaachen.de (C.C.)
* Correspondence: cgoettsch@ukaachen.de; Tel.: +49-241-80-37312
† A.H. and C.C. contributed equally.

Received: 25 February 2020; Accepted: 12 March 2020; Published: 14 March 2020

Abstract: Patients with chronic kidney disease (CKD) are highly susceptible to cardiovascular (CV) complications, thus suffering from clinical manifestations such as heart failure and stroke. CV calcification greatly contributes to the increased CV risk in CKD patients. However, no clinically viable therapies towards treatment and prevention of CV calcification or early biomarkers have been approved to date, which is largely attributed to the asymptomatic progression of calcification and the dearth of high-resolution imaging techniques to detect early calcification prior to the 'point of no return'. Clearly, new intervention and management strategies are essential to reduce CV risk factors in CKD patients. In experimental rodent models, novel promising therapeutic interventions demonstrate decreased CKD-induced calcification and prevent CV complications. Potential diagnostic markers such as the serum T50 assay, which demonstrates an association of serum calcification propensity with all-cause mortality and CV death in CKD patients, have been developed. This review provides an overview of the latest observations and evaluates the potential of these new interventions in relation to CV calcification in CKD patients. To this end, potential therapeutics have been analyzed, and their properties compared via experimental rodent models, human clinical trials, and meta-analyses.

Keywords: chronic kidney disease; cardiovascular disease; vascular calcification; experimental rodent models

Key Contribution: This work provides a comprehensive overview of therapeutic opportunities to combat cardiovascular (CV) calcification in chronic kidney disease (CKD). Novel potential therapeutic approaches have been compared and evaluated in human clinical trials and meta-analyses as well as in experimental rodent models of CV calcification in CKD.

---

1. Introduction

Clinically, interaction between organs is of growing relevance given the increasing number of elderly patients with many comorbidities and the recognition that such comorbidities not only influence the clinical course of a given disease and its prognosis, but also affect treatment options and therapeutic success [1]. To exemplify, impaired kidney function associates with poor outcome mainly due to a high burden of cardiovascular (CV) comorbidity, with its manifestations of ischemic heart disease, heart failure, or CV death—a major public health burden in developed countries [2]. Patients with chronic kidney disease (CKD) exhibit a more than four-fold (CKD stage > 3) higher CV risk compared to the non-CKD cohort [2]. Traditional strategies to reduce this risk are largely ineffective in CKD and end-stage renal disease (ESRD) patients, underscoring the importance of non-traditional CKD-specific CV risk factors that are hitherto unknown [2]. In the general population, classical atherosclerotic endpoints such as stroke or myocardial infarction are the dominant cause of death. Importantly, CKD patients mostly die from sudden cardiac death or ischemic heart disease due to premature vascular and cardiac aging [2].

CKD impairs the removal of harmful substances from the body. Therefore dialysis therapy is required to supplant the most important functions of the kidney. During dialysis, waste products like uremic toxins and excess salts and liquids are discharged via diffusion through a semipermeable dialysis membrane. Because of the small pore size of currently used dialysis membranes, protein-bound uremic toxins cannot be filtered during dialysis [3,4], leading to their presence in the blood of CKD patients, which might play a role in the development of cardiovascular disease (CVD). The protein-bound uremic toxin indoxyl sulfate is associated with CV death, and its levels correlate positively with CV calcification [5]. Thus, the existent dialysis therapy remains insufficient, which may explain the poor prognosis of ESRD patients [3].

These patients suffer from abnormalities in mineral metabolism, caused by an imbalance of calcification promoters (e.g., calcium and phosphate) and inhibitors (e.g., matrix Gla protein (MGP) and fetuin-A) [6] and termed 'mineral bone disorder' (MBD). The interconnection of phosphate, calcium, 1,25-dihydroxycholecalciferol (1,25(OH)2D), and fibroblast growth factor 23 (FGF-23) affects the kidney–parathyroid gland–bone axis [7]. In early CKD stages, physiological phosphate serum levels can be sustained. Renal phosphate is restricted by a decreasing glomerular filtration rate (GFR), causing hyperphosphatemia—a major challenge in CKD–MBD. In response to high serum phosphate, osteoblasts produce FGF-23, which inhibits 1,25(OH)2D production. Deficiency in 1,25(OH)2D lowers the serum calcium levels that stimulate the parathyroid gland to produce parathyroid hormone (PTH). The secondary hyperparathyroidism (sHPT) induces calcium efflux from the bone, leading to low bone mineral density. Vitamin D analogs and calcimimetics are used to suppress PTH. Bisphosphonates inhibit osteoclast activity and are applied to treat the dysregulated bone metabolism in CKD–MBD (Figure 1) [8]. Alterations of the bone mineral density are associated with the progression of aortic calcification in women but not in men [9]. Especially, postmenopausal women exhibit an increased risk for CV events [10]. The International Society of Nephrology (ISN) recommends frequent monitoring of serum levels of calcium, phosphate, and PTH, starting in CKD stage 3 patients [11]. If necessary, patients should be treated to maintain an age-appropriate physiological range of serum parameters.

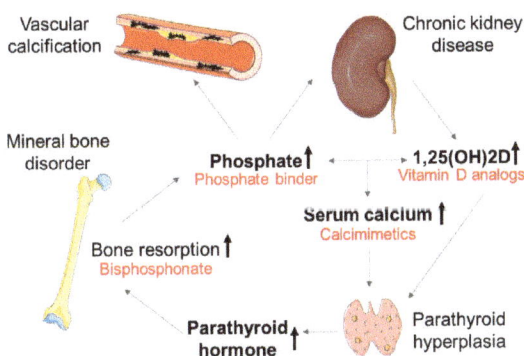

Figure 1. Pathogenesis of chronic kidney disease–mineral bone disorder (CKD–MBD). Targets for therapeutic strategies are written in red; 1,25(OH)2D: 1,25-dihydroxycholecalciferol (calcitriol). The figure was partially created using Servier Medical Art, licensed under a Creative Commons Attribution 3.0 Unported License. Black arrows indicate an increase.

Modifications in the circulation as well as in the myocardium are crucially involved in the increased CV risk in CKD patients. However, both the mediators and the underlying molecular mechanisms remain largely unexplored [12]. CV calcification—both in the tunica intima and in the media—is massively increased in CKD patients and is an independent risk factor for CV morbidity and mortality [13]. CV calcification could be one of the key mechanisms leading to increased CVD in CKD. CV calcification results from active cellular processes in which smooth muscle cells undergo phenotypic changes to build a mineralized matrix [14]. This process is supported by an imbalance of promoters and inhibitors of calcification, which promotes calcium and phosphate precipitation [15,16]. CKD patients with CV risk suffer from mineral deposits in the tunica media (arteriosclerosis) and tunica intima (atherosclerosis). The extent of CV calcification depends on the CKD stage [16,17]. Both traditional and non-traditional risk factors of CV calcification lead to the manifestation of CVD in CKD (Figure 2) [18,19].

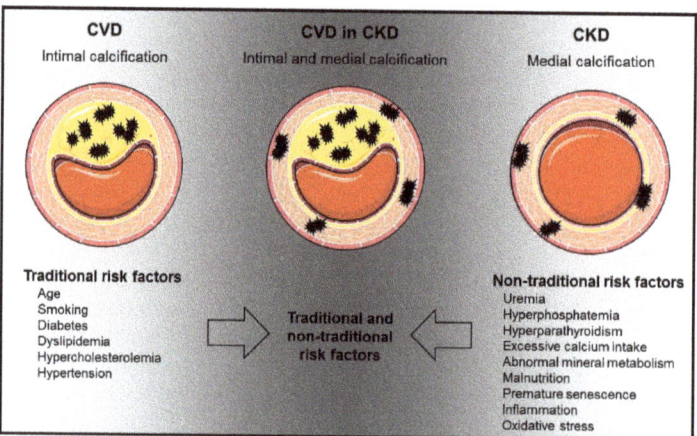

Figure 2. Traditional and non-traditional CVD risk factors affect uremia-induced calcification. Calcification in CKD can result within the tunica intima and tunica media. CVD, cardiovascular disease; The figure was partially created using Servier Medical Art, licensed under a Creative Commons Attribution 3.0 Unported License. Arrows indicate risk factors, which are present in CKD patients suffering from CVD.

Current treatments induce no adequate reduction of CV calcification in CKD, rendering the identification and development of promising therapeutic targets essential. Experimental rodent CKD models proffer novel promising treatments; for example, the hexasodium salt of myo-inositol hexaphosphate SNF472 has been suggested as a potent ectopic calcification inhibitor both in vitro and in vivo [20,21]. Recent studies suggest the peroxisome proliferator-activated receptor-gamma (PPARγ) and the mineralocorticoid receptor (MR) as novel molecular targets for CV complications in CKD. This review focuses on new potential treatments and compares their benefits in non-transgenic animal models with those in human clinical trials and meta-analyses.

2. Animal Models of CKD

Animal models invariably provide valuable insights into the molecular mechanisms of diseases and their underlying pathology. However, none of the prevailing models reproduces the complexity of CVD in CKD [22]. While few non-transgenic rodent models are employed to study CV calcification in CKD [23], one such variant method is the reduction of renal mass via nephrectomy (Figure 3). Five-sixths nephrectomy is limited by the variability in CV calcification, the high mortality rate in patients with advanced CKD, and the necessity for surgery as an irreversible method [24]. Administration of dietary adenine is another strategy to initiate CKD in animal models (Figure 3); adenine is transformed to 2,8-hydroxyadenine, which precipitates in the urinary tract due to its low water solubility [25]. This causes nephrotoxicity, which is similar to clinical CKD [24]. The main disadvantage of this model is the weight loss of the animals due to reduced food intake. The adenine model is a reversible CKD model, because there is no need for surgery, which eases its implementation and handling. As neither five-sixths nephrectomy nor adenine diet alone initiate CV calcification, either high-phosphate or high-fat diet are used as a second trigger (Figure 3) [26]. Both models show similarities—hyperphosphatemia, increased plasma creatinine, and enhanced blood urea nitrogen, but the CV calcification outcome is not consistent. The reasons for this are differences in trial times and the high variability in diet phosphate and calcium concentrations [24]. The sensitivity to CV calcification also depends on the genetic background, age, and gender of the animals [27]. Female mice show higher susceptibility to CV calcification than males [28], which is the opposite to what observed in humans, wherein men tend to have higher average coronary artery calcium scores than women [29]. This might suggest that the hormone status affects vascular calcification and should be considered when planning experiments. CV calcification variabilities in CKD are mostly seen in mice but tend to be strain-dependent [22]. The most commonly used mouse strain is C57Bl/6, which is resistant to the development of hypertension, glomerulosclerosis, and proteinuria. In addition, it shows decreased activity in the renin–angiotensin–aldosterone system, which is important for fibrosis development after five-sixths nephrectomy [27,30]. In summary, compromises have to be made in choosing the right CKD animal model. Therefore, it is essential to agree on standards using rodent models within the CVD–CKD research field.

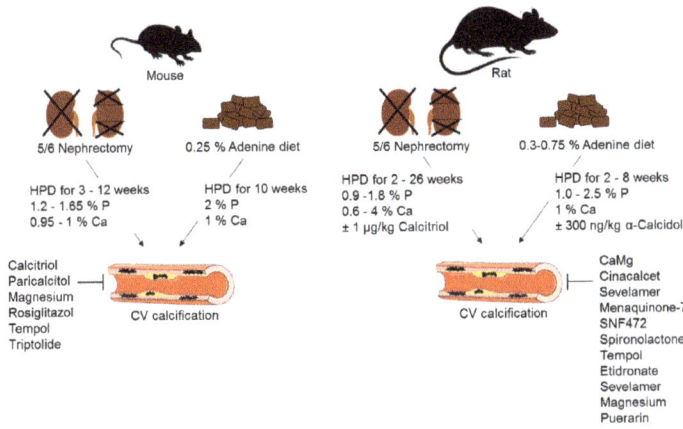

Figure 3. Schematic presentation of rodent non-transgenic animal models of cardiovascular calcification in CKD. HFD: high-phosphate diet; CV: cardiovascular; P: phosphate; Ca: calcium. The figure was partially created using Servier Medical Art, licensed under a Creative Commons Attribution 3.0 Unported License. Arrows indicate CV calcification induced by 5/6 nephrectomy and 0.25 % adenine diet. Fork indicates kidney areas, which are removed during 5/6 nephrectomy.

3. Therapeutic Concepts of CV Calcification in CKD

3.1. Phosphate Binder

Hyperphosphatemia is a major clinical challenge in CKD–MBD. Phosphate binders (PB) are classified into calcium-based PB (CBB; e.g., calcium acetate, calcium carbonate) and non-calcium-based PB (e.g., sevelamer, lanthanum). The administration of PB reduces serum phosphate levels, thereby improving hyperphosphatemia in CKD patients. In two independent experimental CKD models, treatment with sevelamer attenuated vascular calcification (Table 1) [31,32]. The PB calcium acetate/magnesium carbonate (CaMg) reduced CV calcification without affecting bone mineral density in adenine-induced CKD rats (Table 1) [33].

In CKD patients, a meta-analysis of eight different PB (sevelamer, lanthanum, iron, calcium, colestilan, bixalomer, nicotinic acid, magnesium) showed that the PB reduced serum phosphate levels compared to placebo controls, but had no effect on all-cause mortality and CV events [34]. Another systematic review and meta-analysis revealed decreased all-cause mortality by non-calcium-based PB, compared to CBB in CKD patients [35]. A Cochrane systematic review and meta-analysis of randomized clinical trials (RCT) showed that sevelamer compared to CBB decreased all-cause mortality in ESRD patients [36], while sevelamer had no effect on CV mortality [37].

Table 1. Therapeutic strategies that attenuate CV calcification in non-transgenic animal CKD models.

Treatment	Substance	Dosis	Medication	Experimental Model	Species, Strain	Ref.
Phosphate binder	Sevelamer	750 mg/kg	Daily oral gavage, 4 weeks	Adenine diet	Wistar rat	[32]
Phosphate binder	Sevelamer	3%	Diet, 6 months	5/6 nephrectomy	Sprague-Dawley rat	[31]
Phosphate binder	CaMg	185 mg/kg	Daily oral gavage, 6 weeks	Adenine diet	Wistar rat	[33]
Calcimimetic	Cinacalcet	10 mg/kg	Daily oral gavage, 12 weeks	Adenine diet	Wistar rat	[38]

CaMg: acetate/magnesium carbonate; Ref: Reference.

Based on these findings, the Kidney Disease: Improving Global Outcomes (KDIGO) 2017 guideline recommends PB treatment for progressively elevated phosphate and a restriction of CBB treatment [11], with a limited dietary phosphate intake [11]. Given a lack of evidence that PB reduce all-cause mortality, longer placebo-controlled trials are required. It also remains uncertain to which extent pre-dialysis patients would benefit from PB treatment, since adverse effects like nausea, constipation, diarrhea, and abdominal pain are reported [34].

3.2. Calcimimetics

Calcimimetics act on the calcium-sensing receptor and increase its sensitivity to calcium, thereby lowering the PTH level as a result of the feedback mechanism. Two generations of calcimimetics have been developed, the first of which—calcimimetic cinacalcet—is taken orally once daily. The second generation—calcimimetic etecalcetide—is applied intravenously three times per week after hemodialysis (HD) sessions [39].

In an experimental CKD model of adenine-fed rats, cinacalcet ameliorated aortic calcification (Table 1) [38]. The prospective RCTs EVOLVE and ADVANCE treated HD patients with sHPT daily with 30 to 180 mg cinacalcet [40,41]. In the ADVANCE trial, patients additionally received a low-dose vitamin D therapy. Cinacalcet reduced the progression of aortic valve calcification compared to the vitamin D control group, while it had no effect on aortic calcification [41]. Similar results were found in the EVOLVE trial. In both trials, cinacalcet bore no effect on all-cause mortality and CV event rate [40,41]. A meta-analysis of RCTs considering (pre)-dialysis patients and kidney transplant recipients (KTR) revealed that cinacalcet had no effect on all-cause mortality [42]. An observational study confirmed that cinacalcet is not associated with all-cause mortality but is related to reduced CV events [43]. A variety of adverse effects like diarrhea, hypocalcemia, and nausea have been reported [44]. While calcimimetics are quite effective in lowering serum PTH, the effect on all-cause mortality, CV risk, and calcification is uncertain [37]. Especially in pre-dialysis patients, further studies focusing on clinical rather than biochemical outcomes are needed.

4. Novel Therapeutic Strategies—from Experimental Models to the Clinic

4.1. Bisphosphonates

Bisphosphonates, also known as pyrophosphate analogs, are antiresorptive drugs that are administered to treat diseases with high-turnover bone resorption, like osteoporosis, Paget's disease, and multiple myeloma. In CKD–MBD, they are applied to treat the dysregulated bone metabolism [8].

Bisphosphonates inhibit osteoclast activity. There are two groups of bisphosphonates, with different nitrogen content. Non-nitrogen-containing bisphosphonates (e.g., etidronate) cause osteoclast apoptosis, while nitrogen-containing equivalents (e.g., alendronate; pamidronate) inhibit osteoclast activity. Nitrogen-containing bisphosphonates show 10–10,000 times increased potency in inhibiting bone resorption [45]. Bisphosphonate-associated nephrotoxicity has been reported [46,47]. Especially, intravenously applied bisphosphonates can cause acute kidney injury [47–49]. Therefore, doses and treatment period has to be adjusted in patients with pre-existing CKD [46]. Other known side effects are focal segmental glomerulosclerosis, hypocalcemia, and pathological fractures like bisphosphonate-related osteonecrosis of the jaw [46,50]. Still, bisphosphonates are in generally well tolerated, and severe side effects are rare [50–52]. The mechanisms of action and pharmacokinetics of bisphosphonates have recently been reviewed [53].

Etidronate reduced aortic calcification in five-sixths nephrectomy-induced CKD rats (Table 2), as well as in HD and CKD patients [54,55]. Alendronate did not alter aortic calcification in CKD stages 3 and 4 [56]. These results suggest that the nitrogen content of bisphosphonates may affect the potency of bisphosphonates to alter CV calcification. A systematic review summarized 20 performed trials and illustrated contrasting results of the existing bisphosphonate studies [55]. In CKD patients, coronary artery calcification (CAC) and aortic calcification were increased after 12–24 months of bisphosphonate treatment. In a non-CKD cohort of postmenopausal osteoporotic women, intima–media thickening was reduced under bisphosphonate therapy [55]. Evidence remains unclear regarding the effect on arterial stiffness and atherosclerotic plaques in humans. In a retrospective study, female CKD patients had a 22% reduced risk for all-cause mortality when treated with bisphosphonates. However, there was no benefit regarding CV mortality [57]. In different cohorts, beneficial effects were found on arterial calcification, but not on arterial stiffness. CV events were not improved by bisphosphonate therapy [58]. Due to the small amount of studies performed in CKD patients, evidence for a beneficial effect of bisphosphonates on vascular calcification in CKD–MBD is still unclear.

A novel strategy to alter osteoclast activity is the use of a neutralizing antibody against receptor activator of NFκB-ligand (RANKL), called denosumab, which inhibits bone resorption and reduces fracture risk [59]. RANKL is crucial for proper osteoclast function [60] and was shown to promote vascular calcification in vitro and in vivo [61,62]. In contrast to bisphosphonates, denosumab is not eliminated by the kidney [63] and appeared to be safe in HD patients. Nevertheless, a recent study revealed a denosumab-associated increased risk of renal function decline in male patients, patients with renal insufficiency, and patients with acute kidney injury [63]. In HD patients, neither alendronate nor denosumab treatment improved vascular function and CAC score [63].

Clinically and in animal models, there is an association between osteoporosis and CV calcification—the so called osteoporosis–vascular calcification paradox [64,65]. However, current evidence suggests that improving bone mineral density does not alter CV calcification.

Table 2. Novel therapeutic strategies that attenuate CV calcification in non-transgenic animal CKD models.

Treatment	Substance	Dosis	Application	Experimental Model	Species, Strain	Ref.
Bisphospho-nate	Etidronate	5 or 10 mg/kg	s.c., daily, 3 weeks	5/6 nephrectomy	Wistar rat	[54]
Vitamin K	Mena-quinone-7	50 µg/kg	Oral gavage, daily 4 weeks	Adenine diet	Sprague-Dawley rat	[66]
Omega-3 fatty acid	Eicosapenta-enoic acid	300 mg/kg	Oral gavage, daily 4 weeks	Adenine diet	Sprague-Dawley rat	[66]
Vitamin D receptor agonist	Calcitriol	30 ng/kg	i.p., 3 times/week, 3 weeks	5/6 nephrectomy	DBA/2J mouse	[26]
	Paricalcitol	100 or 300 ng/kg				
Dietary supplement	Magnesium	0.1–1.1%	Food intake, 14 days	5/6 nephrectomy	Wistar rat	[67]
Dietary supplement	Magnesium	3%	Food intake, 7 weeks	5/6 nephrectomy	Non-agouti mouse	[68]
Hexasodium salt	SNF472	50 mg/kg	i.v., daily, 19 days	Adenine diet	Wistar rat	[20]

S.c: subcutaneous; i.p.: intraperitoneal; i.v.: intravenous; Ref: Reference.

4.2. Vitamin K

Vitamin K is a cofactor for post-translational γ-carboxylation of calcification inhibitors and activators that plays a role in mineralization and osteogenic differentiation of vascular smooth muscle cells. More importantly, in CKD, vitamin K serves for the carboxylation of the calcification inhibitor MGP and the vitamin K-dependent calcium binder osteocalcin [69,70]. Vitamin K deficiency causes reduced carboxylation of uncarboxylated MGP (ucMGP) to carboxylated MGP (cMGP). Therefore, the inhibiting effect of cMGP is attenuated. The inactive form of ucMGP, which is dephosphorylated (dp-ucMGP), can be measured as a representative for the vitamin K status. In medial calcification (Mönckeberg's sclerosis), which is associated with renal disease, MGP is expressed in all calcified areas in human tissue samples [71]. There are two naturally occurring vitamers of vitamin K, that differ in bioavailability and distribution in the human body: vitamin K1 (phylloquinone) and vitamin K2 (menaquinone, MK). While the former is mainly retained in the liver to serve as a cofactor for the carboxylation of clotting factors, circulating vitamin K2 is available for the extrahepatic tissue and the vascular system [72] and thereby is more capable of acting in the vascular calcification process [70]. Due to its bioavailability, the vitamer MK-7 is mainly used in clinical trials [72]. A single-MK-7 treatment, as well as the combination of MK-7 and eicosapentaenoic, reduced the development of vascular calcification in an experimental model of adenine-induced CKD rats (Table 2) [66].

HD patients show low vitamin K intake, accompanied by increased levels of serum dp-ucMGP [73]. One explanation for this result could be the recommendation for CKD patients to avoid phosphate- and potassium-rich food, which often contains vitamin K [74]. Consequently, vitamin K deficiency increases the risk for vascular calcification in already calcification-prone CKD patients. A prospective cohort study of patients in CKD stages 4 to 5D revealed a positive correlation between serum dp-ucMGP levels and aortic calcification (Table 3) [75]. All-cause mortality was higher in patients with dp-ucMGP levels above the median [75]. HD patients did not reveal a positive correlation of the dp-ucMGP levels with the extent of vascular calcification [75]. After adjustment, low dp-cMGP levels were associated with a higher all-cause and CV mortality risk [75]. In a cohort with stable KTR, all-cause mortality was increased in patients in the highest dp-ucMGP quartile compared to the lowest quartile, after adjustment and exclusion of vitamin K antagonists [76].

Table 3. Observational studies investigating the role of vitamin K in CKD.

Patients	Follow-up	Main Results	Ref.
CKD stages 4 to 5D ($n = 107$)	2.2 years	dp-ucMGP: positive association with progressive CKD stages and increased all-cause mortality	[75]
HD patients ($n = 188$)	3 years	- 6.5-fold elevated dp-ucMGP - dp-cMGP associated with increased all-cause and CV mortality	[75]
KTR ($n = 518$)	9.8 years	dp-ucMGP: association with increased all-cause mortality	[76]

HD: hemodialysis; KTR: kidney transplant recipients; dp-ucMGP: dephosphorylated-uncarboxylated matrix Gla protein; dp-cMGP: dephosphorylated-carboxylated matrix Gla protein.

In vitro studies showed the binding of vitamin K by PB [77]. Therefore, PB inhibit the gastrointestinal uptake of vitamin K2, thus aggravating vitamin K deficiency in CKD patients [78]. In a study, calcium acetate and magnesium carbonate bound to vitamin K2, independent of the presence of phosphate, while sevelamer carbonate did not bind to vitamin K2 in vitro [64]. This could be one additional explanation as to why non-calcium-based PB are favored in the studies mentioned above. Interestingly, the non-calcium-based PB lanthanum bound to vitamin K2 only in the absence of phosphate [78]. In order to investigate the effect of PB on vitamin K deficiency in vivo, a cross-sectional study with HD patients, patients with peritoneal dialysis, and KTR was performed. Dp-ucMGP levels were significantly lower in KTR compared to dialysis patients. No association between the use of any PB and dp-ucMGP was observed, while sevelamer monotherapy was associated with elevated dp-ucMGP levels [79]. This evidence does not fit the in vitro observation that sevelamer did not bind to vitamin K2 [64]. The clinical relevance of the influence of PB on vitamin K deficiency remains unclear.

Clinical interventional trials investigated the effect of vitamin K2 supplementation in CKD patients with vitamin K deficiency (Table 4). In HD patients, MK-7 treatment reduced dp-ucMGP levels, while dp-cMGP did not alter them [75,80,81]. In CKD patients stage 3–5, a combined treatment of MK-7 and vitamin D reduced dp-ucMGP levels and carotid–intima–media thickness, compared to vitamin D therapy only [82]. The CAC score was increased in both groups. Due to the growing interest in vitamin K biology and the role in preventing CV calcification, ongoing randomized controlled trials on vitamin K supplementation in CKD patients are taking place [82]; according to the status update on clinicaltrials.gov, results have yet to be published.

Table 4. Interventional studies investigating the effect of vitamin K in CKD.

Patients	Treatment	Study Design	Main Results	Ref.
CKD stage 3–5 ($n = 42$)	90 µg/d MK-7 + 10 µg/d cholecalciferol, or 10 µg/d cholecalciferol (control), 38.5 weeks	Prospective, randomized, double-blind	Decrease of dp-ucMGP, smaller increase of CAC and CCA-IMT compared to control	[83]
HD patients ($n = 50$)	360 µg/d MK-7, 4 weeks	Prospective, pre-post intervention clinical trial	86% decrease of dp-ucMGP	[80]
HD patients ($n = 17$)	135 µg/d MK-7, 6 weeks	Interventional pilot study	Decrease of dp-ucMGP but not dp-cMGP	[75]
HD patients ($n = 53$), Healthy controls ($n = 50$)	45, 135, 360 µg/d MK-7, 6 weeks	Interventional, randomized, non-placebo-controlled trial	Dose-dependent decrease of dp-ucMGP	[81]

MK-7: menaquinone-7 (vitamin K2); CAC: coronary artery calcification; Vit.K: vitamin K2; CCA–IMT: common carotid artery–intima media thickness.

4.3. Vitamin D

Vitamin D deficiency and sHPT are common comorbidities in progressive CKD stages. Vitamin D application lowers PTH levels in the body. TheKidney Disease: Improving Global Outcomes KDIGO guideline from 2017 recommends vitamin D analogs for both CKD pre-dialysis patients stage 4 and 5 and dialysis patients with sHPT [11].

In a mouse model of CKD with electrocoagulation of the right renal cortex and left nephrectomy, treatment with the vitamin D receptor agonists calcitriol and paricalcitol prevented calcification (Table 2) [26]. A meta-analysis of 20 observational studies revealed an association of vitamin D supplementation in pre-dialysis and HD patients with decreased all-cause and CV mortality [84]. The association between vitamin D deficiency and endothelial dysfunction supports the hypothesis that vitamin D supplementation could attenuate vascular calcification in CKD patients [85]. Therefore, interventional studies investigated the effect of vitamin D analogs on arterial stiffness. A double-blind RCT compared the effect of calcifediol (25-hydroxyvitamin D3) and calcitriol (1,25-dihydroxyvitamin D3) to placebo by analyzing pulse wave velocity (PWV) as a parameter for vascular stiffness [86]. PWV was decreased in the calcifediol group, while it stagnated in the calcitriol group and was increased in the placebo control. Furthermore, cholecalciferol improved vascular stiffness in pre-dialysis patients compared to placebo, suggesting a beneficial effect of cholecalciferol on endothelial function [87]. However, treatment with cholecalciferol did not significantly attenuate CAC in CKD [88]. Evidence for a beneficial effect of vitamin D supplementation on CV calcification progression remains uncertain. The informative value is also limited by the use of different vitamin D analogs and dosages. Further RCT are necessary to evaluate the potential of vitamin D supplementation in CKD. Findings demonstrated a vitamin D level decline prior to the occurrence of changes in PTH and phosphate. Therefore, earlier vitamin D supplementation should be considered in patients without sHPT [89].

4.4. Magnesium

Magnesium is a micronutrient with various functions in the body. In vitro studies revealed an inhibiting role of magnesium in phosphate-induced calcification [90]. Dietary magnesium supplementation reduced and reversed vascular calcification in five-sixths nephrectomized rats (Table 2) [67]. These findings were supported by Kaesler et al., showing that magnesium treatment reduces vascular calcification in five-sixths nephrectomized mice (Table 2) [68].

A negative association of serum magnesium with vascular calcification was shown in CKD patients [91]. In a meta-analysis encompassing 532,979 patients from 19 prospective cohort studies of the general population, serum magnesium as well as dietary magnesium intake was inversely associated with the risk of CV events [92]. This observation was confirmed in different observational studies in HD and peritoneal dialysis patients. Lower serum magnesium levels were associated with higher all-cause and CV mortality [93–96]. However, hypomagnesemia was not an independent predictor for mortality in end-stage renal disease [93,96]. CAC and vessel stiffness occurred in patients with high magnesium serum levels [97]. Although these observations encourage the assumption that magnesium supplementation might attenuate vascular calcification in CKD, few interventional studies have been performed. In HD patients, magnesium treatment reduced carotid intima–media thickness compared to placebo control [98]. Carotid intima–media thickness was also improved in a small trial with magnesium citrate, compared to treatment with the PB calcium acetate [99]. In the ongoing MAGiCAL-CKD trial, pre-dialysis patients ($n = 250$) are treated with 360 mg/day magnesium hydroxide for one year. The change in CAC will be evaluated by CT scans [100]. Results of this study might provide new evidence concerning the role of magnesium in the prevention of CV calcification in CKD.

4.5. Hexasodium Salt of Myo-Inositol Hexaphosphate

A novel therapeutic option is the hexasodium salt of myo-inositol hexaphosphate SNF472, a potent calcification inhibitor in vitro [20]. SNF472 binds to the growth sites of hydroxyapatite crystals, the main constituent part of calcification deposits, thereby reducing the progression of ectopic calcification [20]. SNF472 inhibited CV calcification in adenine-induced CKD rats by up to 90% (Table 2) [20]. In ex vivo analysis using plasma from HD patients, hydroxyapatite crystallization potential was reduced by SNF472 [101,102]. The first phase 2 study CaLIPSO with 274 HD patients demonstrated attenuated progression of CAC and aortic valve calcification compared to placebo control, after 52 weeks of SNF472 treatment [21].

5. Promising Treatments of CV Calcification in Experimental CKD Models

Opportunities for renal transplantation are low, and many patients suffer from progressive CKD and its comorbidities. Existing drug therapies offer no adequate solution to treat/prevent CV calcification in CKD patients. In experimental non-transgenic CKD models, new promising therapeutic interventions and potential drug targets to decrease CKD-induced calcification and prevent or reverse pathophysiological complications have recently been shown. The isoflavonoid compound puerarin, found in the root of *Pueraria lobata*, has anti-inflammatory effects [103] and inhibited calcification in mouse vascular smooth muscle cells [76] and five-sixths nephrectomized rats (Table 5) [104].

PPARγ plays an important role in CVD and is closely connected to atherosclerosis [105,106]. Rosiglitazol, a PPARγ agonist, reduced vascular calcification in five-sixths nephrectomized mice (Table 5) [107]. Another potential drug target for CV calcification in CKD could be the nuclear factor kappa-light-chain-enhancer of activated B cells (NF-κB), which is active in calcified vessels [108]. The NF-κB inhibitors tempol and triptolide reduced vascular calcification in an adenine-induced CKD mouse model [109], as well as in adenine-induced CKD rats (Table 5) [110]. Further, different studies have shown that MR signaling can promote CV calcification [92]. Blockage of MR is increasingly applied as a therapy for improvement of CV outcomes in CKD, diabetes mellitus, hypertension, and heart failure. The MR antagonist spironolactone improved CV outcomes in patients with heart diseases [92] and inhibited dose-dependent vascular calcification and kidney damage in adenine-induced CKD rats (Table 5) [111].

Table 5. Potential therapeutic strategies that attenuate CV calcification in non-transgenic animal CKD models.

Treatment	Substance	Dosis	Application	Experimental Model	Species, Strain	Ref.
Isoflavonoid	Puerarin	400 mg/kg	Oral gavage, daily; 4 weeks	5/6 nephrectomy	Sprague-Dawley rat	[104]
PPARγ agonist	Rosiglitazol	10 mg/kg	Oral gavage, daily; 12 weeks	5/6 nephrectomy	DBA/2J mouse	[107]
NF-κB inhibitor	Tempol	3 mmol/L	Drinking water; 10 weeks	Adenine diet	DBA/2J mouse	[109]
NF-κB inhibitor	Tempol	3 mmol/L	Drinking water; 6 weeks	Adenine diet	Sprague-Dawley rat	[110]
NF-κB inhibitor	Triptolide	70 µg/kg	i.p., daily; 10 weeks	Adenine diet	DBA/2J mouse	[109]
MR antagonist	Spirono-lactone	100 mg/kg	Food intake, daily; 2 weeks	Adenine diet	Sprague-Dawley rat	[111]

MR: mineralocorticoid.

6. Potential Diagnostic Tools for CV Calcification in CKD

6.1. Development of the T_{50} Assay

Circulating biomarkers associated with progression of vascular calcification and mortality in CKD patients lack predictive value. For example, serum levels of fetuin-A and osteoprotegerin positively correlate with mortality of dialysis patients, and soluble klotho is associated with aortic calcification progression [112,113]. In 2012, Pasch et al. introduced a novel concept for the risk assessment for CKD patients. The T_{50} assay is a measure of the propensity for calcification in blood serum [114], based on the time-dependent shape change of calcium-phosphate precipitation particles. Colloidal spherical-shaped primary calciprotein particles (CPP) convert to crystalline secondary CPPs with radial growth of crystalline needles [115]. Nephelometry allows the determination of the transition step from primary to secondary CPPs. The amount of precipitation depends on the capacity of serum to inhibit this process by calcification inhibitors like fetuin-A. In this assay, the patient's serum is supersaturated by adding 6 mM phosphate and 10 mM calcium to accelerate precipitation. This allows the analysis of the half-maximal transition time (T_{50}). Higher T_{50} values reflect longer transition times, thereby less propensity for calcification. A potential clinical use needs to be evaluated [114].

6.2. Clinical Association

An association of shorter T_{50} times with increased all-cause and CV mortality, as well as CV events, could be demonstrated in pre-dialysis CKD patients, HD patients, and KTR (Table 6) [76,107,116–118]. Aortic pulse wave velocity (APWV), as a quantification tool of progressive arterial stiffness and vascular calcification, showed conflicting results in association with T_{50} [116,118]. In KTR, baseline APWV was not associated with T_{50} values [118], while an association of lower T_{50} values with increasing APWV was found in patients with CKD stage 3 and 4 [116]. T_{50} values are not associated with CAC prevalence but rather with greater CAC severity (Table 6) [97]. Further investigations considering clinical parameters that represent the progression of vascular calcification should be made to estimate the predictive value of T_{50} with respect to calcification in CKD patients.

Table 6. Clinical assessment of calcification propensity based on half-maximal transition time (T_{50}) in CKD patients.

Patients	Mean/Median T_{50} (Baseline)	Follow up, Years	Findings	Ref.
CKD stages 2 to 4 (n = 1274), In follow up n = 780	Median: 321 min	3.2	Association of low T50 with increased CAC prevalence and progression	[97]
CKD stages 3 and 4 (n = 184)	Mean: 329 ± 95 min	5.3	Association of low T50 with increased all-cause mortality and APWV	[116]
HD patients (n = 2785), control group (n = 1366)	Mean: 212 min (10th–90th percentile: 109–328 min)	1.7	Association of low T50 with increased all-cause mortality and CVD	[117]
HD patients (n = 188)	Mean: 246 ± 64 min	3.7	Association of low T50 and T50 decline with all-cause and CV mortality	[117]
KTR (n = 699)	Mean: 286 ± 62 min	3.1	Association of low T50 with increased all-cause and CV mortality and graft failure	[76]
KTR (n = 433)	Mean: 340 ± 70 min	3.7	Association of low T50 with increased CVD event risk	[107]
KTR during 10 weeks after transplantation (n = 1435), Follow-up: APWV after 1 year (n = 589)	Median: 188 min (25th–75th percentile: 139–248 min)	5.1	Association of low T50 with increased all-cause and CV mortality APWV not associated with T50 baseline	[118]

APWV: aortic pulse wave velocity.

7. Outlook

Pharmaceutical treatments currently applied in clinical routine offer no adequate solution to treating or preventing CV calcification in CKD. Currently, we have no clear evidence that direct targeting CV calcification leads to an improvement in CV outcomes in CKD and ESRD patients. Still, vitamin K supplementation diminished the progression of aortic valve calcification and subsequently affected the cardiac and clinical outcomes in CVD patients without CKD [119], giving hope that future developments will yield the must needed treatment option to reduce CV risk in CKD patients. In experimental CKD rodent models, new promising therapeutic interventions and potential drug targets to decrease CKD-induced calcification and prevent or reverse pathophysiological CV complications have recently been shown. However, no single animal model thoroughly reproduces the complexity of CV calcification in CKD and all attendant comorbidities. For this reason, it is essential to agree on a consistent animal model within this research area to maintain comparability.

Author Contributions: Designed the review, performed literature search, carried out interpretation, and drafted the manuscript, A.H. and C.C.; contributed to the review concept, participated in interpretation, and aided in overall manuscript development, C.G. All authors have read and agreed to the published version of the manuscript.

Funding: This research was funded by grants from the German Research Foundation (GO1801/5-1 SFB/TRR219 C02 to CG) and the START-Program of the Faculty of Medicine, RWTH Aachen (to CG).

Conflicts of Interest: The authors declare no conflict of interest.

References

1. Metra, M.; Zaca, V.; Parati, G.; Agostoni, P.; Bonadies, M.; Ciccone, M.; Cas, A.D.; Iacoviello, M.; Lagioia, R.; Lombardi, C.; et al. Cardiovascular and noncardiovascular comorbidities in patients with chronic heart failure. *J. Cardiovasc. Med.* **2011**, *12*, 76–84. [CrossRef]
2. Noels, H.; Boor, P.; Goettsch, C.; Hohl, M.; Jahnen-Dechent, W.; Jankowski, V.; Kindermann, I.; Kramann, R.; Lehrke, M.; Linz, D.; et al. The new SFB/TRR219 Research Centre. *Eur. Heart J.* **2018**, *39*, 975–977. [CrossRef]
3. Ito, S.; Yoshida, M. Protein-bound uremic toxins: New culprits of cardiovascular events in chronic kidney disease patients. *Toxins* **2014**, *6*, 665–678. [CrossRef]
4. Lekawanvijit, S.; Kompa, A.R.; Wang, B.H.; Kelly, D.J.; Krum, H. Cardiorenal syndrome: The emerging role of protein-bound uremic toxins. *Circ. Res.* **2012**, *111*, 1470–1483. [CrossRef]
5. Barreto, F.C.; Barreto, D.V.; Liabeuf, S.; Meert, N.; Glorieux, G.; Temmar, M.; Choukroun, G.; Vanholder, R.; Massy, Z.A. Serum indoxyl sulfate is associated with vascular disease and mortality in chronic kidney disease patients. *Clin. J. Am. Soc. Nephrol.* **2009**, *4*, 1551–1558. [CrossRef]
6. Schlieper, G.; Schurgers, L.; Brandenburg, V.; Reutelingsperger, C.; Floege, J. Vascular calcification in chronic kidney disease: An update. *Nephrol. Dial. Transplant.* **2016**, *31*, 31–39. [CrossRef]
7. Viegas, C.; Araujo, N.; Marreiros, C.; Simes, D. The interplay between mineral metabolism, vascular calcification and inflammation in Chronic Kidney Disease (CKD): Challenging old concepts with new facts. *Aging (Albany NY)* **2019**, *11*, 4274–4299. [CrossRef]
8. Dayanand, P.; Sandhyavenu, H.; Dayanand, S.; Martinez, J.; Rangaswami, J. Role of Bisphosphonates in Vascular calcification and Bone Metabolism: A Clinical Summary. *Curr. Cardiol. Rev.* **2018**, *14*, 192–199. [CrossRef]
9. Kiel, D.P.; Kauppila, L.I.; Cupples, L.A.; Hannan, M.T.; O'Donnell, C.J.; Wilson, P.W. Bone loss and the progression of abdominal aortic calcification over a 25 year period: The Framingham Heart Study. *Calcif. Tissue Int.* **2001**, *68*, 271–276. [CrossRef]
10. Tanko, L.B.; Christiansen, C.; Cox, D.A.; Geiger, M.J.; McNabb, M.A.; Cummings, S.R. Relationship between osteoporosis and cardiovascular disease in postmenopausal women. *J. Bone miner. Res.* **2005**, *20*, 1912–1920. [CrossRef]
11. Beto, J.; Bhatt, N.; Gerbeling, T.; Patel, C.; Drayer, D. Overview of the 2017 KDIGO CKD-MBD Update: Practice Implications for Adult Hemodialysis Patients. *J. Ren. Nutr.* **2019**, *29*, 2–15. [CrossRef] [PubMed]

12. Marx, N.; Noels, H.; Jankowski, J.; Floege, J.; Fliser, D.; Bohm, M. Mechanisms of cardiovascular complications in chronic kidney disease: Research focus of the Transregional Research Consortium SFB TRR219 of the University Hospital Aachen (RWTH) and the Saarland University. *Clin. Res. Cardiol.* **2018**, *107*, 120–126. [CrossRef] [PubMed]
13. Martin, S.S.; Blaha, M.J.; Blankstein, R.; Agatston, A.; Rivera, J.J.; Virani, S.S.; Ouyang, P.; Jones, S.R.; Blumenthal, R.S.; Budoff, M.J.; et al. Dyslipidemia, coronary artery calcium, and incident atherosclerotic cardiovascular disease: Implications for statin therapy from the multi-ethnic study of atherosclerosis. *Circulation* **2014**, *129*, 77–86. [CrossRef] [PubMed]
14. Hutcheson, J.D.; Goettsch, C.; Bertazzo, S.; Maldonado, N.; Ruiz, J.L.; Goh, W.; Yabusaki, K.; Faits, T.; Bouten, C.; Franck, G.; et al. Genesis and growth of extracellular-vesicle-derived microcalcification in atherosclerotic plaques. *Nat. Mater.* **2016**, *15*, 335–343. [CrossRef]
15. Shroff, R.C.; Shanahan, C.M. The vascular biology of calcification. *Semin. Dial.* **2007**, *20*, 103–109. [CrossRef]
16. Schlieper, G.; Hess, K.; Floege, J.; Marx, N. The vulnerable patient with chronic kidney disease. *Nephrol. Dial. Transplant.* **2016**, *31*, 382–390. [CrossRef]
17. Ketteler, M.; Schlieper, G.; Floege, J. Calcification and cardiovascular health: New insights into an old phenomenon. *Hypertension* **2006**, *47*, 1027–1034. [CrossRef]
18. Shroff, R.; Long, D.A.; Shanahan, C. Mechanistic insights into vascular calcification in CKD. *J. Am. Soc. Nephrol.* **2013**, *24*, 179–189. [CrossRef]
19. Nitta, K.; Ogawa, T.; Hanafusa, N.; Tsuchiya, K. Recent Advances in the Management of Vascular Calcification in Patients with End-Stage Renal Disease. *Contrib. Nephrol.* **2019**, *198*, 62–72. [CrossRef]
20. Ferrer, M.D.; Ketteler, M.; Tur, F.; Tur, E.; Isern, B.; Salcedo, C.; Joubert, P.H.; Behets, G.J.; Neven, E.; D'Haese, P.C.; et al. Characterization of SNF472 pharmacokinetics and efficacy in uremic and non-uremic rats models of cardiovascular calcification. *PLoS ONE* **2018**, *13*, e0197061. [CrossRef]
21. Raggi, P.; Bellasi, A.; Bushinsky, D.; Bover, J.; Rodriguez, M.; Ketteler, M.; Sinha, S.; Salcedo, C.; Gillotti, K.; Padgett, C.; et al. Slowing Progression of Cardiovascular Calcification with SNF472 in Patients on Hemodialysis: Results of a Randomized, Phase 2b Study. *Circulation* **2019**. [CrossRef] [PubMed]
22. Hewitson, T.D.; Holt, S.G.; Smith, E.R. Animal models to study links between cardiovascular disease and renal failure and their relevance to human pathology. *Front. Immunol.* **2015**, *6*. [CrossRef] [PubMed]
23. Becker, G.J.; Hewitson, T.D. Animal models of chronic kidney disease: Useful but not perfect. *Nephrol. Dial. Transplant.* **2013**, *28*, 2432–2438. [CrossRef] [PubMed]
24. Shobeiri, N.; Adams, M.A.; Holden, R.M. Vascular calcification in animal models of CKD: A review. *Am. J. Nephrol.* **2010**, *31*, 471–481. [CrossRef]
25. Yokozawa, T.; Oura, H.; Okada, T. Metabolic effects of dietary purine in rats. *J. Nutr. Sci. Vitaminol.* **1982**, *28*, 519–526. [CrossRef]
26. Lau, W.L.; Leaf, E.M.; Hu, M.C.; Takeno, M.M.; Kuro-o, M.; Moe, O.W.; Giachelli, C.M. Vitamin D receptor agonists increase klotho and osteopontin while decreasing aortic calcification in mice with chronic kidney disease fed a high phosphate diet. *Kidney Int.* **2012**, *82*, 1261–1270. [CrossRef]
27. Rabe, M.; Schaefer, F. Non-Transgenic Mouse Models of Kidney Disease. *Nephron* **2016**, *133*, 53–61. [CrossRef]
28. El-Abbadi, M.M.; Pai, A.S.; Leaf, E.M.; Yang, H.Y.; Bartley, B.A.; Quan, K.K.; Ingalls, C.M.; Liao, H.W.; Giachelli, C.M. Phosphate feeding induces arterial medial calcification in uremic mice: Role of serum phosphorus, fibroblast growth factor-23, and osteopontin. *Kidney Int.* **2009**, *75*, 1297–1307. [CrossRef]
29. Makaryus, A.N.; Sison, C.; Kohansieh, M.; Makaryus, J.N. Implications of gender difference in coronary calcification as assessed by ct coronary angiography. *Clin. Med. Insights Cardiol.* **2014**, *2014*, 51–55. [CrossRef]
30. Ishola, D.A., Jr.; van der Giezen, D.M.; Hahnel, B.; Goldschmeding, R.; Kriz, W.; Koomans, H.A.; Joles, J.A. In mice, proteinuria and renal inflammatory responses to albumin overload are strain-dependent. *Nephrol. Dial. Transplant.* **2006**, *21*, 591–597. [CrossRef]
31. Cozzolino, M.; Staniforth, M.E.; Liapis, H.; Finch, J.; Burke, S.K.; Dusso, A.S.; Slatopolsky, E. Sevelamer hydrochloride attenuates kidney and cardiovascular calcifications in long-term experimental uremia. *Kidney Int.* **2003**, *64*, 1653–1661. [CrossRef] [PubMed]
32. De Schutter, T.M.; Behets, G.J.; Geryl, H.; Peter, M.E.; Steppan, S.; Gundlach, K.; Passlick-Deetjen, J.; D'Haese, P.C.; Neven, E. Effect of a magnesium-based phosphate binder on medial calcification in a rat model of uremia. *Kidney Int.* **2013**, *83*, 1109–1117. [CrossRef] [PubMed]

33. Neven, E.; De Schutter, T.M.; Dams, G.; Gundlach, K.; Steppan, S.; Buchel, J.; Passlick-Deetjen, J.; D'Haese, P.C.; Behets, G.J. A magnesium based phosphate binder reduces vascular calcification without affecting bone in chronic renal failure rats. *PLoS ONE* **2014**, *9*, e107067. [CrossRef] [PubMed]
34. Palmer, S.C.; Gardner, S.; Tonelli, M.; Mavridis, D.; Johnson, D.W.; Craig, J.C.; French, R.; Ruospo, M.; Strippoli, G.F. Phosphate-Binding Agents in Adults With CKD: A Network Meta-analysis of Randomized Trials. *Am. J. Kidney Dis.* **2016**, *68*, 691–702. [CrossRef] [PubMed]
35. Jamal, S.A.; Vandermeer, B.; Raggi, P.; Mendelssohn, D.C.; Chatterley, T.; Dorgan, M.; Lok, C.E.; Fitchett, D.; Tsuyuki, R.T. Effect of calcium-based versus non-calcium-based phosphate binders on mortality in patients with chronic kidney disease: An updated systematic review and meta-analysis. *Lancet* **2013**, *382*, 1268–1277. [CrossRef]
36. Ruospo, M.; Palmer, S.C.; Natale, P.; Craig, J.C.; Vecchio, M.; Elder, G.J.; Strippoli, G.F. Phosphate binders for preventing and treating chronic kidney disease-mineral and bone disorder (CKD-MBD). *Cochrane Database Syst. Rev.* **2018**, *8*, CD006023. [CrossRef]
37. Block, G.A.; Bushinsky, D.A.; Cheng, S.; Cunningham, J.; Dehmel, B.; Drueke, T.B.; Ketteler, M.; Kewalramani, R.; Martin, K.J.; Moe, S.M.; et al. Effect of Etelcalcetide vs Cinacalcet on Serum Parathyroid Hormone in Patients Receiving Hemodialysis With Secondary Hyperparathyroidism: A Randomized Clinical Trial. *JAMA* **2017**, *317*, 156–164. [CrossRef]
38. Wu, M.; Tang, R.N.; Liu, H.; Pan, M.M.; Liu, B.C. Cinacalcet ameliorates aortic calcification in uremic rats via suppression of endothelial-to-mesenchymal transition. *Acta Pharmacol. Sin.* **2016**, *37*, 1423–1431. [CrossRef]
39. Friedl, C.; Zitt, E. Role of etelcalcetide in the management of secondary hyperparathyroidism in hemodialysis patients: A review on current data and place in therapy. *Drug Des. Dev. Ther.* **2018**, *12*, 1589–1598. [CrossRef]
40. Investigators, E.T.; Chertow, G.M.; Block, G.A.; Correa-Rotter, R.; Drueke, T.B.; Floege, J.; Goodman, W.G.; Herzog, C.A.; Kubo, Y.; London, G.M.; et al. Effect of cinacalcet on cardiovascular disease in patients undergoing dialysis. *N. Engl. J. Med.* **2012**, *367*, 2482–2494. [CrossRef]
41. Raggi, P.; Chertow, G.M.; Torres, P.U.; Csiky, B.; Naso, A.; Nossuli, K.; Moustafa, M.; Goodman, W.G.; Lopez, N.; Downey, G.; et al. The ADVANCE study: A randomized study to evaluate the effects of cinacalcet plus low-dose vitamin D on vascular calcification in patients on hemodialysis. *Nephrol. Dial. Transplant.* **2011**, *26*, 1327–1339. [CrossRef] [PubMed]
42. Palmer, S.C.; Nistor, I.; Craig, J.C.; Pellegrini, F.; Messa, P.; Tonelli, M.; Covic, A.; Strippoli, G.F. Cinacalcet in patients with chronic kidney disease: A cumulative meta-analysis of randomized controlled trials. *PLoS Med.* **2013**, *10*, e1001436. [CrossRef] [PubMed]
43. Evans, M.; Methven, S.; Gasparini, A.; Barany, P.; Birnie, K.; MacNeill, S.; May, M.T.; Caskey, F.J.; Carrero, J.J. Cinacalcet use and the risk of cardiovascular events, fractures and mortality in chronic kidney disease patients with secondary hyperparathyroidism. *Sci. Rep.* **2018**, *8*, 2103. [CrossRef] [PubMed]
44. Zhang, Q.; Li, M.; You, L.; Li, H.; Ni, L.; Gu, Y.; Hao, C.; Chen, J. Effects and safety of calcimimetics in end stage renal disease patients with secondary hyperparathyroidism: A meta-analysis. *PLoS ONE* **2012**, *7*, e48070. [CrossRef] [PubMed]
45. Toussaint, N.D.; Elder, G.J.; Kerr, P.G. Bisphosphonates in chronic kidney disease: balancing potential benefits and adverse effects on bone and soft tissue. *Clin. J. Am. Soc. Nephrol.* **2009**, *4*, 221–233. [CrossRef] [PubMed]
46. Perazella, M.A.; Markowitz, G.S. Bisphosphonate nephrotoxicity. *Kidney Int.* **2008**, *74*, 1385–1393. [CrossRef]
47. Bergner, R.; Diel, I.J.; Henrich, D.; Hoffmann, M.; Uppenkamp, M. Differences in nephrotoxicity of intravenous bisphosphonates for the treatment of malignancy-related bone disease. *Onkologie* **2006**, *29*, 534–540. [CrossRef]
48. Markowitz, G.S.; Appel, G.B.; Fine, P.L.; Fenves, A.Z.; Loon, N.R.; Jagannath, S.; Kuhn, J.A.; Dratch, A.D.; D'Agati, V.D. Collapsing focal segmental glomerulosclerosis following treatment with high-dose pamidronate. *J. Am. Soc. Nephrol.* **2001**, *12*, 1164–1172.
49. Verhulst, A.; Sun, S.; McKenna, C.E.; D'Haese, P.C. Endocytotic uptake of zoledronic acid by tubular cells may explain its renal effects in cancer patients receiving high doses of the compound. *PLoS ONE* **2015**, *10*, e0121861. [CrossRef]
50. Otto, S.; Pautke, C.; Hafner, S.; Hesse, R.; Reichardt, L.F.; Mast, G.; Ehrenfeld, M.; Cornelius, C.P. Pathologic fractures in bisphosphonate-related osteonecrosis of the jaw-review of the literature and review of our own cases. *Craniomaxillofac. Trauma Reconstr.* **2013**, *6*, 147–154. [CrossRef]

51. Miller, P.D.; Roux, C.; Boonen, S.; Barton, I.P.; Dunlap, L.E.; Burgio, D.E. Safety and efficacy of risedronate in patients with age-related reduced renal function as estimated by the Cockcroft and Gault method: A pooled analysis of nine clinical trials. *J. Bone miner. Res.* **2005**, *20*, 2105–2115. [CrossRef] [PubMed]
52. Cunningham, J. Bisphosphonates in the renal patient. *Nephrol. Dial. Transplant.* **2007**, *22*, 1505–1507. [CrossRef] [PubMed]
53. Bostrom, K.I.; Rajamannan, N.M.; Towler, D.A. The regulation of valvular and vascular sclerosis by osteogenic morphogens. *Circ. Res.* **2011**, *109*, 564–577. [CrossRef] [PubMed]
54. Tamura, K.; Suzuki, Y.; Matsushita, M.; Fujii, H.; Miyaura, C.; Aizawa, S.; Kogo, H. Prevention of aortic calcification by etidronate in the renal failure rat model. *Eur. J. Pharmacol.* **2007**, *558*, 159–166. [CrossRef] [PubMed]
55. Caffarelli, C.; Montagnani, A.; Nuti, R.; Gonnelli, S. Bisphosphonates, atherosclerosis and vascular calcification: Update and systematic review of clinical studies. *Clin. Interv. Aging* **2017**, *12*, 1819–1828. [CrossRef]
56. Toussaint, N.D.; Lau, K.K.; Strauss, B.J.; Polkinghorne, K.R.; Kerr, P.G. Effect of alendronate on vascular calcification in CKD stages 3 and 4: A pilot randomized controlled trial. *Am. J. Kidney Dis.* **2010**, *56*, 57–68. [CrossRef]
57. Hartle, J.E.; Tang, X.; Kirchner, H.L.; Bucaloiu, I.D.; Sartorius, J.A.; Pogrebnaya, Z.V.; Akers, G.A.; Carnero, G.E.; Perkins, R.M. Bisphosphonate therapy, death, and cardiovascular events among female patients with CKD: A retrospective cohort study. *Am. J. Kidney Dis.* **2012**, *59*, 636–644. [CrossRef]
58. Kranenburg, G.; Bartstra, J.W.; Weijmans, M.; de Jong, P.A.; Mali, W.P.; Verhaar, H.J.; Visseren, F.L.J.; Spiering, W. Bisphosphonates for cardiovascular risk reduction: A systematic review and meta-analysis. *Atherosclerosis* **2016**, *252*, 106–115. [CrossRef]
59. McCloskey, E.V.; Johansson, H.; Oden, A.; Austin, M.; Siris, E.; Wang, A.; Lewiecki, E.M.; Lorenc, R.; Libanati, C.; Kanis, J.A. Denosumab reduces the risk of osteoporotic fractures in postmenopausal women, particularly in those with moderate to high fracture risk as assessed with FRAX. *J. Bone miner. Res.* **2012**, *27*, 1480–1486. [CrossRef]
60. Feng, X.; Teitelbaum, S.L. Osteoclasts: New Insights. *Bone Res.* **2013**, *1*, 11–26. [CrossRef]
61. Panizo, S.; Cardus, A.; Encinas, M.; Parisi, E.; Valcheva, P.; Lopez-Ongil, S.; Coll, B.; Fernandez, E.; Valdivielso, J.M. RANKL increases vascular smooth muscle cell calcification through a RANK-BMP4-dependent pathway. *Circ. Res.* **2009**, *104*, 1041–1048. [CrossRef] [PubMed]
62. Helas, S.; Goettsch, C.; Schoppet, M.; Zeitz, U.; Hempel, U.; Morawietz, H.; Kostenuik, P.J.; Erben, R.G.; Hofbauer, L.C. Inhibition of receptor activator of NF-kappaB ligand by denosumab attenuates vascular calcium deposition in mice. *Am. J. Pathol.* **2009**, *175*, 473–478. [CrossRef] [PubMed]
63. Iseri, K.; Watanabe, M.; Yoshikawa, H.; Mitsui, H.; Endo, T.; Yamamoto, Y.; Iyoda, M.; Ryu, K.; Inaba, T.; Shibata, T.; et al. Effects of Denosumab and Alendronate on Bone Health and Vascular Function in Hemodialysis Patients: A Randomized, Controlled Trial. *J. Bone miner. Res.* **2019**, *34*, 1014–1024. [CrossRef] [PubMed]
64. Hjortnaes, J.; Bouten, C.V.; Van Herwerden, L.A.; Grundeman, P.F.; Kluin, J. Translating autologous heart valve tissue engineering from bench to bed. *Tissue Eng. Part B Rev.* **2009**, *15*, 307–317. [CrossRef]
65. Rajamannan, N.M.; Evans, F.J.; Aikawa, E.; Grande-Allen, K.J.; Demer, L.L.; Heistad, D.D.; Simmons, C.A.; Masters, K.S.; Mathieu, P.; O'Brien, K.D.; et al. Calcific aortic valve disease: Not simply a degenerative process: A review and agenda for research from the National Heart and Lung and Blood Institute Aortic Stenosis Working Group. Executive summary: Calcific aortic valve disease-2011 update. *Circulation* **2011**, *124*, 1783–1791. [CrossRef]
66. An, W.S.; Lee, S.M.; Son, Y.K.; Kim, S.E. Combination of omega-3 fatty acid and menaquinone-7 prevents progression of aortic calcification in adenine and low protein diet induced rat model. *Nephrol. Dial. Transplant.* **2017**, *32*, iii253–iii254. [CrossRef]
67. Diaz-Tocados, J.M.; Peralta-Ramirez, A.; Rodriguez-Ortiz, M.E.; Raya, A.I.; Lopez, I.; Pineda, C.; Herencia, C.; Montes de Oca, A.; Vergara, N.; Steppan, S.; et al. Dietary magnesium supplementation prevents and reverses vascular and soft tissue calcifications in uremic rats. *Kidney Int.* **2017**, *92*, 1084–1099. [CrossRef]
68. Kaesler, N.; Goettsch, C.; Weis, D.; Schurgers, L.; Hellmann, B.; Floege, J.; Kramann, R. Magnesium but not nicotinamide prevents vascular calcification in experimental uraemia. *Nephrol. Dial. Transplant.* **2019**. [CrossRef]

69. O'Young, J.; Liao, Y.; Xiao, Y.; Jalkanen, J.; Lajoie, G.; Karttunen, M.; Goldberg, H.A.; Hunter, G.K. Matrix Gla protein inhibits ectopic calcification by a direct interaction with hydroxyapatite crystals. *J. Am. Chem. Soc.* **2011**, *133*, 18406–18412. [CrossRef]
70. Tesfamariam, B. Involvement of Vitamin K-Dependent Proteins in Vascular Calcification. *J. Cardiovasc. Pharmacol. Ther.* **2019**, *24*, 323–333. [CrossRef]
71. Schurgers, L.J.; Teunissen, K.J.; Knapen, M.H.; Kwaijtaal, M.; van Diest, R.; Appels, A.; Reutelingsperger, C.P.; Cleutjens, J.P.; Vermeer, C. Novel conformation-specific antibodies against matrix gamma-carboxyglutamic acid (Gla) protein: Undercarboxylated matrix Gla protein as marker for vascular calcification. *Arterioscler. Thromb. Vasc. Biol.* **2005**, *25*, 1629–1633. [CrossRef]
72. Halder, M.; Petsophonsakul, P.; Akbulut, A.C.; Pavlic, A.; Bohan, F.; Anderson, E.; Maresz, K.; Kramann, R.; Schurgers, L. Vitamin K: Double Bonds beyond Coagulation Insights into Differences between Vitamin K1 and K2 in Health and Disease. *Int. J. Mol. Sci.* **2019**, *20*, 896. [CrossRef] [PubMed]
73. Cranenburg, E.C.; Schurgers, L.J.; Uiterwijk, H.H.; Beulens, J.W.; Dalmeijer, G.W.; Westerhuis, R.; Magdeleyns, E.J.; Herfs, M.; Vermeer, C.; Laverman, G.D.; et al. Vitamin K intake and status are low in hemodialysis patients. *Kidney Int.* **2012**, *82*, 605–610. [CrossRef] [PubMed]
74. Lee, S.M.; An, W.S. Supplementary nutrients for prevention of vascular calcification in patients with chronic kidney disease. *Korean J. Intern. Med.* **2019**, *34*, 459–469. [CrossRef] [PubMed]
75. Schlieper, G.; Westenfeld, R.; Kruger, T.; Cranenburg, E.C.; Magdeleyns, E.J.; Brandenburg, V.M.; Djuric, Z.; Damjanovic, T.; Ketteler, M.; Vermeer, C.; et al. Circulating nonphosphorylated carboxylated matrix gla protein predicts survival in ESRD. *J. Am. Soc. Nephrol.* **2011**, *22*, 387–395. [CrossRef] [PubMed]
76. Keyzer, C.A.; de Borst, M.H.; van den Berg, E.; Jahnen-Dechent, W.; Arampatzis, S.; Farese, S.; Bergmann, I.P.; Floege, J.; Navis, G.; Bakker, S.J.; et al. Calcification Propensity and Survival among Renal Transplant Recipients. *J. Am. Soc. Nephrol.* **2016**, *27*, 239–248. [CrossRef] [PubMed]
77. Takagi, K.; Masuda, K.; Yamazaki, M.; Kiyohara, C.; Itoh, S.; Wasaki, M.; Inoue, H. Metal ion and vitamin adsorption profiles of phosphate binder ion-exchange resins. *Clin. Nephrol.* **2010**, *73*, 30–35. [CrossRef]
78. Neradova, A.; Schumacher, S.P.; Hubeek, I.; Lux, P.; Schurgers, L.J.; Vervloet, M.G. Phosphate binders affect vitamin K concentration by undesired binding, an in vitro study. *BMC Nephrol.* **2017**, *18*, 149. [CrossRef]
79. Jansz, T.T.; Neradova, A.; van Ballegooijen, A.J.; Verhaar, M.C.; Vervloet, M.G.; Schurgers, L.J.; van Jaarsveld, B.C. The role of kidney transplantation and phosphate binder use in vitamin K status. *PLoS ONE* **2018**, *13*, e0203157. [CrossRef]
80. Aoun, M.; Makki, M.; Azar, H.; Matta, H.; Chelala, D.N. High Dephosphorylated-Uncarboxylated MGP in Hemodialysis patients: Risk factors and response to vitamin K2, A pre-post intervention clinical trial. *BMC Nephrol.* **2017**, *18*, 191. [CrossRef] [PubMed]
81. Westenfeld, R.; Krueger, T.; Schlieper, G.; Cranenburg, E.C.; Magdeleyns, E.J.; Heidenreich, S.; Holzmann, S.; Vermeer, C.; Jahnen-Dechent, W.; Ketteler, M.; et al. Effect of vitamin K2 supplementation on functional vitamin K deficiency in hemodialysis patients: A randomized trial. *Am. J. Kidney Dis.* **2012**, *59*, 186–195. [CrossRef] [PubMed]
82. Caluwe, R.; Pyfferoen, L.; De Boeck, K.; De Vriese, A.S. The effects of vitamin K supplementation and vitamin K antagonists on progression of vascular calcification: Ongoing randomized controlled trials. *Clin. Kidney J.* **2016**, *9*, 273–279. [CrossRef] [PubMed]
83. Kurnatowska, I.; Grzelak, P.; Masajtis-Zagajewska, A.; Kaczmarska, M.; Stefanczyk, L.; Vermeer, C.; Maresz, K.; Nowicki, M. Effect of vitamin K2 on progression of atherosclerosis and vascular calcification in nondialyzed patients with chronic kidney disease stages 3–5. *Pol. Arch. Med. Wewn.* **2015**, *125*, 631–640. [CrossRef]
84. Zheng, Z.; Shi, H.; Jia, J.; Li, D.; Lin, S. Vitamin D supplementation and mortality risk in chronic kidney disease: A meta-analysis of 20 observational studies. *BMC Nephrol.* **2013**, *14*, 199. [CrossRef]
85. Chitalia, N.; Recio-Mayoral, A.; Kaski, J.C.; Banerjee, D. Vitamin D deficiency and endothelial dysfunction in non-dialysis chronic kidney disease patients. *Atherosclerosis* **2012**, *220*, 265–268. [CrossRef] [PubMed]
86. Levin, A.; Tang, M.; Perry, T.; Zalunardo, N.; Beaulieu, M.; Dubland, J.A.; Zerr, K.; Djurdjev, O. Randomized Controlled Trial for the Effect of Vitamin D Supplementation on Vascular Stiffness in CKD. *Clin. J. Am. Soc. Nephrol.* **2017**, *12*, 1447–1460. [CrossRef] [PubMed]
87. Kumar, V.; Yadav, A.K.; Lal, A.; Kumar, V.; Singhal, M.; Billot, L.; Gupta, K.L.; Banerjee, D.; Jha, V. A Randomized Trial of Vitamin D Supplementation on Vascular Function in CKD. *J. Am. Soc. Nephrol.* **2017**, *28*, 3100–3108. [CrossRef]

88. Samaan, F.; Carvalho, A.B.; Pillar, R.; Rocha, L.A.; Cassiolato, J.L.; Cuppari, L.; Canziani, M.E.F. The Effect of Long-Term Cholecalciferol Supplementation on Vascular Calcification in Chronic Kidney Disease Patients With Hypovitaminosis D. *J. Ren. Nutr.* **2019**, *29*, 407–415. [CrossRef]
89. Levin, A.; Le Barbier, M.; Er, L.; Andress, D.; Sigrist, M.K.; Djurdjev, O. Incident isolated 1,25(OH)(2)D(3) deficiency is more common than 25(OH)D deficiency in CKD. *J. Nephrol.* **2012**, *25*, 204–210. [CrossRef]
90. Louvet, L.; Buchel, J.; Steppan, S.; Passlick-Deetjen, J.; Massy, Z.A. Magnesium prevents phosphate-induced calcification in human aortic vascular smooth muscle cells. *Nephrol. Dial. Transplant.* **2013**, *28*, 869–878. [CrossRef]
91. Massy, Z.A.; Drueke, T.B. Magnesium and outcomes in patients with chronic kidney disease: Focus on vascular calcification, atherosclerosis and survival. *Clin. Kidney J.* **2012**, *5*, i52–i61. [CrossRef]
92. Briet, M.; Schiffrin, E.L. Vascular actions of aldosterone. *J. Vasc. Res.* **2013**, *50*, 89–99. [CrossRef] [PubMed]
93. Mizuiri, S.; Nishizawa, Y.; Yamashita, K.; Naito, T.; Ono, K.; Tanji, C.; Usui, K.; Doi, S.; Masaki, T.; Shigemoto, K. Hypomagnesemia is not an independent risk factor for mortality in Japanese maintenance hemodialysis patients. *Int. Urol. Nephrol.* **2019**, *51*, 1043–1052. [CrossRef]
94. Wu, L.; Cai, K.; Luo, Q.; Wang, L.; Hong, Y. Baseline Serum Magnesium Level and Its Variability in Maintenance Hemodialysis Patients: Associations with Mortality. *Kidney Blood Press. Res.* **2019**, *44*, 222–232. [CrossRef] [PubMed]
95. Sakaguchi, Y.; Fujii, N.; Shoji, T.; Hayashi, T.; Rakugi, H.; Iseki, K.; Tsubakihara, Y.; Isaka, Y.; Committee of Renal Data Registry of the Japanese Society for Dialysis Therapy. Magnesium modifies the cardiovascular mortality risk associated with hyperphosphatemia in patients undergoing hemodialysis: A cohort study. *PLoS ONE* **2014**, *9*, e116273. [CrossRef] [PubMed]
96. Cai, K.; Luo, Q.; Dai, Z.; Zhu, B.; Fei, J.; Xue, C.; Wu, D. Hypomagnesemia Is Associated with Increased Mortality among Peritoneal Dialysis Patients. *PLoS ONE* **2016**, *11*, e0152488. [CrossRef]
97. Bundy, J.D.; Cai, X.; Scialla, J.J.; Dobre, M.A.; Chen, J.; Hsu, C.Y.; Leonard, M.B.; Go, A.S.; Rao, P.S.; Lash, J.P.; et al. Serum Calcification Propensity and Coronary Artery Calcification Among Patients With CKD: The CRIC (Chronic Renal Insufficiency Cohort) Study. *Am. J. Kidney Dis.* **2019**, *73*, 806–814. [CrossRef]
98. Mortazavi, M.; Moeinzadeh, F.; Saadatnia, M.; Shahidi, S.; McGee, J.C.; minagar, A. Effect of magnesium supplementation on carotid intima-media thickness and flow-mediated dilatation among hemodialysis patients: A double-blind, randomized, placebo-controlled trial. *Eur. Neurol.* **2013**, *69*, 309–316. [CrossRef]
99. Turgut, F.; Kanbay, M.; Metin, M.R.; Uz, E.; Akcay, A.; Covic, A. Magnesium supplementation helps to improve carotid intima media thickness in patients on hemodialysis. *Int. Urol. Nephrol.* **2008**, *40*, 1075–1082. [CrossRef]
100. Bressendorff, I.; Hansen, D.; Schou, M.; Kragelund, C.; Brandi, L. The effect of magnesium supplementation on vascular calcification in chronic kidney disease-a randomised clinical trial (MAGiCAL-CKD): Essential study design and rationale. *BMJ Open* **2017**, *7*, e016795. [CrossRef]
101. Salcedo, C.; Joubert, P.H.; Ferrer, M.D.; Canals, A.Z.; Maduell, F.; Torregrosa, V.; Campistol, J.M.; Ojeda, R.; Perello, J. A phase 1b randomized, placebo-controlled clinical trial with SNF472 in haemodialysis patients. *Br. J. Clin. Pharmacol.* **2019**, *85*, 796–806. [CrossRef]
102. Perello, J.; Joubert, P.H.; Ferrer, M.D.; Canals, A.Z.; Sinha, S.; Salcedo, C. First-time-in-human randomized clinical trial in healthy volunteers and haemodialysis patients with SNF472, a novel inhibitor of vascular calcification. *Br. J. Clin. Pharmacol.* **2018**, *84*, 2867–2876. [CrossRef] [PubMed]
103. Zhou, Y.X.; Zhang, H.; Peng, C. Puerarin: A review of pharmacological effects. *Phytother. Res.* **2014**, *28*, 961–975. [CrossRef] [PubMed]
104. Liu, H.; Zhang, X.; Zhong, X.; Li, Z.; Cai, S.; Yang, P.; Ou, C.; Chen, M. Puerarin inhibits vascular calcification of uremic rats. *Eur. J. Pharmacol.* **2019**, *855*, 235–243. [CrossRef] [PubMed]
105. Millar, J.S. Novel benefits of peroxisome proliferator-activated receptors on cardiovascular risk. *Curr. Opin. Lipidol.* **2013**, *24*, 233–238. [CrossRef] [PubMed]
106. Ikejima, H.; Imanishi, T.; Tsujioka, H.; Kuroi, A.; Kobayashi, K.; Shiomi, M.; Muragaki, Y.; Mochizuki, S.; Goto, M.; Yoshida, K.; et al. Effects of telmisartan, a unique angiotensin receptor blocker with selective peroxisome proliferator-activated receptor-gamma-modulating activity, on nitric oxide bioavailability and atherosclerotic change. *J. Hypertens.* **2008**, *26*, 964–972. [CrossRef]

107. Bostom, A.; Pasch, A.; Madsen, T.; Roberts, M.B.; Franceschini, N.; Steubl, D.; Garimella, P.S.; Ix, J.H.; Tuttle, K.R.; Ivanova, A.; et al. Serum Calcification Propensity and Fetuin-A: Biomarkers of Cardiovascular Disease in Kidney Transplant Recipients. *Am. J. Nephrol.* **2018**, *48*, 21–31. [CrossRef]
108. Zhao, G.; Xu, M.J.; Zhao, M.M.; Dai, X.Y.; Kong, W.; Wilson, G.M.; Guan, Y.; Wang, C.Y.; Wang, X. Activation of nuclear factor-kappa B accelerates vascular calcification by inhibiting ankylosis protein homolog expression. *Kidney Int.* **2012**, *82*, 34–44. [CrossRef]
109. Yoshida, T.; Yamashita, M.; Horimai, C.; Hayashi, M. Smooth Muscle-Selective Nuclear Factor-kappaB Inhibition Reduces Phosphate-Induced Arterial Medial Calcification in Mice With Chronic Kidney Disease. *J. Am. Heart Assoc.* **2017**, *6*. [CrossRef]
110. Yamada, S.; Taniguchi, M.; Tokumoto, M.; Toyonaga, J.; Fujisaki, K.; Suehiro, T.; Noguchi, H.; Iida, M.; Tsuruya, K.; Kitazono, T. The antioxidant tempol ameliorates arterial medial calcification in uremic rats: Important role of oxidative stress in the pathogenesis of vascular calcification in chronic kidney disease. *J. Bone miner. Res.* **2012**, *27*, 474–485. [CrossRef]
111. Tatsumoto, N.; Yamada, S.; Tokumoto, M.; Eriguchi, M.; Noguchi, H.; Torisu, K.; Tsuruya, K.; Kitazono, T. Spironolactone ameliorates arterial medial calcification in uremic rats: The role of mineralocorticoid receptor signaling in vascular calcification. *Am. J. Physiol. Ren. Physiol.* **2015**, *309*, F967–F979. [CrossRef]
112. Scialla, J.J.; Kao, W.H.; Crainiceanu, C.; Sozio, S.M.; Oberai, P.C.; Shafi, T.; Coresh, J.; Powe, N.R.; Plantinga, L.C.; Jaar, B.G.; et al. Biomarkers of vascular calcification and mortality in patients with ESRD. *Clin. J. Am. Soc. Nephrol.* **2014**, *9*, 745–755. [CrossRef] [PubMed]
113. Cai, H.; Lu, R.; Zhang, M.; Pang, H.; Zhu, M.; Zhang, W.; Ni, Z.; Qian, J.; Yan, Y. Serum Soluble Klotho Level Is Associated with Abdominal Aortic Calcification in Patients on Maintenance Hemodialysis. *Blood Purif.* **2015**, *40*, 120–126. [CrossRef] [PubMed]
114. Pasch, A.; Farese, S.; Graber, S.; Wald, J.; Richtering, W.; Floege, J.; Jahnen-Dechent, W. Nanoparticle-based test measures overall propensity for calcification in serum. *J. Am. Soc. Nephrol.* **2012**, *23*, 1744–1752. [CrossRef] [PubMed]
115. Heiss, A.; DuChesne, A.; Denecke, B.; Grotzinger, J.; Yamamoto, K.; Renne, T.; Jahnen-Dechent, W. Structural basis of calcification inhibition by alpha 2-HS glycoprotein/fetuin-A. Formation of colloidal calciprotein particles. *J. Biol. Chem.* **2003**, *278*, 13333–13341. [CrossRef] [PubMed]
116. Smith, E.R.; Ford, M.L.; Tomlinson, L.A.; Bodenham, E.; McMahon, L.P.; Farese, S.; Rajkumar, C.; Holt, S.G.; Pasch, A. Serum calcification propensity predicts all-cause mortality in predialysis CKD. *J. Am. Soc. Nephrol.* **2014**, *25*, 339–348. [CrossRef]
117. Lorenz, G.; Steubl, D.; Kemmner, S.; Pasch, A.; Koch-Sembdner, W.; Pham, D.; Haller, B.; Bachmann, Q.; Mayer, C.C.; Wassertheurer, S.; et al. Worsening calcification propensity precedes all-cause and cardiovascular mortality in haemodialyzed patients. *Sci. Rep.* **2017**, *7*, 13368. [CrossRef]
118. Dahle, D.O.; Asberg, A.; Hartmann, A.; Holdaas, H.; Bachtler, M.; Jenssen, T.G.; Dionisi, M.; Pasch, A. Serum Calcification Propensity Is a Strong and Independent Determinant of Cardiac and All-Cause Mortality in Kidney Transplant Recipients. *Am. J. Transplant.* **2016**, *16*, 204–212. [CrossRef]
119. Brandenburg, V.M.; Reinartz, S.; Kaesler, N.; Kruger, T.; Dirrichs, T.; Kramann, R.; Peeters, F.; Floege, J.; Keszei, A.; Marx, N.; et al. Slower Progress of Aortic Valve Calcification With Vitamin K Supplementation: Results From a Prospective Interventional Proof-of-Concept Study. *Circulation* **2017**, *135*, 2081–2083. [CrossRef]

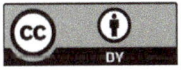

© 2020 by the authors. Licensee MDPI, Basel, Switzerland. This article is an open access article distributed under the terms and conditions of the Creative Commons Attribution (CC BY) license (http://creativecommons.org/licenses/by/4.0/).

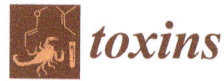

Review

Should We Consider the Cardiovascular System While Evaluating CKD-MBD?

Merita Rroji [1],*, Andreja Figurek [2] and Goce Spasovski [3]

1. University Department of Nephrology, Faculty of Medicine, University of Medicine Tirana, Tirana 1001, Albania
2. Institute of Anatomy, University of Zurich, Zurich 8057, Switzerland; andrejafigurek@yahoo.com
3. University Department of Nephrology, Medical Faculty, University of Skopje, Skopje 1000, North Macedonia; spasovski.goce@gmail.com
* Correspondence: meritarroji@yahoo.com

Received: 6 January 2020; Accepted: 20 February 2020; Published: 25 February 2020

Abstract: Cardiovascular (CV) disease is highly prevalent in the population with chronic kidney disease (CKD), where the risk of CV death in early stages far exceeds the risk of progression to dialysis. The presence of chronic kidney disease-mineral and bone disorder (CKD-MBD) has shown a strong correlation with CV events and mortality. As a non-atheromatous process, it could be partially explained why standard CV disease-modifying drugs do not provide such an impact on CV mortality in CKD as observed in the general population. We summarize the potential association of CV comorbidities with the older (parathyroid hormone, phosphate) and newer (FGF23, Klotho, sclerostin) CKD-MBD biomarkers.

Keywords: chronic kidney disease; uremic cardiopathy; left ventricular hypertrophy; phosphate; PTH; FGF23; klotho; sclerostin

Key Contribution: Although the management of CKD patients was significantly improved, CV mortality continues to be at a higher rate. Here the impact of CKD-MBD has already extended beyond the role in the skeleton, so we tried to go from the candidate mineral disorder to cardiovascular abnormalities. Focusing on such toxins and/or their relevant mediators at early CKD stages might help to interfere on time with the vicious cycle of the cardio–renal connection and improve the outcome of the patients.

1. Introduction

Over the past 25 years, chronic kidney disease (CKD) has become an enormous public health issue with a high risk of morbidity and fatal outcome. Cardiovascular disease (CVD) is the most frequent (39%) cause of mortality in this population of end-stage renal disease (ESRD) [1], whereas the risk of CV mortality in early-stage CKD far exceeds the risk of progressing to dialysis [2]. Cardiovascular involvement is evident, initiates in the early stages of CKD (according to the K/DOQI CKD classification), being present in about 80% of prevalent hemodialysis patients [1]. CKD being recognized as an independent risk factor for CVD is a topic of debate on whether it should be recognized as a coronary disease risk equivalent, independent from the risk of diabetes and hypertension [1].

The complicated relationship between CVD and kidney disease reflects the interaction of traditional, non-traditional cardiovascular risk factors modified by CKD, and new CKD linked risk factors like uremic toxins, CKD-mineral and bone disorder (MBD), anemia, hypervolemia, oxidative stress, inflammation, insulin resistance, etc. [3,4]. Uremic toxins with presumed cardiovascular toxicity including FGF23 and protein-bound uremic toxins (PBUTs) like indoxyl sulfate, p-cresyl sulfate, start to accumulate in the body since early-stages of CKD, and elimination no longer relies on only renal replacement therapy. It is more than clear that CVD in CKD is an accelerated atherosclerosis.

Out of the five subtypes of cardiorenal syndromes classified so far, primary CKD leading to an impairment of cardiac function, can be established in the context of cardiorenal syndrome type 4 [5]. The interrelation between reduced renal function and altered cardiac remodeling in patients with CKD is termed uremic cardiomyopathy [6].

CKD-related cardiomyopathy has multifactorial pathophysiology. Here the effect of CKD-MBD has been already extended beyond the role in the skeleton. The pathogenesis of CKD-MBD has initially been described as a decrease in 1,25-dihydroxy vitamin D [1,25(OH)2 D3] levels leading to increased serum parathyroid hormone (PTH) level, following changes in calcium and phosphorus metabolism [7]. Vitamin D deficiency, together with secondary hyperparathyroidism (sHPTH) and hyperphosphatemia, was defined as the main factor influencing high cardiovascular risks in CKD patients [7]. The identification of new players such as FGF23, klotho [3], and sclerostin has changed what has been portrayed above because of their role not only in the sHPTH pathophysiology but also throughout their direct or indirect involvement in the uremic cardiovascular disease [7]. FGF23, klotho, Fetuin-A/Calciprotein particles, and sclerostin could be used among other old and relevant markers, as biomarkers for CV risk prediction in CKD [8].

We summarize here the potential association of those comorbidities with the older (parathyroid hormone, phosphate, Vit D deficiency) and newer (FGF23, Klotho, sclerostin) CKD-MBD biomarkers [2].

2. Role of Phosphate, Parathyroid Hormone and Vit D Deficiency in Uremic Cardiomyopathy

2.1. Pathophysiology of Uremic Cardiomyopathy in CKD Patients

Uremic cardiomyopathy in patients with CKD or ESRD is a result of the volume and pressure overload, and the uremic state itself, including left ventricular hypertrophy (LVH), the diffuse interstitial fibrosis, and microvascular disease [3,5,6]. Histopathological examination of postmortem cardiac tissue samples in hemodialysis patients showed increased cardiomyocyte diameter, reduced capillary length density, and increased interstitial volume [9].

2.1.1. Left Ventricular Cardiomyopathy

LV hypertrophy is the most frequent cardiac finding in dialysis patients, and it is almost universal [8]. The prevalence of LVH is estimated to be between 16% and 31% in individuals with GFR >30 mL/min; it rises to 60%–75% before renal replacement therapy initiation and increases up to 90% after the dialysis initiation [10]. It is related to chronic volume and pressure overload, neurohormonal activation, and uremic toxin accumulation [11]. The pathophysiological factors involved in LVH of CKD patients are (1) related to afterload, (2) related to preload, and (3) not related to afterload or preload [5,12–14]. The ones in the first group give a picture of an increase in systemic arterial resistance, elevated arterial blood pressure, and reduced large-vessel compliance [11–14] partially correlated to aortic 'calcification', which is specific in CKD patients. LV hypertrophy is a compensatory response that acts to maintain wall stress in the course of long-term loading conditions, where all these factors lead to myocardial cell thickening and concentric LV remodeling. Among the preload-related factors, the role of intravascular volume expansion (salt and fluid retention), secondary anemia, and the presence of arteriovenous fistulas which result in myocardial cell lengthening and eccentric or asymmetric LV remodeling need to be underlined. Both afterload and preload-related factors act with additive and/or synergistic effects. It is suggested that fluid overload and increased arterial stiffness play a role in LVH even before the start of dialysis therapy [15]. Arteriosclerosis, being a hallmark of arterial remodeling in ESRD, is characterized by diffuse calcification in combination with dilatation, and an increased wall thickness of the medial layer of the aorta and its main branches which drives increased arterial stiffness [11,16,17]. Here, LVH happens regardless of the effective control of hypertension. Blood pressure independent LVH also occurs in diabetics with known diabetic nephropathy [18].

Hypertrophied hearts have reduced coronary blood flow reserve and are at increased risk for myocardial ischemia [19]. The coexistence of left atrial enlargement is common, and atrial fibrillation occurs frequently. Eventually, continuing LV load can promote structural changes in the LV, apoptosis of cardiomyocytes, and triggers metabolic pathways able to increase the extracellular matrix production up to fibrosis [9,10,20,21].

2.1.2. Interstitial Fibrosis

Diffuse interstitial cardiac fibrosis is reported in uremic patients and progresses with advancing of CKD [11,13,20–22]. Recently, it was nicely reported that in early-stage CKD patients, noninvasive imaging biomarkers of myocardial fibrosis do not change if renal function remains stable [22]. Fibrosis alters the architecture of myocardium promoting the progression of cardiac disease (progressive impairment in contractility, systolic and diastolic dysfunction, dilated cardiomyopathy, congestive heart failure) towards heart failure (HF) and increase the risk for sustained atrial and ventricular arrhythmias [9]. This may explain why CKD patients are at increased risk of sudden cardiac death (SCD) [23]. Recent studies have pointed out that not only CKD-MBD well-known biomarkers like phosphate, vit D, and PTH [3,5,7] but also novel and early ones like FGF23 are involved in the regulation, growth, and differentiation of cardiac myocytes being players in the pathogenesis of LVH [3,5,11,12].

2.1.3. Microvascular Disease

The coronary microvascular function is not well studied in CKD. Based on one old report around 30% of dialysis patients with clinical angina have only moderate epicardial coronary artery disease (CAD) [24], possibly explained with endothelial dysfunction associated with microvascular disease [11,25]. The presence of structural and coronary functional changes contributes to myocardium-capillary mismatch which is not specific to uremia [9]. Under the condition of disbalance between high oxygen demand and a low oxygen supply microvascular coronary disease exposes cardiomyocytes to the risk of hypoxemia and beyond in possible ischemic myocardial injury at the microvascular level, which could be an explanation for persistently elevated serum troponin levels found in these patients [3,26].

Coronary artery calcification (CAC) as measured by computed tomography is noninvasive with excellent accuracy measurement of the burden of coronary atherosclerosis. CKD patients have higher CAC scores compared with age-matched controls without CKD, and those without baseline calcification present higher incidence rates of developing future de novo CAC [27]. Besides traditional factors, here, in particular, there are nontraditional risk factors such as hyperphosphatemia, calcium-phosphorus product, homocysteine, osteoprotegerin, and sclerostin which were independently related to the presence and high CAC scores [8,27,28].

2.2. Role of Phosphate in Uremic Cardiomyopathy

Phosphate toxicity is a well described phenomenon in CKD [29,30]. Less than 1% of total phosphate is found in the blood and its balance was regulated by the interplay of bone, the parathyroid glands, intestines, and kidneys. The kidney is the principal organ regulating phosphate homeostasis. Following the loss of glomerular filtration rate (GFR), tubular phosphate reabsorption is significantly decreased by dual effect of compensatory increased concentration of two important hormones, the parathyroid hormone (PTH), and fibroblast growth factor 23 (FGF23). In addition, FGF23 suppresses the activation of vitamin D and acts to decrease parathyroid hormone synthesis and secretion being the major trigger in the path of CKD-MBD. FGF23 needs its cofactor klotho to ensure phosphate clearance [31]. Since the expression of Klotho declines in the kidney in the earlier stage CKD, FGF23 rises due to the resistance to FGF23 signaling in the kidney [31,32]. Although renal α-Klotho levels were significantly reduced and serum FGF23 levels were significantly elevated they can maintain serum phosphate within the normal range in early and intermediate stages of CKD. However, as CKD progresses, these defense mechanisms are ineffective, so phosphate retention may occur, and hyperphosphatemia develops.

Elevated serum phosphate has revealed as a non-traditional risk factor for cardiovascular events in CKD and partially explains the increased mortality risk in CKD [29,31,32].

The role of phosphate in vascular calcification has been the focus of intense investigation in the past decades. In elevated phosphate conditions, the biology of the arterial tunica media is found greatly altered; there is vascular smooth muscle cell (VSMC) transition to bone phenotype, apoptosis inactivation of local anti-calcification factors, and elastin degradation [33,34].

The PiT-1 phosphate transporter seems to be a key mediator in phosphate-induced VSMC, activating bone formation-related gene expression, osteochondrogenic differentiation, and was recently shown to be relevant in cell proliferation and embryonic development, referring more functions for this protein than previously thought [33–35]. Vascular mineralization, especially affecting the coronary artery, is strongly related to mortality of CKD patients independently from the established atherogenic markers. The rate of coronary artery mineralization in CKD patients undergoing hemodialysis treatment was reported to be five times higher than in the non-dialysis CKD patients and is associated with features of valvular calcifications sharing the same changes [16,31,36]. Moreover, valvular heart disease is one of the most common complications observed in patients with CKD [37,38] and hyperphosphatemia directly affects progression of valvular calcification.

The progression of valvular calcification leads to obstruction of left ventricular outflow and inflow from the left atrium to the left ventricle associated with hemodynamic changes resulting in very difficult clinical conditions [39].

Endothelial dysfunction is another early and crucial step in the development of cardiovascular disease apart from vascular calcification. Fewer reports have shown that phosphate level not in the physiologic range directly affects endothelial function and vascular remodeling [40,41]. Elevated phosphate level impairs endothelial function, hence diminishing microvascular function, angiogenic ability, and promoting endothelial stiffness [42].

Endothelial stiffness reflects changes in the structural and functional properties of the endothelium. These include cytoskeleton restructuring, successive mechano-signaling activity, intensified endothelial turnover (apoptosis), and diminished NO bioavailability [42].

High serum phosphate levels in HD patients were found to be independently associated with an increased number of endothelial microparticles (EMPs) and circulating (detached) endothelial cells [43]. These circulating submicron-sized membranous vesicles released by endothelium have a major biological role in the vascular injury; EMPs have been shown to act as primary and secondary messengers of vascular inflammation, thrombosis, vasomotor response, angiogenesis, and endothelial survival.

Phosphate is the major contributor to the level and biological activity of Calciprotein particles (CPPs) which are a new biological marker of CKD-MBD. Reports have shown that phosphate alone is not able to induce VSMCs mineralization, describing a synergistic action of both Ca and P in accelerated mineralization in vitro [16]. Insoluble CaP crystals generate when the concentration of calcium and phosphate exceeds the solubility limit. They can grow over time and finally precipitate as hydroxyapatite. The hepatic plasma protein fetuin-A (a natural calcification inhibitor) stabilizes colloidal protein–mineral complexes in the form of CPPs and mediates their clearance from the circulation. Primary CPPs, further, undergo topological rearrangement to find a more stable structure introduced as secondary CPPs [44]. The formation of CPP can be considered as a defense mechanism that prevents blood vessels from being occluded with insoluble CaP precipitates. The CPP level increases in the early stages of CKD, just before the rise of FGF23 and there are clinical findings that raise the hypothesis that CPPs might induce FGF23 [44,45]. In CKD patients, secondary CPPs have lower levels of calcification inhibitors including fetuin-A, and Gla-rich protein, readily taken up by the VSMCs inducing vascular calcification. While phosphate seems to be the driving force of CPP formation, his partner calcium seems to be a promoter of the inflammation-associated tissue damage forming a circle where increased mineralization triggers inflammation and vice-versa [44]. Recent studies have figured out the physiological and pathological significance of CPPs, its contributions to bone and mineral metabolism, and its role in tissue and organ impairments especially in cardiovascular damage and inflammatory responses [16,46,47] (Figure 1). Based on these findings secondary CPPs could be a new biomarker for the pathological condition of CKD-MBD [47]. More studies are required to further clarify the role of CPPs as an essential mediator of CV damage and as a potential therapeutic target in CKD patients [47]. Recently, Ciceri et al. reported that ferric citrate prevents high Pi-induced calcium deposition by preventing apoptosis. Apoptosis has been proposed to be one of the mechanisms that initiate the calcification process by forming a nidus for the deposition of calcium and Pi crystals. Even in the status where VSMCs are already transformed with a procalcified stimulus being present, reverting apoptosis and inducing autophagy presumably contribute to stopping calcium deposition [48].

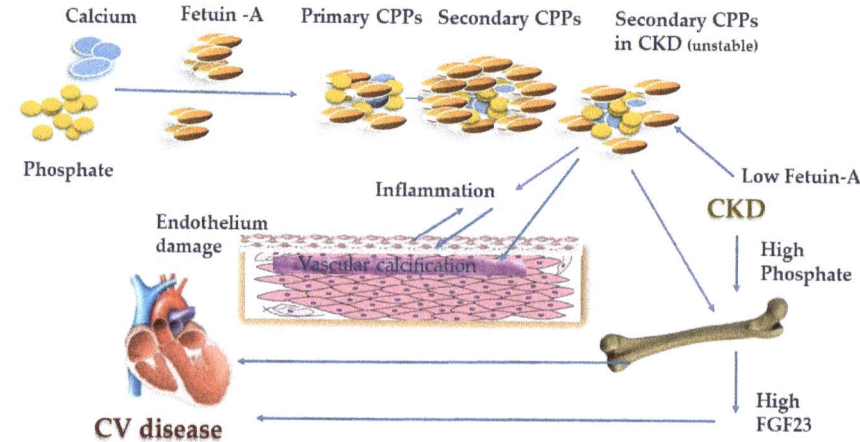

Figure 1. Role of Calciprotein particles in cardiovascular disease. In chronic kidney disease (CKD) patients, secondary Calciprotein particles (CPPs) have lower levels of calcification inhibitors including fetuin-A and were readily taken up by the vascular smooth muscle cells (VSMCs) inducing vascular calcification. Phosphate seems to be the driving force of CPP formation. Figure 1 shows the significance of CPPs, its contributions to bone and mineral metabolism, in an inflammatory response, and its role in the cardiovascular damage.

Animal experimental data suggest that higher dietary phosphate engages multiple mechanisms involved in hypertension, including overactivation of the sympathetic nervous system, increased vascular stiffness, impaired endothelium-dependent vasodilation, together with an increased renal sodium absorption or renal injury [49].

On the other hand, there is limited evidence of a hyperphosphatemia-induced direct effect on cardiomyocytes. Dietary phosphate intake and hyperphosphatemia were frequently associated with abnormalities of the postcoronary arterial vessels in the myocardium and to interstitial fibrosis where hyperphosphatemia accelerate cardiac fibrosis as well as microvascular disease in experimental uremia [9,50]. In vitro studies showed that high Pi alone may not be able to generate cardiac hypertrophy but can initiate fibrosis [51]. Fibrosis, arising from non-myocytes and enhanced by cardiac myocytes, can promote increased wall stiffness and diastolic dysfunction. Moreover, fibrosis interrupts electrical signals, causing the tissue to be more arrhythmogenic [9,23]. Cardio markers and parameters of myocardial function, including Cardiac troponin T (cTnT), left ventricular max index (LVMi), left atrial dimensions (LAD), left ventricular end-systolic dimension (LVDs), left ventricular end-diastolic dimension (LVDd), interventricular septal thickness (IVST), and left ventricular posterior wall thickness (LVPWT), were reported consistently higher in a group of patients with higher serum phosphate (HSP) levels compared to those in the normal serum phosphate group (NSP) group, while left ventricular ejection fraction (LVEF) showed the opposite trend in a CKD cross-sectional study [52]. Furthermore, the lack of difference in mean arterial pressure (MAP) between the two groups suggested that cardiac remodeling including LVH and the declining LVEF might be associated with serum phosphate rather than hypertension and possibly this happens through triggering apoptosis of human cardiomyocytes.

With respect to CV mortality, it is reported that risk assessment varied from 1.09–1.13 for phosphorus (every 1 mg/dL increase) to 1.13–1.28 for calcium (every 1 mg/dL increase) [53].

In conclusion, enhanced phosphate has detrimental effects on the cardiovascular system seriously affecting patient outcomes (brief summary presented in Figure 2). Phosphate is toxic, impairs endothelial cells, promotes the formation of CPPs, induces VSMC transformation to osteogenic phenotype, and initiates cardiac fibrosis that leads to cardiac remodeling.

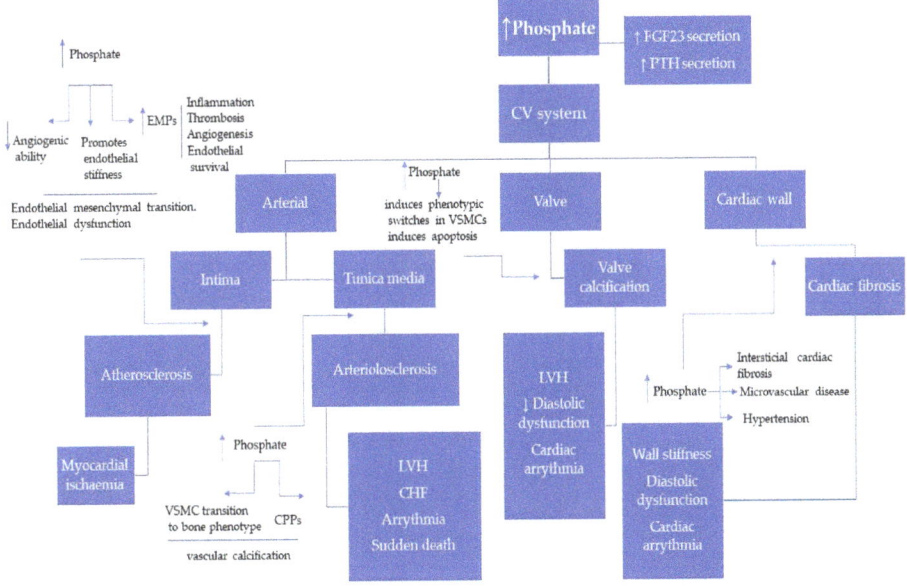

Figure 2. Pathophysiology of phosphate toxicity in the cardiovascular system. In CKD, higher serum phosphate levels are consistently linked with clinical and subclinical cardiovascular disease. Abbreviations: CPPs—Calciprotein particles; EMPs—endothelial microparticles; LVH—left ventricular hypertrophy; CHF—chronic heart failure; VSMCs—vascular smooth muscle cells; ↑ elevate; ↓ decrease.

2.3. Role of Parathyroid Hormone

Secondary hyperparathyroidism is a frequent complication of CKD characterized by an increase in PTH synthesis and secretion and by parathyroid gland hyperplasia. High levels of PTH have an impact on the cardiovascular system apart from the regulation of calcium and phosphate homeostasis [54]. Elevated PTH levels are a common finding in uremic patients which appears much earlier than hyperphosphatemia. PTH and FGF23 have both phosphaturic effects. The difference remains that only PTH has an impact on increased serum calcium. While PTH receptor (PTH1R), is present in bone and kidney, the klotho coreceptor is only expressed in the kidney [7,31]. In addition, PTH stimulates calcitriol synthesis that further contributes to increased serum calcium, whereas FGF23 has an opposite effect on vitamin D and calcium. In the physiologic state, FGF23 acts on the parathyroid gland by reducing gene expression and secretion while in the absence of Klotho, the parathyroid gland shows resistance to FGF23, so enhances PTH secretion.

Experimental data have shown that PTH may directly affect the myocardium although the effect of PTH on the CV system is still under study.

PTH was shown to affect directly rat myocardial cells causing early death of cells by increasing calcium entry into the heart cells [55]. Calcium ions are crucial to myocardial excitation–contraction coupling and cardiac contraction and relaxation [56].

There are early reports by Amman et al. regarding the non-hemodynamic effect of PTH on cardiac fibrosis which was related to diastolic LV function [9]. An experimental rat model of CKD (5/6 nephrectomy) reported that continuous infusion of supraphysiological rates of synthetic PTH in animals with parathyroidectomy was associated with an extensive progression of VC—independently of serum Pi levels or the presence of uremia [57]. Moreover, the higher PTH levels have direct trophic effects on cardiomyocytes, interstitial fibroblasts, and smooth muscle cells of intramyocardial arterioles, promoting cardiac hypertrophy and fibrosis. PTH activates fibroblasts and regulates pro-fibrotic factors, such as aldosterone and angiotensin II (PTH stimulates aldosterone secretion by increasing the calcium concentration in the cells of the adrenal zona glomerulosa directly by binding to the PTH/PTH-rP receptor and indirectly by potentiating angiotensin 2 induced effects) [54,58]. Additionally, PTH potentially would activate protein kinase C, which further on activates other proteins, such as TGF-b, that in turn, promote the proliferation of fibroblasts, collagen synthesis, and fibrosis [59,60]. In vitro studies have found that PTH shows to have chronotropic, inotropic, as well as hypertrophic effects on cardiomyocytes [55] and based on research it was represented that there is a source for a direct role of PTH on cardiac electrophysiology outside of its effect on serum calcium [61].

Furthermore, ex-vivo experiments have shown the interaction between PTH and norepinephrine release in isolated human atria and renal cortex tissue through activation of the PTH1-receptor subtype. This effect would be an explanation for another potential underlying mechanism of the sympathetic overactivity and the associated cardiovascular mortality seen in patients with ESRD [62].

In hemodialysis patients, like in the rat model, the effect of PTH on the myocardium and cardiac fibrosis was well perceived. The hormone was shown to raise the beating rate of myocardial cells and induced their death after prolonged hormonal exposure; PTH stimulates the cyclic AMP production and impairs energy production, transfer, and utilization by myocardial cells [63] and myofibrillar activity of creatine kinase [64]. The presence of sHPTH has also been shown to correlate with enhanced myocardial calcium content and impaired ventricular systolic and diastolic function [65].

Despite a theoretical inverse association between plasma PTH concentration and left ventricular function, parathyroidectomy is not consistently associated with improvement in cardiac contractile function [66]. This suggests that changes induced by PTH could be irreversible in the case of long-standing severe hyperparathyroidism, or other factors contributing to myocardial dysfunction were more important than PTH excess or PTH interferes with the other risk factors of CVD. Despite a theoretical inverse relation between plasma PTH concentration and left ventricular function, parathyroidectomy is not consistently associated with improvement in cardiac contractile function [66]. This suggests in the case of long-standing severe hyperparathyroidism changes induced by PTH could be irreversible, or other factors with an impact on myocardial dysfunction are more important than PTH excess or PTH interferes with the other risk factors of CVD. Furthermore, the inconclusive results of the EVOLVE trial have been linked with this uncertainty since in intent-to-treat analysis a significant advantage of cinacalcet treatment over best presently available standard treatment in the combined primary endpoint (cardiovascular events plus death) was not shown, despite a marked decrease in serum PTH [67]. However, in the subanalysis, when it was adjusted for major confounders such as age and study drug discontinuation, the better control of hyperparathyroidism correlated with a significant advantage in hard outcomes. It was reported that PTH increases with age, weight, BMI, SBP, and LDL, all risk factors for CVD. Increased SBP would be a hemodynamic effect of PTH on cardiac remodeling [68,69]. Evidence suggests that PTH has vascular effects [68]. Here its potential effects on endothelial dysfunction, and increased serum levels of endothelin-1 and IL-6 could be mentioned. In addition, PTH may stimulate the vascular smooth muscle cells to produce factors including collagen and beta-1 integrin which could, in turn, remodel the peripheral vasculature. Another potential effect of PTH would be the increase of renin release and activation of the renin–angiotensin system, a process mediated by serum calcium and renal 1-alpha hydroxylase [69]. Aman et al. have underlined the effect of PTH as the major determining factor of coronary artery lesions, ranging from the discontinuity of the elastic lamina to the calcification of the medial layer, confirming the agreeable action of PTH [70].

In conclusion, there are clinical and experimental reports which support the hypothesis that PTH behaves as a systemic uremic toxin, with direct and indirect effects on uremic cardiomyopathy. PTH acts through four major cardiovascular effects; contractile disturbance, cardiomyocyte hypertrophy, cardiac interstitial fibrotic, and vasodilator effect. Severe sHPTH is an important threat to CKD patient outcomes affecting CV morbidity and mortality and remains an important therapeutic target to prevent bone and CV complications in such patients.

2.4. Role of Vitamin D

During the last decades, the role of Vit D on CV events has triggered a lot of studies where observational studies (OS) have reported an association of vitamin D deficiency with cardiovascular disease, including carotid intima-media thickness, peripheral vascular disease, and cardiovascular death. Vitamin D supplementation diminishes levels of inflammatory markers and lipids (particularly triglycerides), improves endothelial function (as measured by brachial artery flow-mediated dilatation) and blood pressure (BP) control in the general population with or without vitamin D deficiency [71]. Besides, nephrologists have supported supplementation with 1,25-dihydroxy vitamin D in patients with ESRD since the inactivation of Vit D with the progression of CKD was known. If not managed on time, 1,25(OH)2D deficiency might promote the classic view of mineral and bone disorders (MBDs) such as secondary hyperparathyroidism and osteitis fibrosa cystica. These abnormalities together with endothelial dysfunction and vascular changes from the early stages of CKD [72], results in further vascular calcification and arterial stiffness [73]. Vitamin D has been shown to have anti-inflammatory and anti-oxidative properties and additionally downregulates the expression of renin, correlating with an increased prevalence of hypertension, heart failure, CV events, and a higher CV mortality rate in CKD [74–76].

In vitro data have shown a direct effect of vitamin D on endothelial function, related to decreased oxidative stress and increased levels of endothelial nitric oxide synthase (eNOS). These findings are supported by the promising results of a few randomized clinical trials which represented beneficial effects of nutritional vitamin D supplementation or paracalcitriol on endothelial function (brachial artery flow-mediated dilatation) in CKD stage 3–4 [77,78]. Other positive effects on Vit D supplementation were noticed on inflammation markers, intracellular cell adhesion molecule, vascular cell adhesion molecule, E-selectin parathyroid hormone, and arterial stiffness [79].

A recent meta-analysis supports the positive effect of vitamin D intervention on endothelial function mainly in younger patients, apparently due to an earlier diagnosis, where vascular remodeling has not yet been established. Limitations of this meta-analysis were the small number of studies included, and the short duration of intervention suggesting a need for larger and longer studies on this topic, with sufficient power to assess hard endpoints [80]. The controversies remain also on the impact of Vitamin D on cardiac structure and function.

Experimental studies through a specially engineered mouse model have shown that targeted deletion of the vitamin D receptor gene increased cardiomyocyte size and LV weight without fibrosis [81]. Similarly, an association between vitamin D deficiency and increased myocardial collagen content, impairment of cardiac contractile function, and increased cardiac mass was reported previously [82,83]. On the other hand, beneficial effect of treatment with activated vitamin D on attenuation of myocardial hypertrophy [84] and prevention of heart failure [85] in experimental models were not supported neither by Primo and Opera trials, which showed that 48 or 52 weeks of treatment with paricalcitol, respectively, at a dose that adequately controls secondary hyperparathyroidism did not regress LV hypertrophy or improve LV systolic and diastolic dysfunction in CKD stage 3–5. Moreover, the promising effect of lowering CV-related hospitalizations needs further confirmation [86,87].

In addition, based on the data of the recent meta-analysis including 38 studies involving 223,429 patients (17 RCTs, $n = 1819$ and 21 OSs, $n = 221,610$) it could be concluded that that the existing RCTs that used the intention-to-treat principle do not provide an adequate or conclusive evidence that Vit D supplementation affects the mortality of patients with CKD while in observational studies Vit D treatment was significantly correlated with a 38% reduction in all-cause mortality and 45% reduction in CV mortality. The different findings between the RCTs and OSs demonstrate that confidence on neither should be absolute and the conclusion was that large-size RCTs with a proper dose and sufficient treatment time, in the true vitamin D-deficient patients with CKD are needed in the future to assess, prospectively, any potential differences in survival [88].

3. Importance of New CKD-MBD Biomarkers in Early Cardiovascular Risk Assessment

Considering significant CV risk and mortality in patients with CKD, there is a growing attempt to find a reliable biomarker that would timely detect not only kidney disease but also define patients under higher risk to reduce CV mortality.

Compared to the "older" CKD-MBD biomarkers and already established in clinical routine, phosphate and PTH, which however display increased levels when CKD is already advanced, newer biomarkers, FGF23, Klotho, and sclerostin, give a bit more hope as there is growing evidence suggesting that their disturbed serum levels can detect initial CKD (Table 1).

3.1. Role of FGF23

FGF23, a 32 kDa glycoprotein, has been defined as a phosphaturic hormone produced by osteocytes and osteoblasts [89]. In the physiological state, its main role is to maintain normal phosphate levels in the blood through downregulation of sodium-phosphate (NaPi) cotransporters in kidney proximal tubule and, thus, reducing the phosphate reabsorption in the kidney [89]. In addition, FGF23 downregulates 1-α-hydroxylase in proximal tubules, the enzyme responsible for converting 25-OH-vitamin D into his active form, 1,25(OH)2-vitamin D [89]. In this way, FGF23 regulates phosphate levels both directly, through NaPi cotransporters, and indirectly, through vitamin D metabolism and phosphate absorption in the gut.

FGF23 acts by binding with the transmembrane protein, α-klotho, which is expressed mainly in kidney proximal and distal convoluted tubule, parathyroid and pituitary glands, but also in other organs [90,91]. As FGF23 suppresses α-klotho expression in the kidney, it may decrease levels of secreted klotho in the circulation [90,92].

Studies performed so far confirmed that patients with CKD have increased FGF23 levels even from the early stages of the disease [93,94]. As high mortality in CKD patients is well known, the role of FGF23 in CV mortality was intensively investigated, both in experimental and clinical settings. A recent meta-analysis concluded that elevated FGF23 levels are positively associated with CV events and all-cause mortality in HD patients [95]. Data on repeated measurements of FGF23 levels in patients with CKD may identify subpopulation of patients that have higher mortality risk, as it was shown that those patients with slower rise in FGF23 levels in the course of five years have five times higher risk of death and those with rapid rise in FGF23 levels have 15 times higher risk of death compared to the patients with stabile FGF23 levels [96]. These data indicate that FGF23 acts as a toxin in developed CKD-MBD. Most of the studies investigating the association of FGF23 and mortality in CKD patients analyzed the presence of cardiac hypertrophy, known to be very common in CKD, and activation of the renin–angiotensin–aldosterone (RAAS) system. In patients with diabetic nephropathy and early CKD (stages 2 and 3), lower plasmatic Klotho and higher FGF23 levels were associated with a higher risk of concentric hypertrophy, and, thus, higher cardiovascular hospitalization [97]. It was shown that FGF23 stimulates the renin–angiotensin system by suppressing the expression of angiotensin-converting enzyme-2 (ACE2) in the kidney [98]. The study, which included both in vitro investigation of cardiac fibroblasts and myocytes and myocardial autopsy samples of patients with end-stage CKD, demonstrated that RAAS activation is responsible for the induction of FGF23 expression in cardiac myocytes and stimulation of pro-fibrotic crosstalk between cardiac myocytes and fibroblasts [99]. Besides, FGF23 also increases the production of transforming growth factor-β (TGF-β), lipocalin-2, and tumor necrosis factor-α (TNF-α), which are well known inflammatory markers [98].

Table 1. The importance of the FGF-23–klotho–sclerostin axis in left ventricular hypertrophy in CKD.

FGF-23–Klotho–Sclerostin Axis	Cellular Level	Tissue Level	Circulation	Clinical Observation	Therapeutic Potential
FGF-23	FGF23 directly induces LVH by binding to the FGFR-4 in cardiomyocytes RAAS activation induces FGF23 expression in cardiac myocytes and stimulates pro-fibrotic crosstalk between cardiac myocytes and fibroblasts	FGF23 increases production of TGF-β, lipocalin-2, and TNF-α, and thus promoting the inflammation process	LVH is shown to be associated with an increase in both myocardial and serum intact FGF23 FGF23 contributes to renal anemia development -> contribution to LVH aggravation	FGF23 levels correlate positively with LVH and negatively to left ventricular ejection fraction in patients on hemodialysis	Vitamin D treatment reduces LVH Ferric citrate lowers FGF23 levels and improves cardiac function and patient survival
Klotho	Cardioprotective effect by downregulation of TRPC6 channels in cardiomyocytes, important for angiotensin II-induced hypertrophy signaling Klotho upregulation inhibits TGF-β1-induced fibrosis and pathogenic Wnt/β-catenin signaling in cardiomyocytes	Cardiomyocytes and cardiac fibroblasts express klotho	Uremic serum or TGF-β1 suppressed klotho expression by cardiomyocytes	FGF23/klotho ratio correlates with changes in left ventricular mass Low klotho levels are associated with CV events Serum klotho is an independent biomarker of a left ventricular mass index	Klotho administration attenuates high-phosphate induced renal and cardiac fibrosis and improved both renal and cardiac function
Sclerostin	Lacking data about the association with LVH	Lacking data	Lacking data	Elevated serum sclerostin levels in patients with aortic valve calcification with increased upregulation of sclerostin mRNA	Not yet clear whether therapeutic decrease of sclerostin levels is beneficial or deleterious for CV outcome

Abbreviations: LVH—left ventricular hypertrophy; RAAS—renin–angiotensin–aldosterone system; TRPC6—transient receptor potential canonical type 6; TGF-β—transforming growth factor β; TNF-α—tumor necrosis factor α.

Anemia is an important CKD complication that contributes to higher CV risk and mortality. It is important to underline that FGF23 also contributes to renal anemia development and inhibition of FGF23 signaling may decrease erythroid cell apoptosis, attenuate inflammation, and result in increased serum iron and ferritin levels [100]. Hence, it may be concluded that FGF23 increases CV risk either directly (by action on heart) and/or indirectly (RAAS activation, contribution to renal anemia, and inflammation), and also stimulates other pathophysiological factors that contribute to further disease progression. Regarding the relation to LVH, experimental data indicate that FGF23 can exert its action even if α-klotho is not present and to induce hypertrophy of cardiac myocytes [101]. Indeed, it has been shown that FGF23 directly induces LVH by activation of fibroblast growth factor receptor-4 (FGFR-4) in the absence of membrane α-klotho and that administration of soluble klotho attenuates hypertrophy in mice [102]. LVH, on the other hand, is shown to be associated with an increase in both myocardial and serum intact FGF23 [103].

Clinical data suggest the association of FGF23 levels and increased CV risk throughout the CKD stages. FGF23 is shown to be associated with increased risk of CV events and mortality in diabetic patients even with normal or mildly impaired kidney function [104]. Furthermore, FGF23 levels correlated positively with LVH and negatively to left ventricular ejection fraction in patients on hemodialysis, in whom FGF23 was shown to be an independent predictor of overall mortality [105].

Some authors pointed that predictive potential of FGF23 of CV mortality is more emphasized in patients in intermediate eGFR tercile (with mean value of 60 mL/min) [106].

These clinical data strongly support the role of FGF23 as direct cardiac toxin, which causes hypertrophy of cardiomyocytes that are exposed to less blood supply in the further course of the disease. Apart from the association with CV risk and mortality, the relationship of FGF23 with overall mortality can be explained through the stimulation of other pathways (inflammation for instance) that lead to CKD progression and mortality.

Experimental data, on the other hand, indicate that the progression of LVH in CKD could be ameliorated. It is important to note that specific blockade of FGFR4, as shown in 5/6 nephrectomy rat model, attenuates LVH [107]. Moreover, experimental data in uremic rats indicated that vitamin D treatment reduced LVH, FGFR-4 expression, and calcineurin/nuclear factor of activated T cells (NFAT) signaling activation, and, therefore, showing calcitriol cardioprotective effects [108]. Encouraging experimental data also indicate that early administration of ferric citrate slows CKD progression, lowers FGF23 levels, and improves cardiac function and survival [109]. Hence, LVH can be treated in CKD and CV risk can be reduced, either by lowering FGF23 levels or by inhibiting its effect on the FGFR-4. To conclude, FGF23 acts as a toxin in CKD and has an important role in CKD-MBD development and, most importantly, is associated with increased CV risk in CKD patients. Therapeutic strategies to lower FGF23 serum levels and/or to inhibit its action on FGFR-4 might be beneficial for the CV and overall outcome improvement.

Early diagnosis of CKD-MBD is an appropriate time for prevention of CKD complications and reduction of CV risk. Monitoring FGF-23 levels could detect patients with higher CV risk and suggests more regular visits at nephrology departments.

3.2. Role of Klotho

In close relation to FGF23 levels elevation, it is known that patients with CKD are in klotho-deficiency, which, according to the existing knowledge, contributes to high CV mortality among CKD patients. Decreased soluble klotho levels in the circulation could be detected very early in CKD, from stage 2, and in urine even from CKD stage 1 [110].

On the cellular level, it has been shown that circulating klotho has a cardioprotective effect by downregulation of TRPC6 channels in heart as an antagonist of the Wnt/b-catenin pathway [111]. Klotho-deficient CKD mice had more pronounced cardiac hypertrophy than wild-type CKD mice and even after normalization of serum phosphate and FGF23 levels, cardiac hypertrophy was not improved, meaning that klotho-deficiency is an important cause of cardiac hypertrophy in CKD, independently of FGF23 and phosphate [112]. Klotho deficiency in CKD results not only in cardiac hypertrophy but is involved in cardiac fibrosis development. It has been shown that endogenous klotho is expressed both by human cardiomyocytes (HCMs) and cardiac fibroblasts (HCFs) and that uremic serum or TGF-β1 suppressed klotho expression by HCMs [113]. Klotho upregulation inhibits TGF-β1-induced fibrosis and pathogenic Wnt/ β-catenin signaling in HCMs [113].

Clinical studies also support the cardioprotective role of klotho. In patients with CKD 3 stage, a change in FGF23/klotho ratio correlated with the changes in left ventricular mass [114]. In hemodialysis patients, low klotho levels were associated with CV events, independently from other CKD-MBD factors [115]. Analysis of the LURIC (Ludwigshafen Risk and Cardiovascular Health) study did not show any additional predictive power of CV and mortality risk in patients with normal kidney function [116]. On the contrary, in patients with CKD, as presented by the KNOW-CKD study, serum klotho was shown to be an independent biomarker of a left ventricular mass index, but not of arterial stiffness [117].

Klotho deficiency also contributes indirectly to increased CV risk in CKD. Known to be expressed in the vasculature, klotho deficiency is involved in VC and endothelial dysfunction development [118] and, therefore, contributes to increased arterial stiffness and pressure overload.

Experimental data indicate that calcified human aortic valves have lower klotho levels and that treatment with recombinant klotho reduces high phosphate-induced osteogenic activity in human aortic valve interstitial cells [119]. Another study confirmed that klotho administration attenuated high-phosphate induced renal and cardiac fibrosis and improved both renal and cardiac function in the absence of previous kidney disease [120]. Taken together, experimental data encourage that treatment of klotho deficiency in CKD may have a beneficial effect on heart disease in CKD.

Whereas klotho did not predict CV events (death, atherosclerotic events, and decompensated heart failure) in patients CKD stages 2–4, FGF23, on the other hand, was significantly associated with future decompensated heart failure [121].

Bearing in mind klotho/FGF23 axis disturbance, the klotho deficiency, and high FGF23 levels, in patients with CKD, it has been suggested that the klotho/FGF23 axis could be not only diagnostic and prognostic biomarkers of CKD and CV disease but could be treatment targets as they contribute to the CKD progression and development of CV disease as complication [122].

3.3. Role of Sclerostin

Sclerostin, a protein produced by osteocytes, and coded by the SOST gene on chromosome 17q12-q21, is an inhibitor of wingless-type mouse mammary tumor virus integration site (Wnt) pathway in osteoblasts, which is responsible for osteoblastogenesis [123]. In this way, sclerostin inhibits bone formation in a healthy state. Although previously described to be secreted as 27 kDa monomer only by osteocytes [124,125], later research pointed to the secretion also by other cells (osteoblasts, osteoclasts, chondrocytes, cementocytes) [126,127]. Interestingly, the SOST gene is found to be also expressed in other tissues and organs and, besides bone, primarily in heart, lung, aorta, and kidney [128,129]. Based on these data, sclerostin was no longer considered to be a bone-specific protein and marker of bone turnover, but the topic of further research aiming to understand its role in extraosseal tissues and organs. Unfortunately, the exact nature of sclerostin in those are not fully understood, neither in health, nor in a disease. Some of the limiting factors are the weak association between protein expression in the tissue and mRNA levels and different nature of sclerostin in different parts of the same tissue [130].

Clinical data on the association of sclerostin with CV risk and mortality are not very clear. It is known that patients with CKD have increased serum sclerostin levels already from the initial stages [131]. As the SOST gene is present in the heart and vascular tissue, the potential association of serum sclerostin with increased CV risk in CKD patients has also been investigated and is still an important topic in experimental and clinical research. However, compared to the studies investigating the association of FGF23 and klotho with LVH, most studies linked sclerostin with the presence of atherosclerosis and VC in CKD. Studies investigating the heart in CKD referred to the relationship between sclerostin and valvular calcification. In addition, sclerostin may exert an indirect effect on heart disease in CKD, by taking part in VC development and, hence, through increased peripheral vascular resistance and heart failure.

Elevated serum sclerostin levels were seen in patients with aortic valve calcification with increased upregulation of sclerostin mRNA [132]. Sclerostin is shown to be an independent risk factor for heart valve calcification in patients with CKD stages 3–5 and is increased in serum before the increase in serum phosphate and PTH is seen [133]. In addition, in patients with CKD stages 2–5, serum sclerostin was reported to be associated with inflammation markers, phosphate, FGF23, indoxylsulphate and p-cresyl sulphate, β2-microglobulin, and arterial stiffness [134], emphasizing its role in CKD-MBD development.

High sclerostin serum levels (>200 pg/mL) were reported to be associated with increased carotid-femoral pulse wave velocity (>9.5 m/s) in HD patients [135]. Although during 2-year follow-up HD patients who died had higher sclerostin levels, sclerostin did not predict survival [136]. Similarly, to this study, it was reported that higher CV risk in HD patients was associated with sclerostin values above the median (>84pmol/L) during the five-year follow up period [137].

Recent experimental data suggest a positive correlation between the presence of VC in CKD rats and vascular Wnt3a and β-catenin expression together with blood pressure variability, but no association with sclerostin was seen [138]. In CKD patients, sclerostin was positively associated with VC (coronary arteries and thoracic aorta, but not with those at the aortic or mitral valves and it did not predict cardiovascular events) [139]. Meta-analysis performed by Kanbay et al. showed that serum sclerostin was not associated with all-cause and CV mortality [140]. Previously, it has been shown that serum sclerostin values were associated with fatal and nonfatal CV events in non-dialysis CKD patients [141]. On the other hand, the NECOSAD study indicated that incident dialysis patients with higher sclerostin level had better CV survival [142].

Up to now, there are some data suggesting the association of serum sclerostin with vascular and valvular calcification in CKD patients and the number of studies is very scarce with conflicting results. On the other hand, data on the potential relationship of sclerostin with uremic cardiomyopathy are lacking. Taken together, clinical studies on the role of sclerostin in CKD report inconclusive data and the exact role of sclerostin in CKD-MBD and CV risk is yet not clear with a need for further investigation.

At present, it cannot be clearly stated whether serum sclerostin turns into a toxin in CKD and increases CV risk and mortality, or if it is only a marker of disturbed bone and (cardio)vascular and valvular metabolism. The critical point here is the ability to confirm the origin of high serum sclerostin levels and then to explain the reason for such increased values. Similarly, CKD-MBD treatment for reducing sclerostin levels is a double-edged sword. Although it has been shown that the application of anti-sclerostin antibodies improves bone and mineral density and reduces fracture risk in osteoporosis [143], there is also important data indicating that such treatment can increase CV risk in patients with primary osteoporosis [144].

Nevertheless, new studies on this topic should reveal the real physiological and pathophysiological roles of sclerostin in heart and vascular disease in patients with CKD and will direct future therapeutic strategies.

3.4. Role of OPG-RANK-RANKL System in CKD-MBD

Bone disease is an important component of CKD-MBD, that is linked to vascular disease and described as a calcification paradox [145] (depicted in Figure 3).

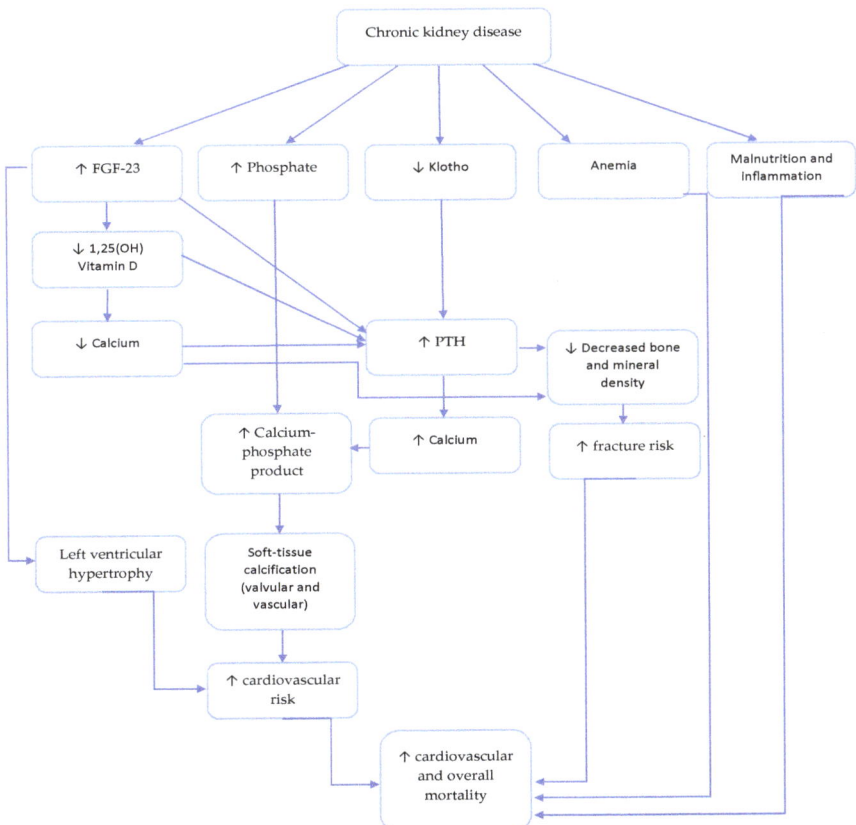

Figure 3. Mechanism of increased mortality in patients with chronic kidney disease. ↑ increases/increased; ↓ decreases/decreased.

The disturbed OPG-RANK-RANKL pathway might be one of the contributors to bone disease and VC development in CKD. In physiological conditions, osteoprotegerin (OPG) is a protein which inhibits activation and differentiation of osteoclasts by blocking the binding of receptor activator of nuclear factor kappa–B ligand (RANKL) to RANK expressed on osteoclast precursors [145]. It has been shown that osteoprotegerin is produced by the arterial wall and other tissues [146].

Experimental data indicate that OPG knockout in mice is responsible for osteoporosis and VC development [147]. Moreover, OPG knockout mice displays higher RANKL and RANK levels, as well as OPG downregulation detected in calcified human arteries [148,149]. An important mediator of the opposite OPG-RANK-RANKL system regulation in bone and vasculature might be TGF-β, as it increases the OPG/RANKL ratio in bone and decreases in vasculature, disabling the VC inhibition by OPG [145]. Clinical data showed that coronary artery calcification score correlated positively with serum osteoprotegerin and negatively with RANKL, and serum osteoprotegerin correlated positively with the progression of coronary artery calcification score in hemodialysis patients [150].

Nevertheless, the calcification paradox seems to be very complex and most likely disturbs several pathways deserving more detailed experimental and clinical explanation.

4. Conclusions

Although the management of CKD patients was significantly improved, we are still faced with a high rate of CV mortality. In this review, we tried to go from each of the candidate mineral disorder to the CV abnormalities (summarized in Table 2). The risks of each mineral disorder from the oldest to the newest one varied with each kind of cardiac abnormality, which means that it is a significant challenge to prevent all cardiac abnormalities, even if CKD-MBD control has been guided in strict compliance with the guidelines. Therefore, we do have CKD-MBD markers acting as toxins: phosphate, PTH, and FGF23, as present important targets for treatment. On the other side, cardioprotective CKD-MBD markers such as vitamin D and klotho could be additional and very helpful points to treat. Finally, the newest CKD-MBD biomarker sclerostin, that interplays in CKD-MBD developing pathways, is still debatable concerning its protective role or acting as a toxin and consequently increasing CV risk development.

Table 2. CKD-mineral and bone disorder (MBD) biomarkers, role in bone metabolism and the cardiovascular system.

CKD-MBD Biomarkers	Role in Bone Metabolism	Vascular Calcification	Uremic Cardiomyopathy
Phosphate	Major trigger in CKD-MBD $\uparrow$P $\rightarrow \uparrow$PTH$\rightarrow \uparrow$Vit D $\rightarrow \uparrow$Ca $\uparrow$P $\rightarrow \uparrow$FGF23$\rightarrow \downarrow$Vit D$\rightarrow \downarrow$Ca	Promotes VC Impairs endothelial function	Cardiac fibrosis
PTH	Key mediator of bone turnover Regulates P and Ca homeostasis	Complex paracrine and systemic effect Promotes VC Impairs endothelial function	Cardiac electrophysiology Cardiomyocyte hypertrophy Cardiac interstitial fibrosis
Vit D	Key role in Ca, P homeostasis Depletion promote sHPTH and osteitis fibrosis cystica	Biphasic curve of Vit D on calcification	Increases collagen $\downarrow$Vit D$\rightarrow$ impairs contractile function Increases cardiac mass
Klotho	Acts as a Wnt-inhibitor Modify bone metabolism	Inhibitor of VC Klotho deficiency$\rightarrow$ impair endothelial function	Klotho deficiency$\rightarrow$ LVH Cardiac fibrosis
FGF23	Posphaturic hormone acts through α-klotho	Is not clear if it has a direct effect on VC	Concentric hypertrophy
Sclerostin	Inhibits bone turnover	Marker of vascular calcification	There are no conclusive data

Abbreviations: VC—vascular calcification; P—Phosphate; LVH—left ventricular hypertrophy; sHPTH—secondary hyperparathyroidism. $\rightarrow$ - brings to; $\downarrow$ decrease; $\uparrow$ increase.

Diagnosis of CKD-MBD in the early development of CKD (stages 1 and 2) would be of great importance in preventing CKD progression, its complications, and would improve patients' survival and quality of life.

Focusing on such toxins and/or their relevant mediators at early CKD stages might help to interfere over time with the vicious cycle of the cardio–renal connection, and improve the outcome of patients. Further clinical studies exploring the beneficial influence of therapy in CKD (vitamin D, iron replacement, anemia treatment, etc.) and the association to FGF-23 and sclerostin levels with the cardiovascular outcome, would be of great help in understanding the complex pathophysiological mechanism of CKD-MBD.

Author Contributions: Conceptualization, M.R.; A.F.; and G.S.; writing—original draft preparation, M.R.; A.F.; writing—review and editing, G.S.; supervision, G.S., M.R.; & A.F; contributed equally in the manuscript. All authors have read and agreed to the published version of the manuscript.

Funding: This research received no external funding.

Conflicts of Interest: The authors declare no conflict of interest.

References

1. *Annual Data Report: Atlas of Chronic Kidney Disease and End-Stage Renal Disease in the United States*; National Institutes of Health, National Institute of Diabetes and Digestive and Kidney Diseases: Bethesda, MD, USA, 2013; Available online: www.usrds.org/atlas (accessed on 21 February 2020).
2. Gargiulo, R.; Suhail, F.; Lerma, E. Cardiovascular disease and chronic kidney disease. *Dis Mon.* **2015**, *61*, 403–413. [CrossRef] [PubMed]
3. De Albuquerque Suassuna, P.G.; Sanders-Pinheiro, H.; De Paula, R.B. Uremic Cardiomyopathy: A New Piece in the Chronic Kidney Disease-Mineral and Bone Disorder Puzzle. *Front. Med.* **2018**, *5*, 206. [CrossRef] [PubMed]
4. Remppis, A.; Ritz, E. Cardiac problems in the dialysis patient: Beyond coronary disease. *Semin. Dial.* **2008**, *21*, 319–325. [CrossRef] [PubMed]
5. Di Lullo, L.; Gorini, A.; Russo, D.; Santoboni, A.; Ronco, C. Left Ventricular Hypertrophy in Chronic Kidney Disease Patients: From Pathophysiology to Treatment. *Cardio Renal. Med.* **2015**, *5*, 254–266. [CrossRef]
6. Wang, X.; Shapiro, J.I. Evolving concepts in the pathogenesis of uraemic cardiomyopathy. *Nat. Rev. Nephrol.* **2019**. [CrossRef]
7. Hruska, K.A.; Seife, M.; Sugatani, T. Pathophysiology of the Chronic Kidney Disease—Mineral Bone Disorder (CKD-MBD). *Curr. Opin. Nephrol. Hypertens.* **2015**, *24*, 303–309.
8. D'Marco, L.; Bellasi, A.; Raggi, P. Cardiovascular biomarkers in chronic kidney disease: State of current research and clinical applicability. *Dis. Markers* **2015**. [CrossRef]
9. Amann, K.; Breitbach, M.; Ritz, E.; Mall, G. Myocyte/capillary mismatch in the heart of uremic patients. *J. Am. Soc. Nephrol.* **1998**, *9*, 1018–1022.
10. Chinnappa, S.; Hothi, S.S.; Tan, L.B. Is uremic cardiomyopathy a direct consequence of chronic kidney disease? *Expert Rev. Cardiovasc. Ther.* **2014**, *12*, 127–130. [CrossRef]
11. Chirakarnjanakorn, S.; Navaneethan, S.D.; Francis, G.S.; Tang, W.H. Cardiovascular impact in patients undergoing maintenance hemodialysis: Clinical management considerations. *Int. J. Cardiol.* **2017**, *232*, 12–23. [CrossRef]
12. Grabner, A.; Faul, C. The Role of FGF23 and Klotho in Uremic Cardiomyopathy. *Curr. Opin. Nephrol. Hypertens* **2016**, *25*, 314–324. [CrossRef] [PubMed]
13. Gross, M.L.; Ritz, E. Hypertrophy and fibrosis in the cardiomyo pathy of uremia—Beyond coronary heart disease. *Semin. Dial.* **2008**, *21*, 308–318. [CrossRef] [PubMed]
14. Ritz, E. Left ventricular hypertrophy in renal disease: Beyond preload and afterload. *Kidney Int.* **2009**, *75*, 771–773. [CrossRef] [PubMed]
15. Fedecostante, M.; Spannella, F.; Cola, G.; Espinosa, E.; Dessì-Fulgheri, P.; Sarzani, R. Chronic kidney disease is characterized by "double trouble" higher pulse pressure plus night-time systolic blood pressure and more severe cardiac damage. *PLoS ONE* **2014**, *9*. [CrossRef]
16. Viegas, C.; Araújo, N.; Marreiros, C.; Simes, D. The interplay between mineral metabolism, vascular calcification and inflammation in Chronic Kidney Disease (CKD): Challenging old concepts with new facts. *Aging* **2019**, *11*, 4274–4299. [CrossRef]
17. Valdivielso, J.M.; Rodríguez-Puyol, D.; Pascua, J.; Barrios, C.; Bermúdez-López, M.; Sánchez-Niño, M.D.; Pérez-Fernández, M.; Ortiz, A. Atherosclerosis in Chronic Kidney Disease: More, Less, or Just Different? *Arterioscler Thromb. Vasc. Biol.* **2019**, *39*, 1938–1966. [CrossRef]
18. Alhaj, E.; Alhaj, N.; Rahman, I.; Niazi, T.O.; Berkowitz, R.; Klapholz, M. Uremic Cardiomyopathy: An Underdiagnosed Disease. *Congest. Heart Fail.* **2013**, *19*, 40–45. [CrossRef]
19. Ikram, H.; Lynn, K.L.; Bailey, R.R.; Little, P.J. Cardiovascular changes in chronic hemodialysis patients. *Kidney Int.* **1983**, *24*, 371–376. [CrossRef]
20. Mall, G.; Huther, W.; Schneider, J.; Lundin, P.; Ritz, E. Diffuse intermyocardiocytic fibrosis in uraemic patients. *Nephrol. Dial. Transpl.* **1990**, *5*, 39–44. [CrossRef]
21. Mall, G.; Rambausek, M.; Neumeister, A.; Kollmar, S.; Vetterlein, F.; Ritz, E. Myocardial interstitial fibrosis in experimental uremia–implications for cardiac compliance. *Kidney Int.* **1988**, *33*, 804–811. [CrossRef]

22. Hayer, M.K.; Price, A.M.; Liu, B.; Baig, S.; Ferro, C.J.; Townend, J.N.; Steeds, R.P.; Edwards, N.C. Diffuse Myocardial Interstitial Fibrosis and Dysfunction in Early Chronic Kidney Disease. *Am. J. Cardiol.* **2018**, *121*, 656–660. [CrossRef] [PubMed]
23. Zoccali, C.; Benedetto, F.A.; Tripepi, G.; Mallamaci, F. Cardiac consequences of hypertension in hemodialysis patients. *Semin. Dial.* **2004**, *17*, 299–303. [CrossRef] [PubMed]
24. Rostand, S.G.; Kirk, K.A.; Rutsky, E.A. The epidemiology of coronary artery disease in patients on maintenance hemodialysis: Implications for management. *Contrib. Nephrol.* **1986**, *52*, 34–41. [PubMed]
25. Mohandas, R.; Segal, M.S.; Huo, T.; Handberg, E.M.; Petersen, J.W.; Johnson, B.D.; Pepine, C.J. Renal Function and Coronary Microvascular Dysfunction in Women with Symptoms/Signs of Ischemia. *PLoS ONE* **2015**, *10*, e0125374. [CrossRef]
26. Schwarz, U.; Buzello, M.; Ritz, E.; Stein, G.; Raabe, G.; Wiest, G.; Mall, G.; Amann, K. Morphology of coronary atherosclerotic lesions in patients with end-stage renal failure. *Nephrol. Dial. Transpl.* **2000**, *15*, 218–223. [CrossRef]
27. Colbert, G.; Jain, N.; De Lemos, J.A.; Hedayati, S.S. Utility of traditional circulating and imaging-based cardiac biomarkers in patients with predialysis CKD. *Clin. J. Am. Soc. Nephrol.* **2015**, *10*, 515–529. [CrossRef]
28. Morena, M.; Jaussent, I.; Dupuy, A.M.; Bargnoux, A.S.; Kuster, N.; Chenine, L.; Leray-Moragues, H.; Klouche, K.; Vernhet, H.; Canaud, B.; et al. Osteoprotegerin and sclerostin in chronic kidney disease prior to dialysis: Potential partners in vascular calcifications. *Nephrol. Dial. Transpl.* **2015**, *30*, 1345–1356. [CrossRef]
29. Lutsey, P.L.; Alonso, A.; Michos, E.D.; Loehr, L.R.; Astor, B.C.; Coresh, J.; Folsom, A.R. Serum magnesium, phosphorus, and calcium are associated with risk of incident heart failure: The Atherosclerosis Risk in Communities (ARIC) Study. *Am. J. Clin. Nutr.* **2014**, *100*, 756–764. [CrossRef]
30. Vervloet, M.G.; Massy, Z.A.; Brandenburg, V.M.; Mazzaferro, S.; Cozzolino, M.; Ureña-Torres, P.; Bover, J.; Goldsmith, D. CKD-MBD Working Group of ERA-EDTA. Bone: A new endocrine organ at the heart of chronic kidney disease and mineral and bone disorders. *Lancet Diabetes Endocrinol.* **2014**, *2*, 427–436. [CrossRef]
31. Vervloet, M. Modifying Phosphate Toxicity in Chronic Kidney Disease. *Toxins* **2019**, *11*, 522. [CrossRef]
32. Hu, M.C.; Shiizaki, K.; Kuro-O, M.; Moe, O.W. Fibroblast growth factor 23 and Klotho: Physiology and pathophysiology of an endocrine network of mineral metabolism. *Annu. Rev. Physiol.* **2013**, *75*, 503–533. [CrossRef] [PubMed]
33. Jono, S.; McKee, M.D.; Murry, C.E.; Shioi, A.; Nishizawa, Y.; Mori, K.; Morii, H.; Giachelli, C.M. Phosphate regulation of vascular smooth muscle cell calcification. *Circ. Res.* **2000**, *87*, 10–17. [CrossRef] [PubMed]
34. Paloian, N.J.; Giachelli, C.M. A current understanding of vascular calcification in CKD. *Am. J. Physiol. Renal. Physiol.* **2014**, *307*, 891–900. [CrossRef] [PubMed]
35. Giachelli, C.M. The emerging role of phosphate in vascular calcification. *Kidney Int.* **2009**, *75*, 890–897. [CrossRef] [PubMed]
36. Razzaque, M.S. Phosphate Toxicity and Vascular Mineralization. *Phosphate and Vitamin D in Chronic Kidney Disease. Contrib. Nephrol.* **2013**, *180*, 74–85.
37. Taniguchi, M.; Fukagawa, M.; Fujii, N.; Hamano, T.; Shoji, T.; Yokoyama, K.; Nakai, S.; Shigematsu, T.; Iseki, K.; Tsubakihara, Y. Serum phosphate and calcium should be primarily and consistently controlled in prevalent hemodialysis patients. *Ther. Apher. Dial.* **2013**, *17*, 221–228. [CrossRef]
38. Rroji, M.; Seferi, S.; Cafka, M.; Petrela, E.; Likaj, E.; Barbullushi, M.; Thereska, N.; Spasovski, G. Is residual renal function and better phosphate control in peritoneal dialysis an answer for the lower prevalence of valve calcification compared to hemodialysis patients? *Int. Urol. Nephrol.* **2014**, *46*, 175–182. [CrossRef]
39. Fujii, H.; Joki, N. Mineral metabolism and cardiovascular disease in CKD. *Clin. Exp. Nephrol.* **2017**, *21*, 53–63. [CrossRef]
40. Peng, A.; Wu, T.; Zeng, C.; Rakheja, D.; Zhu, J.; Ye, T.; Hutcheson, J.; Vaziri, N.D.; Liu, Z.; Mohan, C.; et al. Adverse effects of simulated hyper- and hypo-phosphatemia on endothelial cell function and viability. *PLoS ONE* **2011**, *6*, e23268. [CrossRef]
41. Di Marco, G.S.; Hausberg, M.; Hillebrand, U.; Rustemeyer, P.; Wittkowski, W.; Lang, D.; Pavenstädt, H. Increased inorganic phosphate induces human endothelial cell apoptosis in vitro. *Am. J. Physiol. Renal. Physiol.* **2008**, *294*, 1381–1387. [CrossRef]
42. Di Marco, G.S.; König, M.; Stock, C.; Wiesinger, A.; Hillebrand, U.; Reiermann, S.; Reuter, S.; Amler, S.; Köhler, G.; Buck, F.; et al. High phosphate directly affects endothelial function by downregulating annexin II. *Kidney Int.* **2013**, *83*, 213–222. [CrossRef]

43. Koc, M.; Bihorac, A.; Segal, M.S. Circulating endothelial cells as potential markers of the state of the endothelium in hemodialysis patients. *Am. J. Kidney Dis.* **2003**, *42*, 704–712. [CrossRef]
44. Kuro-O, M. Calciprotein particle (CPP): A true culprit of phosphorus woes? *Nefrologia* **2014**, *34*, 1–4. [PubMed]
45. Akiyama, K. Calciprotein particle contributes to the synthesis and secretion of fibroblast growth factor 23 induced by dietary phosphate intake. *J. Am. Soc. Nephrol.* **2017**, *28*, 210.
46. Viegas, C.S.B.; Santos, L.; Macedo, A.L.; Matos, A.A.; Silva, A.P.; Neves, P.L.; Staes, A.; Gevaert, K.; Morais, R.; Vermeer, C.; et al. Chronic Kidney Disease Circulating Calciprotein Particles and Extracellular Vesicles Promote Vascular Calcification: A Role for GRP (Gla-Rich Protein). *Arterioscler Thromb. Vasc. Biol.* **2018**, *38*, 575–587. [CrossRef]
47. Akiyama, K.; Kimura, T.; Shiizaki, K. Biological and Clinical Effects of Calciprotein Particles on Chronic Kidney Disease-Mineral and Bone Disorder. *Int. J. Endocrinol.* **2018**. [CrossRef]
48. Ciceri, P.; Falleni, M.; Tosi, D.; Martinelli, C.; Cannizzo, S.; Bulfamante, G.; Block, G.A.; Marchetti, G.; Cozzolino, M. Therapeutic Effect of Iron Citrate in Blocking Calcium Deposition in High Pi-Calcified VSMC: Role of Autophagy and Apoptosis. *Int. J. Mol. Sci.* **2019**, *20*, 5925. [CrossRef] [PubMed]
49. Han-Kyul, K.; Masaki, M.; Wanpen, V. Phosphate, the forgotten mineral in hypertension. *Curr. Opin. Nephrol. Hypertens.* **2019**, *28*, 345–351.
50. Amann, K.; Törnig, J.; Kugel, B.; Gross, M.L.; Tyralla, K.; El-Shakmak, A.; Szabo, A.; Ritz, E. Hyperphosphatemia aggravates cardiac fibrosis and microvascular disease in experimental uremia. *Kidney Int.* **2003**, *63*, 1296–1301. [CrossRef]
51. Hu, M.C.; Shi, M.; Cho, H.J.; Adams-Huet, B.; Paek, J.; Hill, K.; Shelton, J.; Amaral, A.P.; Faul, C.; Taniguchi, M.; et al. Klotho and phosphate are modulators of pathologic uremic cardiac remodeling. *J. Am. Soc. Nephrol.* **2015**, *26*, 1290–1302. [CrossRef]
52. Wang, S.; Qin, L.; Wu, T.; Deng, B.; Sun, Y.; Hu, D.; Mohan, C.; Zhou, X.J.; Peng, A.L. Elevated Cardiac Markers in Chronic Kidney Disease as a Consequence of Hyperphosphatemia-Induced Cardiac Myocyte Injury. *Med. Sci. Monit.* **2014**, *20*, 2043–2053. [CrossRef] [PubMed]
53. Covic, A.; Kothawala, P.; Nernal, M.; Robbins, S.; Chalian, A.; Goldsmith, D. Systematic review of the evidence underlying the association between mineral metabolism disturbances and risk of all-cause mortality, cardiovascular mortality and cardiovascular events in chronic kidney disease. *Nephrol. Dial. Transpl.* **2009**, *24*, 1506–1523. [CrossRef] [PubMed]
54. Tomaschitz, A.; Ritz, E.; Pieske, B.; Rus-Machan, J.; Kienreich, K.; Verhyen, N.; Gaksch, M.; Gruber, M.; Fahrleitner-Pammer, A.; Mrak, P.; et al. Aldosterone and parathyroid hormone interactions as mediators of metabolic and cardiovascular disease. *Metabolism* **2014**, *63*, 20–31. [CrossRef] [PubMed]
55. Bogin, E.; Massry, S.G.; Harary, I. Effect of parathyroid-hormone on rat heart cells. *J. Clin. Investig.* **1981**, *67*, 1215–1227. [CrossRef] [PubMed]
56. Silver, J.; Rodriguez, M.; Slatopolsky, E. FGF23 and PTH—Double agents at the heart of CKD. *Nephrol. Dial. Transpl.* **2012**, *27*, 1715–1720. [CrossRef] [PubMed]
57. Neves, K.R.; Graciolli, F.G.; Dos Reis, L.M.; Pasqualucci, C.A.; Moysés, R.M.; Jorgetti, V. Adverse effects of hyperphosphatemia on myocardial hypertrophy, renal function, and bone in rats with renal failure. *Kidney Int.* **2004**, *66*, 2237–2244. [CrossRef]
58. Tomaschitz, A.; Ritz, E.; Pieske, B.; Fahrleitner-Pammer, A.; Kienreich, K.; Horina, J.H.; Drechsler, C.; März, W.; Ofner, M.; Pieber, R.; et al. Aldosterone and parathyroid hormone: A precarious couple for cardiovascular disease. *Cardiovasc. Res.* **2012**, *94*, 10–19. [CrossRef]
59. Schluter, K.D.; Piper, H.M. Trophic effects of catecholamines and parathyroid hormone on adult ventricular cardiomyocytes. *Am. J. Physiol.* **1992**, *263*, 1739–1746. [CrossRef]
60. Custódio, M.R.; Koike, M.K.; Neves, K.R.; Dos Reis, L.M.; Graciolli, F.G.; Neves, C.L.; Batista, D.G.; Magalhães, A.O.; Hawlitschek, P.; Oliveira, I.B.; et al. Parathyroid hormone and phosphorus overload in uremia: Impact on cardiovascular system. *Nephrol. Dial. Transpl.* **2012**, *27*, 1437–1445. [CrossRef]
61. Palmeri, N.O.; Walker, M.D. Parathyroid Hormone and Cardiac Electrophysiology: A Review. *Cardiol. Rev.* **2019**, *27*, 182–188. [CrossRef]
62. Potthoff, S.A.; Janus, A.; Hoch, H.; Frahnert, M.; Tossios, P.; Reber, D.; Giessing, M.; Klein, H.M.; Schwertfeger, E.; Quack, I.; et al. PTH-receptors regulate norepinephrine release in human heart and kidney. *Regul. Pept.* **2011**, *171*, 35–42. [CrossRef] [PubMed]

63. Drüeke, T.; Fauchet, M.; Fleury, J.; Lesourd, P.; Toure, Y.; Le Pailleur, C.; De Vernejoul, P.; Crosnier, J. Effect of parathyroidectomy on left-ventricular function in haemodialysis patients. *Lancet* **1980**, *1*, 112–114. [CrossRef]
64. London, G.M.; Fabiani, F.; Marchais, S.J.; De Vernejoul, M.C.; Guerin, A.P.; Safar, M.E.; Metivier, F.; Llach, F. Uremic cardiomyopathy: An inadequate left ventricular hypertrophy. *Kidney Int.* **1987**, *31*, 973–980. [CrossRef] [PubMed]
65. Coratelli, P.; Buongiorno, E.; Petrarulo, F.; Corciulo, R.; Giannattasio, M.; Passavanti, G.; Antonelli, G. Pathogenetic aspects of uremic cardiomyopathy. *Miner Electrolyte Metab.* **1989**, *15*, 246–253.
66. Fellner, S.K.; Lang, R.M.; Neumann, A.; Bushinsky, D.A.; Borow, K.M. Parathyroid hormone and myocardial performance in dialysis patients. *Am. J. Kidney Dis.* **1991**, *18*, 320–325. [CrossRef]
67. Evolve Trial Investigators; Chertow, G.M.; Block, G.A.; Correa-Rotter, R.; Drüeke, T.B.; Floege, J.; Goodman, W.G.; Herzog, C.A.; Kubo, Y.; London, G.M.; et al. Effect of cinacalcet on cardiovascular disease in patients undergoing dialysis. *N. Engl. J. Med.* **2012**, *367*, 2482–2494.
68. Jorde, R.; Svartberg, J.; Sundsfjord, J. Serum parathyroid hormone as a predictor of increase in systolic blood pressure in men. *J. Hypertens.* **2005**, *23*, 1639–1644. [CrossRef]
69. Pascale, A.V.; Inelli, R.; Giannotti, R.; Visco, V.; Fabbricatore, D.; Matula, I.; Mazzeo, P.; Ragosa, N.; Massari, A.; Izzo, R.; et al. Vitamin D, parathyroid hormone and cardiovascular risk: The good, the bad and the ugly. *J. Cardiovasc. Med.* **2018**, *19*, 62–66. [CrossRef]
70. Noce, A.; Canale, M.P.; Capria, A.; Rovella, V.; Tesauro, M.; Splendiani, G.; Annicchiarico-Petruzzelli, M.; Manzuoli, M.; Simonetti, G.; Di Daniele, N.; et al. Coronary artery calcifications predict long term cardiovascular events in nondiabetic Caucasian hemodialysis patients. *Aging* **2015**, *7*, 269–279. [CrossRef]
71. Baigent, C.; Landray, M.J.; Reith, C.; Emberson, J.; Wheeler, D.C.; Tomson, C.; Wanner, C.; Krane, V.; Cass, A.; Craig, J.; et al. SHARP Investigators: The effects of lowering LDL cholesterol with simvastatin plus ezetimibe in patients with chronic kidney disease (study of heart and renal protection): A randomized placebo-controlled trial. *Lancet* **2011**, *377*, 2181–2192. [CrossRef]
72. Schlieper, G.; Schurgers, L.; Brandenburg, V.; Reutelingsperger, C.; Floege, J. Vascular calcification in chronic kidney disease: An update. *Nephrol. Dial. Transpl.* **2016**, *31*, 31–39. [CrossRef] [PubMed]
73. Stam, F.; Van Guldener, C.; Becker, A.; Dekker, J.M.; Heine, R.J.; Bouter, L.M.; Stehouwer, C.D. Endothelial dysfunction contributes to renal function associated cardiovascular mortality in a population with mild renal insufficiency: The Hoorn study. *J. Am. Soc. Nephrol.* **2006**, *17*, 537–545. [CrossRef] [PubMed]
74. Vimaleswaran, K.S.; Cavadino, A.; Berry, D.J.; Jorde, R.; Dieffenbach, A.K.; Lu, C.; Jorde, R.; Dieffenbach, A.K.; Lu, C.; Alves, A.C.; et al. Association of vitamin D status with arterial blood pressure and hypertension risk: A mendelian randomisation study. *Lancet Diabetes Endocrinol.* **2014**, *2*, 719–729. [CrossRef]
75. Jiang, W.L.; Gu, H.B.; Zhang, Y.F.; Xia, Q.Q.; Qi, J.; Chen, J.C. Vitamin D supplementation in the treatment of chronic heart failure: A meta-analysis of randomized controlled trials. *Clin. Cardiol.* **2016**, *39*, 56–61. [CrossRef]
76. Mann, M.C.; Hobbs, A.J.; Hemmelgarn, B.R.; Roberts, D.J.; Ahmed, S.B.; Rabi, D.M. Effect of oral vitamin D analogs on mortality and cardiovascular outcomes among adults with chronic kidney disease: A meta-analysis. *Clin. Kidney J.* **2015**, *8*, 41–48. [CrossRef]
77. Kumar, V.; Yadav, A.K.; Singhal, M.; Kumar, V.; Lal, A.; Banerjee, D.; Gupta, K.L.; Jha, V. Vascular function and cholecalciferol supplementation in CKD: A self-controlled case series. *J. Steroid Biochem. Mol. Biol.* **2018**, *180*, 19–22. [CrossRef]
78. Chitalia, N.; Ismail, T.; Tooth, L.; Boa, F.; Hampson, G.; Goldsmith, D.; Kaski, J.C.; Banerjee, D. Impact of vitamin D supplementation on arterial vasomotion, stiffness and endothelial biomarkers in chronic kidney disease patients. *PLoS ONE* **2014**, *9*, e91363. [CrossRef]
79. Löfman, I.; Szummer, K.; Dahlström, U.; Jernberg, T.; Lund, L.H. Associations with and prognostic impact of chronic kidney disease in heart failure with preserved, mid-range, and reduced ejection fraction. *Eur. J. Heart Fail.* **2017**, *19*, 1606–1614. [CrossRef]
80. Lundwall, K.; Jacobson, S.H.; Jörneskog, G.; Spaak, J. Treating endothelial dysfunction with vitamin D in chronic kidney disease: A metaanalysis. *BMC Nephrol.* **2018**, *19*, 247. [CrossRef]
81. Chen, S.; Law, C.S.; Grigsby, C.L.; Olsen, K.; Hong, T.T.; Zhang, Y.; Yeghiazarians, Y.; Gardner, D.G. Cardiomyocyte-specific deletion of the vitamin D receptor gene results in cardiac hypertrophy. *Circulation* **2011**, *124*, 1838–1847. [CrossRef]

82. Weishaar, R.E.; Simpson, R.U. Involvement of vitamin D3 with cardiovascular function. II. Direct and indirect effects. *Am. J. Physiol.* **1987**, *253*, 675–683. [CrossRef] [PubMed]
83. Weishaar, R.E.; Simpson, R.U. Vitamin D3 and cardiovascular function in rats. *J. Clin. Investig.* **1987**, *79*, 1706–1712. [CrossRef] [PubMed]
84. Wu, J.; Garami, M.; Cheng, T.; Gardner, D.G. 1.25 (OH)2 vitamin D3, and retinoic acid antagonize endothelin-stimulated hypertrophy of neonatal rat cardiac myocytes. *J. Clin. Investig.* **1996**, *97*, 1577–1588. [CrossRef] [PubMed]
85. Bae, S.; Yalamarti, B.; Ke, Q.; Choudhury, S.; Yu, H.; Karumanchi, S.A.; Kroeger, P.; Thadhani, R.; Kang, P.M. Preventing progression of cardiac hypertrophy and development of heart failure by paricalcitol therapy in rats. *Cardiovasc. Res.* **2011**, *91*, 632–639. [CrossRef]
86. Wang, A.Y.; Fang, F.; Chan, J.; Wen, Y.Y.; Qing, S.; Chan, I.H.; Lo, G.; Lai, K.N.; Lo, W.K.; Lam, C.W.; et al. Effect of paricalcitol on left ventricular mass and function in CKD—The OPERA trial. *J. Am. Soc. Nephrol.* **2014**, *25*, 175–186. [CrossRef]
87. Thadhani, R.; Appelbaum, E.; Pritchett, Y.; Chang, Y.; Wenger, J.; Tamez, H.; Bhan, I.; Agarwal, R.; Zoccali, C.; Wanner, C.; et al. Vitamin D therapy and cardiac structure and function in patients with chronic kidney disease: The PRIMO randomized controlled trial. *JAMA* **2012**, *307*, 674–684. [CrossRef]
88. Lu, R.J.; Zhu, S.M.; Tang, F.L.; Zhu, X.S.; Fan, Z.D.; Wang, G.L.; Jiang, Y.F.; Zhang, Y. Effects of vitamin or its analogues on the mortality of patients with chronic kidney disease: An updated systematic review and meta-analysis. *Eur. J. Clin. Nutr.* **2017**, *71*, 683–693. [CrossRef]
89. Shimada, T.; Yamazaki, Y.; Takahashi, M.; Hasegawa, H.; Urakawa, I.; Oshima, T.; Kakitani, M.; Tomizuka, K.; Fujita, T.; Fukumoto, S.; et al. Vitamin D receptor-intependent FGF23 actions in regulating phosphate and vitamin D metabolism. *Am. J. Physiolol. Ren. Physiol.* **2005**, *289*, 1088–1095. [CrossRef]
90. Zhou, L.; Li, Y.; Zhou, D.; Tan, R.J.; Liu, Y. Loss of Klotho contributes to kidney injury by derepression of Wnt/β-catenin signaling. *J. Am. Soc. Nephrol.* **2013**, *24*, 771–785. [CrossRef]
91. Lindberg, K.; Olauson, H.; Amin, R.; Ponnusamy, A.; Goetz, R.; Taylor, R.F.; Mohammadi, M.; Canfield, A.; Kublickiene, K.; Larsson, T.E. Arterial Klotho expression and FGF23 effects on vascular calcification and function. *PLoS ONE* **2013**, *8*, e60658. [CrossRef]
92. Xie, J.; Cha, S.K.; An, S.W.; Kuro, O.M.; Birnbaumer, L.; Huang, C.L. Cardioprotection by Klotho through downregulation of TRPC6 channels in the mouse heart. *Nat. Commun.* **2012**, *3*, 1238. [CrossRef] [PubMed]
93. Isakova, T.; Wahl, P.; Vargas, G.S.; Gutierrez, O.-M.; Scialla, J.; Xie, H.; Appleby, D.; Nessel, L.; Bellovich, K.; Chen, J.; et al. Fibroblast growth factor 23 is elevated before parathyroid hormone and phosphate in chronic kidney disease. *Kidney Int.* **2011**, *79*, 1370–1378. [CrossRef] [PubMed]
94. Figurek, A.; Spasovski, G.; Popovic-Pejicic, S. FGF23 level and intima-media thickness are elevated from early stages of chronic kidney disease. *Ther. Apher. Dial.* **2018**, *22*, 40–48. [CrossRef] [PubMed]
95. Gao, S.; Xu, J.; Zhang, S.; Jin, J. Meta-Analysis of the association between fibroblast growth factor 23 and mortality and cardiovascular events in hemodialysis patients. *Blood Purif.* **2019**, *47*, 24–30. [CrossRef]
96. Isakova, T.; Cai, X.; Lee, J.; Xie, D.; Wang, X.; Mehta, R.; Allen, N.B.; Scialla, J.J.; Pencina, M.J.; Anderson, A.H.; et al. Longitudinal FGF23 trajectories and mortality in patients with CKD. *J. Am. Soc. Nephrol.* **2018**, *29*, 579–590. [CrossRef]
97. Silva, A.P.; Mendes, F.; Carias, E.; Goncalves, R.B.; Fragoso, A.; Dias, C.; Tavares, N.; Cafe, H.M.; Santos, N.; Rato, F.; et al. Plasmatic Klotho and FGF23 levels as biomarkers of CKD-associated cardiac disease in type 2 diabetic patients. *Int. J. Mol. Sci.* **2019**, *20*, 1536. [CrossRef]
98. Dai, B.; David, V.; Martin, A.; Huang, J.; Li, H.; Jiao, Y.; Gu, W.; Quarles, L.D. A comparative transcriptome analysis identifying FGF23 regulated genes in the kidney of a mouse CKD model. *PLoS ONE* **2012**, *7*, e44161. [CrossRef]
99. Leifheit-Nestler, M.; Kirchhoff, F.; Nespor, J.; Richter, B.; Soetje, B.; Klintschar, M.; Heineke, J.; Haffner, D. Fibroblast growth factor 23 is induced by an activated renin-angiotensin-aldosterone system in cardiac myocytes and promotes the pro-fibrotic crosstalk between cardiac myocytes and fibroblasts. *Nephrol. Dial. Transpl.* **2018**, *33*, 1722–1734. [CrossRef]
100. Agoro, R.; Montagna, A.; Goetz, R.; Aligbe, O.; Singh, G.; Coe, L.M.; Mohammadi, M.; Rivella, S.; Sitara, D. Inhibition of fibroblast growth factor 23 (FGF23) signaling rescues renal anemia. *FASEB J.* **2018**, *32*, 3752–3764. [CrossRef]

101. Faul, C.; Amaral, A.P.; Oskouei, B.; Hu, M.C.; Sloan, A.; Isakova, T.; Gutierrez, O.M.; Aguillon-Prada, R.; Lincoln, J.; Hare, J.M.; et al. FGF23 induces left ventricular hypertrophy. *J. Clin. Investig.* **2011**, *121*, 4393–4408. [CrossRef]
102. Han, X.; Cai, C.; Xiao, Z.; Quarles, L.D. FGF23 induced left ventricular hypertrophy mediated by FGFR4 signaling in the myocardium is attenuated by soluble Klotho in mice. *J. Mol. Cell Cardiol.* **2019**, *21*, 66–74. [CrossRef] [PubMed]
103. Matsui, I.; Oka, T.; Kusunoki, Y.; Mori, D.; Hashimoto, N.; Matsumoto, A.; Shimada, K.; Yamaguchi, S.; Kubota, K.; Yonemoto, S.; et al. Cardiac hypertrophy elevates serum levels of fibroblast growth factor 23. *Kidney Int.* **2018**, *94*, 60–71. [CrossRef] [PubMed]
104. Yeung, S.M.H.; Binnenmars, S.H.; Gant, C.M.; Navis, G.; Gansevoort, R.T.; Bakker, S.J.L.; De Brost, M.H.; Laverman, G.D. Fibroblast growth factor 23 and mortality in patients with type 2 diabetes and normal or mildly impaired kidney function. *Diabetes Care* **2019**, *42*, 2151–2153. [CrossRef] [PubMed]
105. Nielsen, T.L.; Plesner, L.L.; Warming, P.E.; Mortensen, O.H.; Iversen, K.K.; Heaf, J.G. FGF23 in hemodialysis patients is associated with left ventricular hypertrophy and reduced ejection fraction. *Nefrologia* **2019**, *39*, 258–268. [CrossRef]
106. Gruson, D.; Ferracin, B.; Ahn, S.S.; Rousseau, M.F. Comparison of fibroblast growth factor 23, soluble ST2 and Galectin-3 for prognostication of cardiovascular death in heart failure patients. *Int. J. Cardiol.* **2015**, *189*, 185–187. [CrossRef]
107. Grabner, A.; Schramm, K.; Silswal, N.; Hendrix, M.; Yanucil, C.; Czaya, B.; Singh, S.; Wolf, M.; Hermann, S.; Stypmann, J.; et al. FGF23/FGFR4-mediated left ventricular hypertrophy is reversible. *Sci. Rep.* **2017**, *16*, 1993. [CrossRef]
108. Leifheit-Nestler, M.; Grabner, A.; Hermann, L.; Richter, B.; Schmitz, K.; Fischer, D.C.; Yanucil, C.; Faul, C.; Haffner, D. Vitamin D treatment attenuates cardiac FGF23/FGFR4 signaling and hypertrophy in uremic rats. *Nephrol. Dial. Transpl.* **2017**, *32*, 1493–1503. [CrossRef]
109. Francis, C.; Courbon, G.; Gerber, C.; Neuburg, S.; Wang, X.; Dussold, C.; Capella, M.; Qi, L.; Isakova, T.; Mehta, R.; et al. Ferric citrate reduces fibroblast growth factor 23 levels and improves renal and cardiac function in a mouse model of chronic kidney disease. *Kidney Int.* **2019**, *96*, 1346–1358. [CrossRef]
110. Neyra, J.A.; Hu, M.C. Potential application of klotho in human chronic kidney disease. *Bone* **2017**, *100*, 41–49. [CrossRef]
111. Kovesdy, C.P.; Quarles, L.D. The role of fibroblast growth factor-23 in cardiorenal syndrome. *Nephron Clin. Pract.* **2013**, *123*, 194–201. [CrossRef]
112. Xie, J.; Yoon, J.; An, S.W.; Kuro-o, M.; Huang, C.L. Soluble Klotho Protects against Uremic Cardiomyopathy Independently of Fibroblast Growth Factor 23 and Phosphate. *J. Am. Soc. Nephrol.* **2015**, *26*, 1150–1160. [CrossRef] [PubMed]
113. Liu, Q.; Zhu, L.J.; Waaga-Gasser, A.M.; Ding, Y.; Cao, M.; Jadhav, S.J.; Kirollos, S.; Shekar, P.S.; Padera, R.F.; Chang, Y.C.; et al. The axis of local cardiac endogenous Klotho-TGF-β1-Wnt signaling mediates cardiac fibrosis in human. *J. Mol. Cell Cardiol.* **2019**, *136*, 113–124. [CrossRef] [PubMed]
114. Seifert, M.E.; De Las Fuentes, L.; Ginsberg, C.; Ginsberg, C.; Rothstein, M.; Dietzen, D.J.; Cheng, S.C.; Ross, W.; Windus, D.; Davila-Roman, V.G.; et al. Left ventricular mass progression despite stable blood pressure and kidney function in stage 3 chronic kidney disease. *Am. J. Nephrol.* **2014**, *39*, 392–399. [CrossRef] [PubMed]
115. Memmos, E.; Sarafidis, P.; Pateinakis, P.; Tsiantoulas, A.; Faitatzidou, D.; Giamalis, P.; Vasilikos, V.; Papagianni, A. Soluble Klotho is associated with mortality and cardiovascular events in hemodialysis. *BMC Nephrol.* **2019**, *11*, 217. [CrossRef] [PubMed]
116. Brandenburg, V.M.; Kleber, M.E.; Vervloet, M.G.; Larsson, T.E.; Tomaschitz, A.; Pilz, S.; Stojakovic, T.; Delgado, G.; Grammer, T.B.; Marx, N.; et al. Soluble klotho and mortality: The Ludwigshafen Risk and Cardiovascular Health Study. *Atherosclerosis* **2015**, *242*, 483–489. [CrossRef] [PubMed]
117. Kim, H.J.; Kang, E.; Oh, Y.K.; Kim, Y.H.; Han, S.H.; Yoo, T.H.; Chae, D.W.; Lee, J.; Ahn, C.; Oh, K.H.; et al. The association between soluble klotho and cardiovascular parameters in chronic kidney disease: Results from the KNOW-CKD study. *BMC Nephrol.* **2018**, *5*, 51. [CrossRef]
118. Smith, E.R.; Holt, S.G.; Hewitson, T.D. αKlotho-FGF23 interactions and their role in kidney disease: A molecular insight. *Cell Mol. Life Sci.* **2019**, *76*, 4705–4724. [CrossRef]

119. Li, F.; Yao, Q.; Ao, L.; Cleveland, J.C., Jr.; Dong, N.; Fullerton, D.A.; Meng, X. Klotho suppresses high phosphate-induced osteogenic responses in human aortic valve interstitial cells through inhibition of Sox9. *J. Mol. Med.* **2017**, *95*, 739–751. [CrossRef]
120. Hu, M.C.; Shi, M.; Gillings, N.; Flores, B.; Takahashi, M.; Kuro-O, M.; Moe, O.W. Recombinant α-Klotho may be prophylactic and therapeutic for acute to chronic kidney disease progression and uremic cardiomyopathy. *Kidney Int.* **2017**, *91*, 1104–1114. [CrossRef]
121. Seiler, S.; Rogacev, K.S.; Roth, H.J.; Shafein, P.; Emrich, I.; Neuhaus, S.; Floege, J.; Fliser, D.; Heine, G.H. Associations of FGF-23 and sKlotho with cardiovascular outcomes among patients with CKD stages 2-4. *Clin. J. Am. Soc. Nephrol.* **2014**, *6*, 1049–1058. [CrossRef]
122. Lu, X.; Hu, M.C. Klotho/FGF23 Axis in Chronic Kidney Disease and Cardiovascular Disease. *Kidney Dis.* **2017**, *3*, 15–23. [CrossRef] [PubMed]
123. Winkler, D.G.; Sutherland, M.K.; Geoghegan, J.C.; Yu, C.; Hayes, T.; Skonier, J.E.; Shpektor, D.; Jonas, M.; Kovacevich, B.R.; Staehling-Hampton, K.; et al. Osteocyte control of bone formation via sclerostin, a novel BMP antagonist. *EMBO J.* **2003**, *22*, 6267–6276. [CrossRef] [PubMed]
124. Chen, X.X.; Baum, W.; Dwyer, D.; Stock, M.; Schwabe, K.; Ke, H.Z.; Stolina, M.; Schett, G.; Bozec, A. Sclerostin inhibition reverses systemic periarticular and local bone loss in arthritis. *Ann. Rheum. Dis.* **2013**, *72*, 1732–1736. [CrossRef] [PubMed]
125. Van Bezooijen, R.L.; Ten Dijke, P.; Papapoulos, S.E.; Lowik, C.W. SOST/sclerostin, an osteocyte-derived negative regulator of bone formation. *Cytokine Growth Factor Rev.* **2005**, *6*, 319–327. [CrossRef]
126. Van Bezooijen, R.L.; Bronckers, A.L.; Gortzak, R.A.; Hogendoorn, P.C.W.; Van der Wee-Pals, L.; Balemans, W.; Oostenbroek, H.J.; Van Hul, W.; Hamersma, H.; Dikkers, F.G.; et al. Sclerostin in mineralised matrices and van Buchem disease. *J. Dent. Res.* **2009**, *88*, 569–574. [CrossRef]
127. Winkler, D.G.; Sutherland, M.S.; Ojala, E.; Turcott, E.; Geoghegan, J.C.; Shpektor, D.; Skonier, J.E.; Yu, C.; Latham, J.A. Sclerostin inhibition of Wnt-3a-induced C3H10T1/2 cell differentiation is indirect and mediated by bone morphogenetic proteins. *J. Biol. Chem.* **2005**, *280*, 2498–2502. [CrossRef]
128. Brunkow, M.E.; Gardner, J.C.; Van Ness, J.; Paeper, B.W.; Kovacevich, B.R.; Proll, S.; Skonier, J.E.; Zhao, L.; Sabo, P.J.; Fu, Y.; et al. Bone dysplasia sclerosteosis results from loss of the SOST gene product, a novel cystine knot containing protein. *Am. J. Hum. Genet.* **2001**, *68*, 577–589. [CrossRef]
129. Balemans, W.; Ebeling, M.; Patel, N.; Van Hul, E.; Olson, P.; Dioszegi, M.; Lacza, C.; Wuyts, W.; Van Den Ende, J.; Willems, P.; et al. Increased bone density in sclerosteosis is due to the deficiency of a novel secreted protein (SOST). *Hum. Mol. Genet.* **2001**, *10*, 537–543. [CrossRef]
130. Anderson, L.; Seilhamer, J. A comparison of selected mRNA and protein abundances in human liver. *Electrophoresis* **1997**, *18*, 533–537. [CrossRef]
131. Figurek, A.; Spasovski, G. Is serum sclerostin a marker of atherosclerosis in patients with chronic kidney disease-mineral and bone disorder? *Int. Urol. Nephrol.* **2018**, *50*, 1863–1870. [CrossRef]
132. Koos, R.; Brandenburg, V.; Mahnken, A.H.; Schneider, R.; Dohmen, G.; Autschbach, R.; Marx, N.; Kramann, R. Sclerostin as a potential novel biomarker for aortic valve calcification: An in-vivo and ex-vivo study. *J. Heart Valve Dis.* **2013**, *22*, 317–325. [PubMed]
133. Ji, Y.Q.; Guan, L.N.; Yu, S.X.; Yin, P.Y.; Shen, X.Q.; Sun, Z.W.; Liu, J.; Lv, W.; Yu, G.P.; Ren, C.; et al. Serum sclerostin as a potential novel biomarker for heart valve calcification in patients with chronic kidney disease. *Eur. Rev. Med. Pharmacol. Sci.* **2018**, *22*, 8822–8829. [PubMed]
134. Desjardins, L.; Liabeuf, S.; Oliveira, R.B.; Louvet, L.; Kamel, S.; Lemke, H.D.; Vanholder, R.; Choukroun, G.; Massy, Z.A.; European Uremic Toxin (EuTox) Work Group. Uremic toxicity and sclerostin in chronic kidney disease patients. *Nephrol. Ther.* **2014**, *10*, 463–470. [CrossRef] [PubMed]
135. Stavrinou, E.; Sarafidis, P.A.; Koumaras, C.; Loutradis, C.; Giamalis, P.; Tziomalos, K.; Karagiannis, A.; Papagianni, A. Increased Sclerostin, but Not Dickkopf-1 Protein, Is Associated with Elevated Pulse Wave Velocity in Hemodialysis Subjects. *Kidney Blood Press. Res.* **2019**, *44*, 679–689. [CrossRef]
136. Kirkpantur, A.; Balci, M.; Turkvatan, A.; Afsar, B. Serum sclerostin levels, arteriovenous fistula calcification and 2-years all-cause mortality in prevalent hemodialysis patients. *Nefrologia* **2016**, *36*, 24–32. [CrossRef]
137. Kalousova, M.; Dusilova-Sulkova, S.; Kubena, A.A.; Zakiyanov, O.; Tesar, V.; Zima, T. Sclerostin levels predict cardiovascular mortality in long-term hemodialysis patients: A prospective observational cohort study. *Physiol. Res.* **2019**, *29*, 547–558. [CrossRef]

138. Liao, R.; Wang, L.; Li, J.; Sun, S.; Xiong, Y.; Li, Y.; Han, M.; Jiang, H.; Anil, M.; Su, B.; et al. Vascular calcification is associated with Wnt-signaling pathway and blood pressure variability in chronic kidney disease rats. *Nephrology* **2019**. [CrossRef]
139. Jorgensen, H.S.; Winther, S.; Dupont, L.; Bottcher, M.; Rejnmark, L.; Hauge, E.M.; Svensson, M.; Ivarsen, P. Sclerostin is not associated with cardiovascular event or fracture in kidney transplantation candidates. *Clin. Nephrol.* **2018**, *90*, 18–26. [CrossRef]
140. Kanbay, M.; Solak, Y.; Siriopol, D.; Aslan, G.; Afsar, B.; Yazici, D.; Covic, A. Sclerostin, cardiovascular disease and mortality: A systematic review and meta-analysis. *Int. Urol. Nephrol.* **2016**, *48*, 2029–2042. [CrossRef]
141. Kanbay, M.; Siriopol, D.; Saglam, M.; Kurt, Y.G.; Gok, M.; Cetinkay, H.; Karaman, M.; Unal, H.U.; Oguz, Y.; Sari, S.; et al. Serum sclerostin and adverse outcomes in nondialyzed chronic kidney disease patients. *J. Clin. Endocrinol. Metab.* **2014**, *99*, E1854–E1861. [CrossRef]
142. Drechsler, C.; Evenepoel, P.; Vervloet, M.G.; Wanner, C.; Ketteler, M.; Marx, N.; Floege, J.; Dekker, F.W.; Brandenburg, V.M. NECOSAD Study Group. High levels of circulating sclerostin are associated with better cardiovascular survival in incident dialysis patients: Results from the NECOSAD study. *Nephrol. Dial. Transpl.* **2015**, *30*, 288–293. [CrossRef] [PubMed]
143. McClung, M.R. Sclerostin antibodies in osteoporosis: Latest evidence and therapeutic potential. *Ther. Adv. Musculoskelet Dis.* **2017**, *9*, 263–270. [CrossRef] [PubMed]
144. Lv, F.; Cai, X.; Yang, W.; Gao, L.; Chen, L.; Wu, J.; Lingong, J. Denosumab or romosozumab therapy and risk of cardiovascular events in patients with primary osteoporosis: Systematic review and meta-analysis. *Bone* **2020**, *130*, 115121. [CrossRef] [PubMed]
145. Persy, V.; D'Haese, P. Vascular calcification and bone disease: The calcification paradox. *Trends Mol. Med.* **2009**, *15*, 405–406. [CrossRef]
146. Collin-Osdoby, P. Regulation of vascular calcification by osteoclast regulatory factors RANKL and osteoprotegerin. *Circ. Res.* **2004**, *95*, 1046–1057. [CrossRef]
147. Bucay, N.; Sarosi, I.; Dunstan, C.R.; Morony, S.; Tarpley, J.; Capparelli, C.; Scully, S.; Tan, H.L.; Xu, W.; Lacey, D.L.; et al. Osteoprotegerin-deficient mice develop early onset osteoporosis and arterial calcification. *Genes. Dev.* **1998**, *12*, 1260–1268. [CrossRef]
148. Min, H.; Morony, S.; Sarosi, I.; Dunstan, C.R.; Capparelli, C.; Scully, S.; Van, G.; Kaufman, S.; Kostenuik, P.J.; Lacey, D.L.; et al. Osteoprotegerin reverses osteoporosis by inhibiting endosteal osteoclasts and prevents vascular calcification by blocking a process resembling osteoclastogenesis. *J. Exp. Med.* **2000**, *192*, 463–474. [CrossRef]
149. Tyson, K.L.; Reynolds, J.L.; McNair, R.; Zhang, Q.; Weissberg, P.L.; Shanahan, C.M. Osteo/chondrocytic transcription factors and their target genes exhibit distinct patterns of expression in human arterial calcification. *Arterioscler. Thromb. Vasc. Biol.* **2003**, *23*, 489–494. [CrossRef]
150. Ozkok, A.; Caliskan, Y.; Sakaci, T.; Erten, G.; Karahan, G.; Ozel, A.; Unsal, A.; Yildiz, A. Osteoprotegerin/RANKL axis and progression of coronary artery calcification in hemodialysis patients. *Clin. J. Am. Soc. Nephrol.* **2012**, *7*, 965–973. [CrossRef]

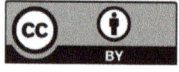

© 2020 by the authors. Licensee MDPI, Basel, Switzerland. This article is an open access article distributed under the terms and conditions of the Creative Commons Attribution (CC BY) license (http://creativecommons.org/licenses/by/4.0/).

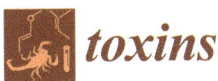

Review

Klotho/FGF23 and Wnt Signaling as Important Players in the Comorbidities Associated with Chronic Kidney Disease

Juan Rafael Muñoz-Castañeda [1,2,3,4,†], **Cristian Rodelo-Haad** [1,2,3,4,†], **Maria Victoria Pendon-Ruiz de Mier** [1,2,3,4,*], **Alejandro Martin-Malo** [1,2,3,4], **Rafael Santamaria** [1,2,3,4,‡] and **Mariano Rodriguez** [1,2,3,4,‡]

1. Maimonides Institute for Biomedical Research (IMIBIC), 14005 Cordoba, Spain; juanr.munoz.exts@juntadeandalucia.es (J.R.M.-C.); crisroha@yahoo.com (C.R.-H.); alejandro.martin.sspa@juntadeandalucia.es (A.M.-M.); rsantamariao@gmail.com (R.S.); marianorodriguezportillo@gmail.com (M.R.)
2. School of Medicine, Department of Medicine, University of Cordoba, 14005 Cordoba, Spain
3. Nephrology Service, Reina Sofia University Hospital, 14005 Cordoba, Spain
4. Spanish Renal Research Network (REDinREN), Institute of Health Carlos III, 28029 Madrid, Spain
* Correspondence: mvictoriaprm@gmail.com
† These authors share first authorship.
‡ These authors share last authorship.

Received: 15 January 2020; Accepted: 11 March 2020; Published: 16 March 2020

Abstract: Fibroblast Growth Factor 23 (FGF23) and Klotho play an essential role in the regulation of mineral metabolism, and both are altered as a consequence of renal failure. FGF23 increases to augment phosphaturia, which prevents phosphate accumulation at the early stages of chronic kidney disease (CKD). This effect of FGF23 requires the presence of Klotho in the renal tubules. However, Klotho expression is reduced as soon as renal function is starting to fail to generate a state of FGF23 resistance. Changes in these proteins directly affect to other mineral metabolism parameters; they may affect renal function and can produce damage in other organs such as bone, heart, or vessels. Some of the mechanisms responsible for the changes in FGF23 and Klotho levels are related to modifications in the Wnt signaling. This review examines the link between FGF23/Klotho and Wnt/β-catenin in different organs: kidney, heart, and bone. Activation of the canonical Wnt signaling produces changes in FGF23 and Klotho and vice versa; therefore, this pathway emerges as a potential therapeutic target that may help to prevent CKD-associated complications.

Keywords: FGFG23; Klotho; Wnt/β-catenin; CKD; cardiorenal syndrome

Key Contribution: FGF23, Klotho, and the activation of the Wnt/β-catenin pathway play a critical role in the progression of CKD, but also on different comorbidities associated with CKD such as cardiovascular disease, cardiac fibrosis, bone frailty among others. The interactions between FGF23/Klotho axis and Wnt elements could contribute to pathological processes such as renal hypertension, mineral metabolism alterations, vascular calcification, renal and cardiac fibrosis, cardiac hypertrophy or arrhythmias.

1. Introduction

Chronic kidney disease (CKD) causes alterations in mineral metabolism, which worsens as the renal disease progresses. It is observed that with only a marginal decrease of glomerular filtration, there is a downregulation of renal α-Klotho (Klotho) [1]. Renal Klotho is the co-receptor of Fibroblast Growth Factor Receptor-1 (FGFR1), the specific receptor of the phosphaturic hormone Fibroblast

Growth Factor-23 (FGF23). Thus, FGF23 promotes urinary excretion of phosphate and prevents hyperphosphatemia until the glomerular filtration rate falls below 15–20 mL/min. In addition to α-Klotho, expressed in tubular cell membranes, there are two other types of Klotho: soluble (sKlotho) and secreted Klotho, with additional effects in other organs. Actually, there are studies showing the pleiotropic effects of Klotho in the cardiovascular system [2], bone [3], and even as a tumor suppressor molecule [4,5]. The mechanisms behind this reduction of renal α-Klotho during CKD are unclear, and they are attributed mainly to kidney function deterioration, although Wnt/β-catenin activation has also been suggested as a key factor leading to Klotho reduction [6].

FGF23 is a hormone produced mainly in mature osteoblasts and osteocytes, and in addition to its phosphaturic effect, it also inhibits $1,25(OH)_2D$ and PTH production [7]. In CKD patients, the concentration of plasma FGF23 increases progressively in part due to kidney resistance to the action of FGF23 generated by the lack of the co-receptor α-Klotho. An experiment in animals demonstrated that the reduction of α-Klotho is precipitated by an excessive tubular load of phosphate [6,8]. In fact, the increase in FGF23 levels is accompanied by a marked decrease in Klotho. Drueke et al. showed a descriptive illustration where it is collected through progressive changes in the parameters of mineral metabolism, and through CKD parameters during renal disease progression [1]. It is interesting to note that in parallel to the decrease of Klotho, and the increase of FGF23, there are also changes in the levels of Wnt inhibitors, such as sclerostin or Dickkopf-related proteins (Dkk1). However, the relationship between the FGF23/Klotho axis and Wnt signaling has not been sufficiently explored.

Works from different researchers have described an interrelationship between alterations in mineral metabolism and changes in Wnt signaling in the kidney, vessels, heart, bone, and brain, among others. This review will summarize the relationship between Wnt signaling, FGF23, and Klotho expression.

2. The Wnt/β-Catenin Cell Signaling Pathway

The Wnt pathway is highly conserved in the evolution of animal life. It is classified into several sub-pathways called canonical and non-canonical. The non-canonical Wnt pathways are not dependent on the β-catenin-T-cell factor/lymphoid enhancer-binding factor (TCF/LEF), such as the Wnt/Ca^{2+} pathway and the non-canonical Wnt planar cell polarity [9]. The canonical Wnt pathway involves the nuclear translocation of β-catenin and the activation of the target genes via TCF/LEF transcription factors (Figure 1). The activation of the canonical Wnt pathway requires the binding of the Wnt ligands to the receptors of the Frizzled family, and the interaction with co-receptors lipoprotein-receptor related protein 5 (LRP5) and LRP6. The binding of ligand and receptor stimulates the sequestration of Axin protein by the Disheveled protein, which prevents the formation of the complex necessary for the degradation of β-catenin. In this setting, β-catenin is not phosphorylated, became stabilized, and is translocated into the nucleus. Into the nucleus, it activates the transcription of the Wnt target genes through the interaction with the transcription factors TCF/LEF [10] (Figure 1A).

In the absence of soluble Wnt protein ligands, the protein Axin forms a complex with the proteins adenomatous polyposis coli (APC), Casein kinase 1 isoform α (CK1α), and glycogen synthase kinase 3α (GSK3α). Axin and APC act as scaffold proteins for GSK3β that binds and phosphorylates β-catenin, which is degraded by the proteasome (Figure 1B).

Some proteins regulate the Wnt/β-catenin pathway by blocking the Wnt ligands and co-receptors. The members of the secreted Frizzled-related protein (sFRP) are proteins that contain a cysteine-rich domain homologous to the putative Wnt-binding site of Frizzled proteins, which inhibit Wnt activation (Figure 1B). Other proteins as sclerostin (the product of the SOST gene) and Dkk1 interact with LRP5/6, and they function as Wnt signaling inhibitors. Sclerostin binds the LRP5/6 receptors, impairs the LRP5/6-Frizzled interaction, and the interaction of the Wnt signaling proteins with the receptors [11,12]. Dkk1 also binds the LRP5/6 receptor and prevents the activation of the Wnt/β-catenin pathway [13] (see Figure 1).

Although there is not much evidence about the direct interaction of FGF23 or Klotho with Wnt elements, it has been shown that the extracellular domain of Klotho binds to multiple Wnt ligands, inhibiting their ability to activate Wnt signaling [14,15]. It is also known that there is a reciprocal relationship between Klotho, FGF23, and Wnt signaling; thus, Wnt signaling dysregulation affects to FGF23 and Klotho levels and vice versa. There is data suggesting potential crosstalk between Wnt/β-catenin signaling and the regulation of Klotho and FGF23. In CKD patients, uremic toxins, phosphate overload, sclerostin, Dkk1, and inflammation may affect Wnt signaling, thus contributing to the progression of CKD-associated comorbidities [16]. This subject will be exposed in the following sections.

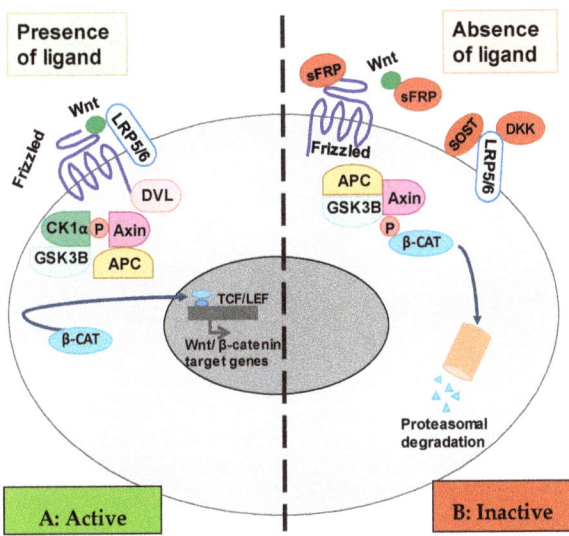

Figure 1. Simplified scheme of the Wnt/β-catenin signaling pathway. (**A**) Wnt ligand interaction with Frizzled protein and LRP5/6. Disheveled (DVL) protein binds the Frizzled receptor and sequester the protein complex CK1a-GSK3-Axin-APC blocking β-catenin phosphorylation and degradation. β-catenin activates TCF/LEF transcription factor in the nucleus. (**B**) Interference of Wnt ligand–Frizzled protein interaction by sFRP, SOST, or DKK1. Disheveled (DVL) protein does not bind to the Frizzled receptor. Protein complex GSK3-Axin-APC phosphorylates β-catenin. Phosphorylated β-catenin is led to proteasomal degradation. Abbreviations: GSK3β: glycogen synthase kinase 3; APC: adenomatous polyposis coli; TCF/LEF: T-cell factor/lymphoid enhancer-binding factor; sFRP: secreted Frizzled-related proteins; SOST: sclerostin; DKK1: Dickkopf-related proteins.

3. Klotho-FGF23 and Wnt in Chronic Kidney Disease

3.1. Regulation of Klotho Expression in the Kidney: The Effect of the Tubular Load of Phosphate

Our group has studied the factors associated with a reduction of renal Klotho expression in rats. Administration of recombinant FGF23 (rFGF23) produced phosphaturia and reduced renal Klotho expression in healthy rats [6]. In 5/6 nephrectomized rats, circulating levels of FGF23 were markedly increased, and Klotho was found to be reduced. In these rats, the administration of anti-FGF23 antibodies further reduced the renal Klotho expression. These results suggest that the increased tubular load of phosphate causes a reduction in Klotho expression. In vitro, HEK-293 cells incubated in high phosphate medium produced nuclear translocation of β-catenin that was followed by a reduction in Klotho expression [6]. We concluded that high phosphate levels decreased renal Klotho expression via activation of the Wnt/β-catenin pathway (Figure 2). The administration of calcitriol to cultured HEK-293 cells prevented Klotho reduction induced by high phosphate.

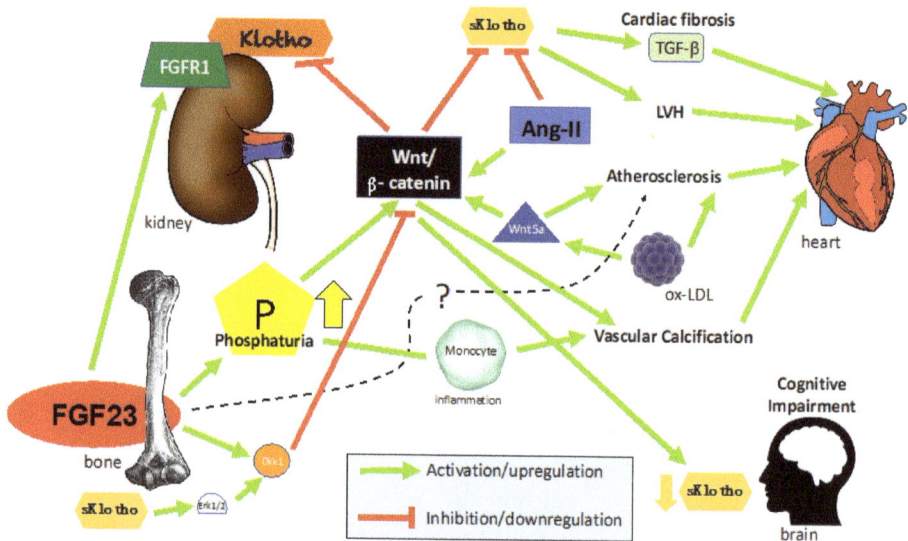

Figure 2. Schematic representation of FGF23/Klotho interactions with the Wnt/β-catenin pathway in the bone, kidney, and heart.

3.2. Klotho, Wnt/β-Catenin, and Renal Damage

Albuminuria downregulates tubular expression of Klotho even in the early stages of CKD [17]. Klotho deficiency induces Wnt activation, which, in turn, is associated with podocyte injury in mice models of diabetic nephropathy and patients with diabetes [18]. Podocyte injury is reduced after the deletion of β-catenin [18]. Although not fully elucidated, Snail-1, a transcription factor induced by Wnt through GSK3β, reduces nephrin expression playing a pivotal role in podocyte injury [19]. The opposite effect is observed with the overexpression of the Wilms Tumor 1 (WT1), which actively suppresses the Wnt pathway through the inhibition of Disheveled protein in podocytes [20].

In the mature kidney, Wnt is suppressed, allowing the podocyte to perform its physiological function. Interestingly, Wnt/β-catenin activity may be affected by high glucose; thus, a pathogenic role of Wnt/β-catenin in diabetic nephropathy cannot be ruled out [21]. In this regard, in a mice model of diabetic nephropathy, Klotho seems to protect glomerular and podocyte injury by inhibiting glomerular hypertrophy and reducing albuminuria [22]. Klotho may also reduce proteinuria by blocking the transient receptor potential cation channel (TRPC6) in podocytes [23], and in the heart, Klotho attenuates stress-induced cardiac hypertrophy via inhibition of TRPC6 [24].

3.3. Klotho, Wnt/β-Catenin, and Polycystic Kidney Disease (PKD)

The Wnt/β-catenin pathway activation is also involved in the development of polycystic kidney disease (ADPKD) [25,26]. These patients show increased plasma levels of FGF23 as compared to GFR-matched CKD patients or healthy volunteers irrespective of the renal function, age, and serum levels of PTH and vitamin D [27]. Furthermore, ADPKD patients exhibit resistance to the renal effect of FGF23 that could be explained by the reduction in Klotho [28]. ADPKD patients show significantly reduced circulating sKlotho, as well as higher FGF23 with a superior FGF23-to-Klotho ratio as compared to healthy volunteers and GFR-matched CKD 1 and 2 patients [28]. Interestingly, sKlotho levels inversely correlate with the total cyst volume and the annual growth of the kidney.

Cardiovascular disease (CVD) is apparent in ADPKD patients. Indeed, a high incidence of intracranial aneurysms, mitral and aortic valvular prolapse, aortic regurgitation, left ventricular hypertrophy (LVH), and coronary artery disease has been reported, all of which may culminate in heart failure (HF) [29–31]. Although some of these manifestations have a genetic background, such as aneurysms, it is also possible that the dysregulation of the FGF23–Klotho complex could play a role in the development of these complications, mainly those that directly affect the heart. However, to our knowledge, no study has described crosstalk between FGF23 increase and Klotho reduction as responsible for ADPKD cardiac and vascular disease.

3.4. Consequences of the Close Relationship between Wnt and Klotho

Since Klotho is downregulated in CKD, it is important to delineate this relationship. The fall of renal Klotho is postulated as one of the most important effects of Wnt signaling activation. Therefore, the design of new strategies directed to increase Klotho levels should be considered as a strategy to reduce morbidity and mortality associated with kidney and heart diseases.

sKlotho binds to multiple Wnt ligands suppressing a variety of gene transcription. The upregulation of Klotho halts the activation of Wnt, which reduces the deposition of the extracellular matrix and decreases the transcription of cytokines [32]. The contrary is observed in Klotho heterozygous mutant mice in which Wnt is overexpressed together with an increment of Transforming Growth Factor-β (TGF-β) and collagen type III (Col3); the extracellular matrix deposition and interstitial fibrosis are remarkable as compared to the wild type. Hence, in vivo models have demonstrated that sKlotho attenuates renal fibrosis by halting Wnt signaling [33].

3.5. Kidney Fibrosis

Recently, the Wnt pathway in the kidney has gained attention because of its association with renal fibrosis. In the kidney, pericytes are recognized as collagen-producing cells [34]. Once a kidney injury is established, pericytes migrate to the interstitial space where they differentiate into scar-forming myofibroblasts [34]. In this context, the Wnt pathway is markedly activated in pericytes at the time they differentiate into myofibroblasts, which may cause fibrosis of the kidney interstitium [35].

3.6. Cardiorenal Syndrome

Cardiorenal syndromes have been defined as "disorders of the heart and kidneys whereby acute or chronic dysfunction in one organ may induce acute or chronic dysfunction of the other [36]. There are five subcategories of cardiorenal syndrome based on the primary damaged organ (heart or kidney) and the time course of progression (acute or chronic) [36]. Type 2 cardiorenal syndrome (CRS2) is where HF causes renal dysfunction, and type 4 CRS (CRS4) is where advanced CKD promotes heart dysfunction.

With respect to CRS4, clinical reports have substantiated a relationship between heart and kidney disease [37]. It appears that Klotho deficiency may contribute to the generation of cardiac hypertrophy observed in patients CKD stages G3a–b and G4; however, publications on this issue are limited [38].

In the case of CRS2, a study on a mice model of HF has shed light on the potential mechanisms connecting cardiac and renal dysfunction [39]. In these mice, the constriction of the aorta induced LVH and HF. The increased cardiac remodeling was associated with a significant reduction of Klotho and activation of the Wnt/β-catenin and renin–angiotensin system (RAS). The Wnt/β-catenin activation mediates the injury in both organs, heart, and kidney. Once HF is established, the renal expression of podocalyxin was reduced while fibronectin and Snail1 expression increased, resulting in kidney interstitial fibrosis and albuminuria [39].

Furthermore, different cardiac Wnt ligands increased together with β-catenin, angiotensin-converting enzyme (ACE), renin, and angiotensin I (AT1) expression. Perhaps, the most important finding of this research is that the inhibition of the cardiac-secreted Wnt/β-catenin/RAS axis prevented kidney injury by a downregulation of the expression of fibronectin, Snail1, ACE, renin, and AT1 in the kidney with a consequent reduction of kidney interstitial fibrosis. All the cardiac lesions worsened in association with renal-dependent Klotho depletion. The presence of sKlotho partially inhibited Wnt/β-catenin signaling, which in turn promoted the downregulation of cardiac fibronectin and α-smooth muscle actin. Therefore, the activity of Wnt/β-catenin in the heart is accompanied by kidney injury. Concomitantly, Klotho deficiency resulting from kidney failure worsens cardiac remodeling and function. This finding is not surprising since Klotho deficiency, high serum phosphate, and elevated FGF23 have been demonstrated to modulate cardiac remodeling [40] (Figure 2).

In CKD patients, more information on the relationship between serum Klotho and FGF23 levels and the values of the Wnt ligands, such as Wnt1, Wnt3a, or Wnt10b, could be useful to assess the comorbidities dependent on the Wnt signaling system, such as renal and cardiac fibrosis.

4. FGF23/Klotho/Wnt in Cardiovascular Disease (CVD)

The involvement of Wnt signaling activation in the pathogenesis of CVD has been widely documented. In addition to the cardiovascular development during embryogenesis, Wnt signaling participates in many cardiac and vascular pathological processes such as RAS alterations, cardiac fibrosis and hypertrophy, atherosclerosis, vascular calcification, endothelial dysfunction, myocardial infarction, or arrhythmias [41] (Figure 2).

4.1. Klotho, Wnt/β-Catenin, and RAS

Another point of interest is the association between Wnt/β-catenin signaling and the Pro-Renin Receptor (PRR), a component of the RAS, and critical regulator of blood pressure [42]. In the kidney, PRR is involved in nephron formation, podocytes instability, blood pressure regulation, and sodium transport [42,43]. PRR increases as CKD progress; however, the mechanisms leading are not fully understood. A recent study has demonstrated that Wnt/β-catenin stimulates PRR mRNA expression of in a dose-dependent manner [42]. Similarly, PRR overexpression triggers Wnt gene transcription, perpetuating a cycle that exacerbates kidney fibrosis and a decline of renal function. Multiple RAS genes are direct targets of Wnt/β-catenin signaling [44].

However, to date, there is no evidence showing the relationship between Klotho reduction and PRR expression. Given that CKD and Wnt/β-catenin signaling regulate PRR expression, and FGF23 enhances sodium reabsorption through sodium/chloride cotransporter in the distal tubule [45,46], it can be hypothesized that increased FGF23, Wnt activation, and the downregulation of Klotho in CKD may promote volume overload and an elevation in blood pressure, two well-known risk factors for heart failure. Nevertheless, this remains speculative and requires further investigation. Therefore, FGF23, Klotho, and the Wnt pathway may have relevance in the control of blood pressure and RAS.

4.2. FGF23/Klotho and Cardiac Hypertrophy

An increase in the FGF23/Klotho ratio is present since the early stages of CKD, and it is associated with CVD, especially with LVH [47] and vascular calcification [48,49]. Studies by Myles Wolf's group demonstrated that high levels of FGF23 caused LVH [50]. It is reasonable to speculate that FGF23 through a Wnt signaling activation might be a cause of LVH. In the experimental setting, and with respect to left ventricular remodeling, it is observed that Wnt signaling inhibition improves cardiac function; sFRP or Disheveled, both Wnt inhibitors, attenuate left ventricular remodeling [51].

Experimental studies have shown a cardioprotective effect of Klotho, although the mechanisms are unknown. Yu et al. [52] observed that Klotho reduced the Angiotensin II-induced hypertrophic growth of neonatal cardiomyocytes. In these cells, Angiotensin-II promoted Wnt/β-catenin activation while Klotho decreased it. Klotho administration also suppressed the expression of Angiotensin-II receptor type I showing that Klotho might be considered as an antihypertrophic factor useful in heart diseases.

A recent study has shown in hemodialysis patients that higher serum FGF23 and lower sKlotho and sclerostin (an endogenous Wnt inhibitor) levels were associated with chronic inflammation, malnutrition, secondary hyperparathyroidism, and may be considered as predictors of cardiovascular complications, such as LVH, acute coronary syndrome, or rhythm disturbances [53].

4.3. FGF23–Klotho–Wnt and Cardiac Fibrosis

During cardiac fibrosis some of the evidences showing a crosstalk of FGF23 and Klotho with Wnt signaling are described. Cardiac fibrosis is characterized as an excessive accumulation of fibroblasts, myofibroblasts, and extracellular matrix proteins in the myocardium [54]. Human hearts with severe epicardial fibrosis show increased activation of β-catenin and TCF/LEF [55]. Additionally, TGF-β is a key profibrotic cytokine in the development of cardiac fibrogenesis. It has been proposed that TGF-β activates Wnt/β-catenin signaling through the production of Wnt proteins, and by direct deactivation of GSK3β. Activated Wnt/β-catenin, in turn, stabilizes the TGF-β/Smad response. It appears that the co-activation of these two pathways is required to trigger the effective fibrotic response [56]. Akhmetshina et al. showed that canonical Wnt signaling activation is required for TGF-β-mediated fibrosis [57]. Recently, Liu Q et al. showed through in vitro studies that the loss of endogenous cardiac Klotho in CKD patients, specifically in cardiomyocytes, intensifies TGF-β1 signaling, which enables more vigorous cardiac fibrosis through upregulation of Wnt signaling. Moreover, the upregulation of endogenous Klotho inhibited Wnt/β-catenin signaling [58], a desirable strategy for the prevention and treatment of cardiac fibrosis in CKD patients.

Other authors have shown that secreted Klotho can inhibit TGF-β1 signaling through its interaction with TGF-β1 cell-surface receptors [59].

With respect to FGF23, Hao et al. observed that in cultured adult mouse cardiac fibroblasts, rFGF23 increased active β-catenin, procollagen I, and procollagen III expression [60]. Schumacher et al. showed that FGF23 increased the expression of Collagen 1, MMP8, and fibronectin in cardiac fibroblasts; in addition, they showed that high levels of FGF23 increased the expression of TGF-β1 in M2 polarized macrophages [61]. So, FGF23 might be involved also in cardiac fibrosis generation.

These studies reveal a close association between Klotho, TGF-β, and Wnt signaling activation in the generation of cardiac fibrosis. The evaluation of these parameters in the context of clinical studies will determine if modulation of Wnt signaling could be a potential therapeutic target.

4.4. FGF23/Klotho and Atherosclerosis

Vascular endothelial dysfunction is one of the first events in the atherosclerotic process. The endothelial injury allows monocyte adhesion with subsequent infiltration into the subintimal space. Subsequently, these monocytes are differentiated into macrophages, beginning an inflammatory process with the release of proinflammatory cytokines and nuclear translocation of NF-kB. This inflammatory process produces changes in vascular smooth muscle cells (VSMC) from contractile to a synthetic phenotype with a higher capability to migrate from the media to the intima layer in arteries. In this space, both macrophages and VSMC accumulate lipids resulting in the formation of an atherosclerotic plaque with a fibrous cap on the luminal side of the vessel [62].

The atherosclerotic process is also associated with Wnt signaling activation. There is a positive correlation between the severity of the atherosclerotic lesion and serum Wnt5a levels. Moreover, Wnt5a staining has been detected in intimal areas of macrophage accumulation in atherosclerotic lesions of apolipoprotein-deficient mice, and human endarterectomy samples. Christman et al. showed that oxidized LDL induced Wnt5a expression, a potential mechanism to activate Wnt signaling (Figure 2) [63]. Other authors have shown that elevated concentrations of oxidized LDL induce a decrease in renal Klotho expression [64].

Similarly, in human umbilical vein endothelial cell (HUVEC), recombinant Klotho supplementation can attenuate oxidized-LDL-induced oxidative stress through upregulating oxidative scavengers (SOD and NO) [65]. Certainly, more studies are necessary to confirm the potential interaction between oxidized LDL, Klotho, Wnt, and atherosclerosis progression.

In a recent publication, we have reported a significant association between FGF23 levels and carotid intimal media thickness. In 939 subjects with coronary heart disease without CKD enrolled in the CORDIOPREV study, we found that FGF23 was independently associated with intima-media thickness of both common carotid arteries [66].

Chen et al. observed that in hemodialysis patients, sclerostin was also positively associated with carotid intima-media thickness, and patients with low baseline serum sclerostin displayed a better survival. Interestingly, in this study, the authors found a negative association of sclerostin with sKlotho [67]. Although in these patients, low sKlotho levels are caused by the advanced state of CKD, it is unknown if low sKlotho levels also cause high levels of sclerostin. At the moment, it is unknown whether FGF23 through the Wnt signaling might promote the atherosclerotic process.

4.5. FGF23/Klotho and Vascular Calcification

Vascular calcifications are common in patients with advanced CKD, and at present, it is responsible for the high CVD-related mortality [68]. Vascular calcification is the final consequence of a process where VSMC are transdifferentiated into osteoblast-like cells [69].

Patients with end-stages CKD have an important disbalance of mineral metabolism with high levels of serum phosphate, which have been associated in vivo, and in vitro, with the generation of vascular calcification [70]. Different authors and our group have shown that high phosphate levels can activate Wnt signaling in VSMC [71,72]. Interestingly other studies have shown that Klotho supplementation may prevent VSMC calcification through inhibition of the Wnt/β-catenin pathway [73].

We have investigated the relationship between vascular calcification, inflammation, and Wnt signaling. The administration of lipopolysaccharide (LPS) to healthy rats produced inflammation and a parallel increase in serum FGF23 levels and a reduction in renal Klotho expression. Subsequently, ex vivo experiments using slices of kidney tissue showed that LPS and also high phosphate-induced nuclear translocation of β-catenin and p65-NF-kB, with a decrease in Klotho. Inhibition of both inflammation and Wnt signaling activation decreased FGF23 levels and increased renal Klotho [74] (Figure 2). These results support the close relationship between inflammation, impairment in phosphate regulation, calcification, Klotho, and Wnt signaling.

The potential direct effect of FGF23 on VSMC to promote or inhibit calcification remains controversial. Some authors have found that FGF23 directly increases VSMC calcifications, while other authors emphasized that FGF23 is not involved in this process [75–77]. Similarly, it is unknown if FGF23 might or might not promote changes on the VSMC phenotype, with loss of vascular function, atherosclerosis, or even arterial stiffness [78].

5. FGF23-Klotho and Wnt in Bone

Historically, the participation of the Wnt/β-catenin pathway in bone disorders has been widely documented. SOST gene produces sclerostin that modulates the Wnt activity. Without sclerostin, Wnt activity is unrestricted, producing increased bone mineral density with hyperostosis. Thus, the canonical Wnt pathway is critical in bone formation, and its modulation could be a target in the treatment of bone disorders.

In relation to CKD, two inhibitors of the canonical Wnt pathway have been investigated: Dkk1 and sclerostin [79]. Paradoxically, despite both molecules inhibiting the Wnt ligand–LRP5/6–Frizzled interaction, the downstream responses are different, illustrating the complexity of this pathway. In CKD patients, the correlation of serum Dkk1 with mineral and bone parameters is nonexistent in most studies [80,81], suggesting that Dkk1 might have a weak relation with renal osteodystrophy. Nevertheless, the serum sclerostin levels increase early in CKD before renal osteodystrophy is established. Sclerostin is produced and secreted by osteocytes, suggesting an essential role in the relationship between bone, kidney, and Wnt in CKD patients [82]. Serum sclerostin levels are higher in males than females, and the levels do not correlate with age. In CKD patients, plasma sclerostin increases progressively as the glomerular filtration rate declines, and it correlates with serum phosphate [83]. The cause of increased plasma levels of sclerostin in CKD patients is unknown. Osteocytes produce sclerostin, and VSMC transdifferentiated into osteoblast in calcified vessels. Likewise, there is limited information about the relationship between sclerostin levels and bone in CKD. Paradoxically, there is a positive association between serum sclerostin levels and bone mineral density in hemodialysis patients [84]. Additionally, the administration of neutralizing antibodies against sclerostin in a murine model of CKD resulted in beneficial only in low PTH conditions [85].

There are many questions in relation to sclerostin and CKD that remain to be answered. It is unknown if high levels of sclerostin protect against vascular calcification where Wnt/β-catenin promotes osteogenic transdifferentiation of VSMC; it is also unclear to what extent high sclerostin affects bone turnover and renal osteodystrophy. The relationship between sclerostin and other mineral metabolism parameters, such as PTH, FGF23, vitamin D, or Klotho, is also unclear. Perhaps more studies are necessary to characterize the effects of Wnt activity on bone metabolism in CKD.

With respect to FGF23, Carrillo et al. identified that FGF23 directly inhibits Wnt signaling through the increase of Dkk1 levels. This action occurs in bone with the participation of soluble Klotho (sKlotho) [86]. This work provides evidence of the autocrine effects of FGF23, which could contribute to the generation of renal osteodystrophy (Figure 2). These results would be aligned with those indicating that an increase of sclerostin would contribute to the inhibition of osteogenesis. A recent study has shown a positive correlation between FGF23 and sclerostin levels in patients with rheumatic arthritis, suggesting a link between FGF23, reduced Wnt activity, and bone demineralization in these patients [87]. Evenepoel et al. found that sclerostin but not Dkk1 participate in alterations of mineral metabolism related to CKD [79,81].

In vitro studies have shown an interaction between FGF23, Klotho, and Wnt signaling in bone cells. The presence of Klotho in osteocytes and osteoblasts [88], suggests that the bone is another target organ for FGF23. Several studies indicate that Klotho is a negative modulator of bone formation [3]. The mechanisms are not clear, but it is speculated that Klotho allows FGF23 to enhance Dkk1 expression resulting in inhibition of Wnt signaling and osteogenesis. This hypothesis is supported by previous observations showing that Wnt activity is increased in Klotho knockout mice [89]. Ma et al. observed that in UMR-106, a bone cell line, the addition of β-glycerophosphate increased the expression of Wnt target genes; the co-administration of β-glycerophosphate and sKlotho led to a decrease in FGF23 levels and a reduction in Wnt activation, suggesting that sKlotho could modulate osteogenesis and FGF23 production [90]. In this line, other authors have observed that secreted Klotho, through the inhibition of FGFR1 and ERK phosphorylation, can delay human mesenchymal stem cell differentiation into osteoblasts [91,92] (Figure 2).

6. Wnt and the Central Nervous System

FGF23, FGF receptors (FGFR), and the co-receptor Klotho are also expressed in the central nervous system. The biological relevance of the FGF23/Klotho system in the brain is uncertain, but there is some evidence that FGF23 directly acts on hippocampal neurons reducing memory functions and learning capacity in CKD patients [93,94]. Low serum Klotho levels have been reported to be associated with cognitive impairment [95]; however, the mechanisms are unknown. Given that Klotho is an antagonist of endogenous Wnt/β-catenin activity [32], it is reasonable to speculate that if Klotho reduces Wnt activity, upregulation of Wnt could be associated with cognitive impairment. Klotho-deficient mouse models rapidly develop cognitive impairment and show some evidence of neurodegeneration. In humans, there are reports showing a correlation between Klotho deficiency with dementia and Alzheimer's [96]. Different explanations may support this association. First, both FGF23 increase and Klotho deficiency are associated with a vascular disease, which may cause cognitive deterioration because based on vascular dysfunction. Second, Vitamin D deficiency is highly prevalent in CKD patients, and alterations mainly mediate in the FGF23/Klotho axis. Vitamin D deficiency has also been related to cognitive decline in older adults. Third, Klotho plays a critical role in life-extension by regulating telomere length and telomerase activity. Both Klotho and telomeres regulate the stem cell aging process through Wnt signaling [97] (Figure 2). Klotho deficiency results in continuous activation of Wnt signaling and senescence of stem cells [98]. Long-lasting activation of Wnt signaling may cause rapid exhaustion and depletion of neural stem cells. Since stem cell dysfunction limits tissue regeneration and potentially affects aging processes, the ability of secreted Klotho protein to inhibit Wnt signaling may reduce aging-like phenotypes in Klotho-deficient mice. Li et al. have shown that Klotho improves memory performance but disturbs some aspects of social behavior [99]. This has been proven in in vivo experiments, in which the addition of only the secreted Klotho protein improves the learning and memory capabilities of old animals [100]. Klotho is also being considered a new therapeutic target of neurodegenerative diseases [101]. Since CKD patients have an increase of FGF23 and a reduction of vitamin D and Klotho levels, it could be hypothesized that CKD patients may also show a decrease in the production of cerebral Klotho, which would upregulate Wnt signaling and produce the cognitive dysfunction frequently observed in these patients.

7. FGF23/Klotho and Wnt in Other Organs

In the lungs, low Klotho may contribute to the development of idiopathic pulmonary fibrosis [102]. The co-administration of Klotho with rFGF23 reduced fibrosis and inflammation through the inhibition of the TGF-β signaling and the decrease in SMAD3 phosphorylation. Klotho relevance on pulmonary disease is reinforced by recent evidence suggesting that less circulating Klotho correlates negatively with lung function parameters, such as the forced vital capacity (FVC), the forced expiratory volume in 1 s (FEV1), and the diffusing capacity of the lung for carbon monoxide (DL_{CO}) [102,103].

Chronic obstructive pulmonary disease (COPD) is associated with the downregulation of Klotho expression in the airways and an increase in circulating FGF23 levels [104]. Oxidative stress produced by cigarette smoking may be responsible for Klotho deficiency in such a population. Moreover, COPD patients also show elevated inflammatory parameters that may increase FGF23 production, which in turn induce the expression of locally secreted IL-1β in bronchial epithelial cells [105]. Interestingly, the instillation of sKlotho protects bronchial epithelial cells from the pro-inflammatory actions associated with cigarette smoke and FGF23 [105]. Nevertheless, the precise mechanisms whereby pulmonary Klotho expression is downregulated remain undefined. Wnt/β-catenin signaling has recently gained relevance after the demonstration of enhanced noncanonical Wnt-5a activation in human fibroblasts from COPD patients, causing enlargement and destruction of alveolar space and contributing to emphysema development [106]. The inhibition of the Wnt-5a pathways in the lung helps to recover alveolar cell functions, perhaps through the regulation of TGF-β activity by Wnt-5a [107]. Upregulation of Wnt signaling is also associated with an increment in pulmonary vascular resistance, leading to the development of pulmonary arterial hypertension [41]; upregulation of the Wnt/β-catenin pathway has been associated with the proliferation of pulmonary artery smooth muscle cells, pulmonary artery resistance, and heart failure.

Our opinion is that the evidence is limited, and further investigation to define whether deficiency of lung Klotho and Wnt/β-catenin signaling plays a role in pulmonary fibrosis and emphysema is required.

Concerning the liver, a specific effect of α-Klotho in the liver is only partially defined. To date, there is no evidence of a detrimental effect of the FGF23/Klotho complex in the liver. In fact, FGF23 promotes hepatocytes proliferation and cytokine production [94,108], despite the lack of expression of Klotho in hepatocytes [94]. Thus, FGF23 action on the liver is Klotho independent, and it is mediated by FGFR4 [46,108]. The Wnt/β-catenin, together with different FGFs, are pivotal in hepatobiliary development; early in embryonal development, β-catenin warrants hepatoblast proliferation and conversion into hepatocytes [109].

The liver is tightly associated with multiple endocrine functions, such as energy homeostasis. In this line, it seems that sKlotho improves insulin sensitivity and insulin release, and it reduces lipid accumulation in the liver [110]. Reciprocally, β-Klotho likely preserves liver integrity by serving as co-receptor for endocrine FGF21, a liver-derived hormone and member of the FGF family that promotes thermogenesis and glucose uptake in adipose tissue [111]. Chronic liver injuries frequently evolve liver fibrosis with a loss of function. There is data suggesting that the Wnt/β-catenin pathway is the main regulator of liver fibrosis. Both Wnt-5a and TGF-β are related to myofibroblast proliferation, collagen deposition, and fibrosis of the liver [41,112]. Nonetheless, dysregulation of Klotho has not been identified as responsible for liver fibrosis.

In summary, a consequence of the deterioration of kidney function is the modification of regulatory systems in an attempt to restore homeostasis. However, the "price to pay" is that these adaptations may disrupt the physiology, and comorbidities may become apparent. The Wnt/β-catenin cell signaling pathway has gained attention, given the demonstrated role in the development of different CKD-associated comorbidities. Phosphate overload downregulates renal Klotho expression through the activation of the Wnt/β-catenin signaling pathway, thus contributing to the development of vascular calcification and the alteration of the regulation of mineral metabolism.

The activation of Wnt/β-catenin has other consequences; it promotes tissue fibrosis in both kidney and heart and, more importantly, the upregulation of Wnt/β-catenin may facilitate the crosstalk between the heart and kidney playing a critical role in the development of the cardiorenal syndrome. It is important to note that activation of FGF23/Klotho/Wnt signaling correlates with the severity of atherosclerotic plaques, carotid intimal media thickness, and VSMC calcification. As such, the current evidence suggests that Wnt/β-catenin activation plays an essential role in CKD progression and cardiovascular disease. Therefore, the Wnt/β-catenin pathway may deserve future evaluation as a potential therapeutic target aiming to reduce the prevalence of CKD-associated comorbidities.

Author Contributions: J.R.M.-C., C.R.-H., and M.V.P.-R.d.M. wrote the draft. R.S., A.M.-M., and M.R. provided expertise and feedback. All authors edited and confirmed the manuscript. All authors have read and agreed to the published version of the manuscript.

Funding: This work was supported by a Spanish government grant from the Programa Nacional I+D+I 2013–2016 and Instituto de Salud Carlos III (ISCIII) Grants PI18/0138, PI17/01010 cofinancing from European Funds (FEDER), Consejería de Salud (Grant PI-0136) from the Junta de Andalucía, Framework Programme 7 Syskid UE Grant FP7-241544, and EUTOX and REDinREN from the ISCIII. J.R.M.-C. is senior researcher supported by the Nicolás Monardes Programme, Consejería de Salud-Servicio Andaluz de Salud (Junta de Andalucía).

Conflicts of Interest: M.R. has received honorarium for lectures from Abbott, Amgen, Inc., Fresenius, and Shire. The remaining authors declare no conflicts of interest.

Abbreviations

FGF23	Fibroblast Growth Factor 23
CKD	Chronic kidney disease
FGFR1	Fibroblast Growth Factor Receptor-1
1,25(OH)$_2$D	1,25 hydroxyvitamin D
PTH	Parathyroid Hormone
Dkk1	Dickkopf-related protein-1
TCF/LEF	T-cell factor/lymphoid enhancer-binding factor
LRP5	Lipoprotein-receptor related protein 5
APC	Adenomatous Polyposis Coli
CK1α	Casein kinase 1 isoform α
GSK3β	Glycogen Synthase Kinase 3β
sFRP	Secreted Frizzled-Related Protein
SOST	Sclerostin
DVL	Disheveled
TRPC6	Transient Receptor Potential Cation Channel
CRS	Cardiorenal Syndrome
PKD	Polycystic kidney disease
ADPKD	Autosomal Polycystic kidney disease
CVD	Cardiovascular disease
LVH	Left Ventricular Hypertrophy
HF	Heart Failure
ACE	Angiotensin-Converting Enzyme
AT1	Angiotensin I

PRR   Pro-Renin Receptor
RAS   Renin-angiotensin system
VSMC   Vascular Smooth Muscle Cells
HUVEC   Human Umbilical Vein Endothelial Cell
CIMT   Carotid Intima-Media Thickness
LPS   Lipopolysaccharide
COPD   Chronic Obstructive Pulmonary Disease

References

1. Drüeke, T.B.; Massy, Z.A. Changing bone patterns with progression of chronic kidney disease. *Kidney Int.* **2016**, *89*, 289–302. [CrossRef]
2. Donato, A.J.; Machin, D.R.; Lesniewski, L.A. Mechanisms of Dysfunction in the Aging Vasculature and Role in Age-Related Disease. *Circ. Res.* **2018**, *123*, 825–848. [CrossRef]
3. Komaba, H.; Kaludjerovic, J.; Hu, D.Z.; Nagano, K.; Amano, K.; Ide, N.; Sato, T.; Densmore, M.J.; Hanai, J.-I.; Olauson, H.; et al. Klotho expression in osteocytes regulates bone metabolism and controls bone formation. *Kidney Int.* **2017**, *92*, 599–611. [CrossRef] [PubMed]
4. Wolf, I.; Levanon-Cohen, S.; Bose, S.; Ligumsky, H.; Sredni, B.; Kanety, H.; Kuro-o, M.; Karlan, B.; Kaufman, B.; Koeffler, H.P.; et al. Klotho: A tumor suppressor and a modulator of the IGF-1 and FGF pathways in human breast cancer. *Oncogene* **2008**, *27*, 7094–7105. [CrossRef]
5. Abramovitz, L.; Rubinek, T.; Ligumsky, H.; Bose, S.; Barshack, I.; Avivi, C.; Kaufman, B.; Wolf, I. KL1 internal repeat mediates klotho tumor suppressor activities and inhibits bFGF and IGF-I signaling in pancreatic cancer. *Clin. Cancer Res. Off. J. Am. Assoc. Cancer Res.* **2011**, *17*, 4254–4266. [CrossRef] [PubMed]
6. Muñoz-Castañeda, J.R.; Herencia, C.; Pendón-Ruiz de Mier, M.V.; Rodriguez-Ortiz, M.E.; Diaz-Tocados, J.M.; Vergara, N.; Martínez-Moreno, J.M.; Salmerón, M.D.; Richards, W.G.; Felsenfeld, A.; et al. Differential regulation of renal Klotho and FGFR1 in normal and uremic rats. *FASEB J. Off. Publ. Fed. Am. Soc. Exp. Biol.* **2017**, *31*, 3858–3867. [CrossRef] [PubMed]
7. Bacchetta, J.; Bardet, C.; Prié, D. Physiology of FGF23 and overview of genetic diseases associated with renal phosphate wasting. *Metabolism* **2020**, *103S*, 153865. [CrossRef] [PubMed]
8. John, G.B.; Cheng, C.-Y.; Kuro-o, M. Role of Klotho in aging, phosphate metabolism, and CKD. *Am. J. Kidney Dis.* **2011**, *58*, 127–134. [CrossRef]
9. Niehrs, C. The complex world of WNT receptor signalling. *Nat. Rev. Mol. Cell Biol* **2012**, *13*, 767–779. [CrossRef]
10. Krishnan, V.; Bryant, H.U.; Macdougald, O.A. Regulation of bone mass by Wnt signaling. *J. Clin. Investig.* **2006**, *116*, 1202–1209. [CrossRef]
11. Semënov, M.; Tamai, K.; He, X. SOST is a ligand for LRP5/LRP6 and a Wnt signaling inhibitor. *J. Biol. Chem.* **2005**, *280*, 26770–26775. [CrossRef]
12. Li, X.; Zhang, Y.; Kang, H.; Liu, W.; Liu, P.; Zhang, J.; Harris, S.E.; Wu, D. Sclerostin binds to LRP5/6 and antagonizes canonical Wnt signaling. *J. Biol. Chem.* **2005**, *280*, 19883–19887. [CrossRef] [PubMed]
13. Mao, B.; Wu, W.; Li, Y.; Hoppe, D.; Stannek, P.; Glinka, A.; Niehrs, C. LDL-receptor-related protein 6 is a receptor for Dickkopf proteins. *Nature* **2001**, *411*, 321–325. [CrossRef] [PubMed]
14. Wang, Y.; Sun, Z. Current understanding of klotho. *Ageing Res. Rev.* **2009**, *8*, 43–51. [CrossRef] [PubMed]
15. Liu, H.; Fergusson, M.M.; Castilho, R.M.; Liu, J.; Cao, L.; Chen, J.; Malide, D.; Rovira, I.I.; Schimel, D.; Kuo, C.J.; et al. Augmented Wnt signaling in a mammalian model of accelerated aging. *Science* **2007**, *317*, 803–806. [CrossRef] [PubMed]
16. Hruska, K.A.; Sugatani, T.; Agapova, O.; Fang, Y. The chronic kidney disease—Mineral bone disorder (CKD-MBD): Advances in pathophysiology. *Bone* **2017**, *100*, 80–86. [CrossRef] [PubMed]
17. Fernandez-Fernandez, B.; Izquierdo, M.C.; Valiño-Rivas, L.; Nastou, D.; Sanz, A.B.; Ortiz, A.; Sanchez-Niño, M.D. Albumin downregulates Klotho in tubular cells. *Nephrol. Dial. Transplant. Off. Publ. Eur. Dial. Transpl. Assoc. Eur. Ren. Assoc.* **2018**, *33*, 1712–1722. [CrossRef]
18. Dai, C.; Stolz, D.B.; Kiss, L.P.; Monga, S.P.; Holzman, L.B.; Liu, Y. Wnt/beta-catenin signaling promotes podocyte dysfunction and albuminuria. *J. Am. Soc. Nephrol. JASN* **2009**, *20*, 1997–2008. [CrossRef]

19. Matsui, I.; Ito, T.; Kurihara, H.; Imai, E.; Ogihara, T.; Hori, M. Snail, a transcriptional regulator, represses nephrin expression in glomerular epithelial cells of nephrotic rats. *Lab. Investig. J. Tech. Methods Pathol.* **2007**, *87*, 273–283. [CrossRef]
20. Kim, M.S.; Yoon, S.K.; Bollig, F.; Kitagaki, J.; Hur, W.; Whye, N.J.; Wu, Y.-P.; Rivera, M.N.; Park, J.Y.; Kim, H.-S.; et al. A novel Wilms tumor 1 (WT1) target gene negatively regulates the WNT signaling pathway. *J. Biol. Chem.* **2010**, *285*, 14585–14593. [CrossRef]
21. Lin, C.-L.; Wang, J.-Y.; Huang, Y.-T.; Kuo, Y.-H.; Surendran, K.; Wang, F.-S. Wnt/beta-catenin signaling modulates survival of high glucose-stressed mesangial cells. *J. Am. Soc. Nephrol. JASN* **2006**, *17*, 2812–2820. [CrossRef] [PubMed]
22. Oh, H.J.; Nam, B.Y.; Wu, M.; Kim, S.; Park, J.; Kang, S.; Park, J.T.; Yoo, T.-H.; Kang, S.-W.; Han, S.H. Klotho plays a protective role against glomerular hypertrophy in a cell cycle-dependent manner in diabetic nephropathy. *Am. J. Physiol. Renal Physiol.* **2018**, *315*, F791–F805. [CrossRef] [PubMed]
23. Kim, J.-H.; Xie, J.; Hwang, K.-H.; Wu, Y.-L.; Oliver, N.; Eom, M.; Park, K.-S.; Barrezueta, N.; Kong, I.-D.; Fracasso, R.P.; et al. Klotho May Ameliorate Proteinuria by Targeting TRPC6 Channels in Podocytes. *J. Am. Soc. Nephrol. JASN* **2017**, *28*, 140–151. [CrossRef] [PubMed]
24. Xie, J.; Cha, S.-K.; An, S.-W.; Kuro-O, M.; Birnbaumer, L.; Huang, C.-L. Cardioprotection by Klotho through downregulation of TRPC6 channels in the mouse heart. *Nat. Commun.* **2012**, *3*, 1238. [CrossRef]
25. Wang, Y.; Zhou, C.J.; Liu, Y. Wnt Signaling in Kidney Development and Disease. *Prog. Mol. Biol. Transl. Sci.* **2018**, *153*, 181–207.
26. Wuebken, A.; Schmidt-Ott, K.M. WNT/β-catenin signaling in polycystic kidney disease. *Kidney Int.* **2011**, *80*, 135–138. [CrossRef]
27. Pavik, I.; Jaeger, P.; Kistler, A.D.; Poster, D.; Krauer, F.; Cavelti-Weder, C.; Rentsch, K.M.; Wüthrich, R.P.; Serra, A.L. Patients with autosomal dominant polycystic kidney disease have elevated fibroblast growth factor 23 levels and a renal leak of phosphate. *Kidney Int.* **2011**, *79*, 234–240. [CrossRef]
28. Pavik, I.; Jaeger, P.; Ebner, L.; Poster, D.; Krauer, F.; Kistler, A.D.; Rentsch, K.; Andreisek, G.; Wagner, C.A.; Devuyst, O.; et al. Soluble klotho and autosomal dominant polycystic kidney disease. *Clin. J. Am. Soc. Nephrol. CJASN* **2012**, *7*, 248–257. [CrossRef]
29. Perrone, R.D. Extrarenal manifestations of ADPKD. *Kidney Int.* **1997**, *51*, 2022–2036. [CrossRef]
30. Perrone, R.D.; Malek, A.M.; Watnick, T. Vascular complications in autosomal dominant polycystic kidney disease. *Nat. Rev. Nephrol.* **2015**, *11*, 589–598. [CrossRef]
31. Krishnappa, V.; Vinod, P.; Deverakonda, D.; Raina, R. Autosomal dominant polycystic kidney disease and the heart and brain. *Cleve. Clin. J. Med.* **2017**, *84*, 471–481. [CrossRef] [PubMed]
32. Zhou, L.; Li, Y.; Zhou, D.; Tan, R.J.; Liu, Y. Loss of Klotho contributes to kidney injury by derepression of Wnt/β-catenin signaling. *J. Am. Soc. Nephrol. JASN* **2013**, *24*, 771–785. [CrossRef] [PubMed]
33. Satoh, M.; Nagasu, H.; Morita, Y.; Yamaguchi, T.P.; Kanwar, Y.S.; Kashihara, N. Klotho protects against mouse renal fibrosis by inhibiting Wnt signaling. *Am. J. Physiol. Renal Physiol.* **2012**, *303*, F1641–F1651. [CrossRef] [PubMed]
34. Kida, Y.; Duffield, J.S. Pivotal role of pericytes in kidney fibrosis. *Clin. Exp. Pharmacol. Physiol.* **2011**, *38*, 467–473. [CrossRef] [PubMed]
35. He, W.; Dai, C.; Li, Y.; Zeng, G.; Monga, S.P.; Liu, Y. Wnt/beta-catenin signaling promotes renal interstitial fibrosis. *J. Am. Soc. Nephrol. JASN* **2009**, *20*, 765–776. [CrossRef]
36. Ronco, C.; McCullough, P.; Anker, S.D.; Anand, I.; Aspromonte, N.; Bagshaw, S.M.; Bellomo, R.; Berl, T.; Bobek, I.; Cruz, D.N.; et al. Cardio-renal syndromes: Report from the consensus conference of the acute dialysis quality initiative. *Eur. Heart J.* **2010**, *31*, 703–711. [CrossRef]
37. Ishigami, J.; Cowan, L.T.; Demmer, R.T.; Grams, M.E.; Lutsey, P.L.; Carrero, J.-J.; Coresh, J.; Matsushita, K. Incident Hospitalization with Major Cardiovascular Diseases and Subsequent Risk of ESKD: Implications for Cardiorenal Syndrome. *J. Am. Soc. Nephrol. JASN* **2020**. [CrossRef]
38. Tanaka, S.; Fujita, S.-I.; Kizawa, S.; Morita, H.; Ishizaka, N. Association between FGF23, α-Klotho, and Cardiac Abnormalities among Patients with Various Chronic Kidney Disease Stages. *PLoS ONE* **2016**, *11*, e0156860. [CrossRef]
39. Zhao, Y.; Wang, C.; Hong, X.; Miao, J.; Liao, Y.; Hou, F.F.; Zhou, L.; Liu, Y. Wnt/β-catenin signaling mediates both heart and kidney injury in type 2 cardiorenal syndrome. *Kidney Int.* **2019**, *95*, 815–829. [CrossRef]

40. Hu, M.C.; Shi, M.; Cho, H.J.; Adams-Huet, B.; Paek, J.; Hill, K.; Shelton, J.; Amaral, A.P.; Faul, C.; Taniguchi, M.; et al. Klotho and Phosphate Are Modulators of Pathologic Uremic Cardiac Remodeling. *J. Am. Soc. Nephrol.* **2015**, *26*, 1290–1302. [CrossRef]
41. Foulquier, S.; Daskalopoulos, E.P.; Lluri, G.; Hermans, K.C.M.; Deb, A.; Blankesteijn, W.M. WNT Signaling in Cardiac and Vascular Disease. *Pharmacol. Rev.* **2018**, *70*, 68–141. [CrossRef] [PubMed]
42. Li, Z.; Zhou, L.; Wang, Y.; Miao, J.; Hong, X.; Hou, F.F.; Liu, Y. (Pro)renin Receptor Is an Amplifier of Wnt/β-Catenin Signaling in Kidney Injury and Fibrosis. *J. Am. Soc. Nephrol. JASN* **2017**, *28*, 2393–2408. [CrossRef] [PubMed]
43. Ramkumar, N.; Stuart, D.; Mironova, E.; Bugay, V.; Wang, S.; Abraham, N.; Ichihara, A.; Stockand, J.D.; Kohan, D.E. Renal tubular epithelial cell prorenin receptor regulates blood pressure and sodium transport. *Am. J. Physiol. Renal Physiol.* **2016**, *311*, F186–F194. [CrossRef] [PubMed]
44. Zhou, L.; Li, Y.; Hao, S.; Zhou, D.; Tan, R.J.; Nie, J.; Hou, F.F.; Kahn, M.; Liu, Y. Multiple genes of the renin-angiotensin system are novel targets of Wnt/β-catenin signaling. *J. Am. Soc. Nephrol. JASN* **2015**, *26*, 107–120. [CrossRef]
45. Andrukhova, O.; Slavic, S.; Smorodchenko, A.; Zeitz, U.; Shalhoub, V.; Lanske, B.; Pohl, E.E.; Erben, R.G. FGF23 regulates renal sodium handling and blood pressure. *EMBO Mol. Med.* **2014**, *6*, 744–759. [CrossRef]
46. Rodelo-Haad, C.; Santamaria, R.; Muñoz-Castañeda, J.R.; Pendón-Ruiz de Mier, M.V.; Martin-Malo, A.; Rodriguez, M. FGF23, Biomarker or Target? *Toxins* **2019**, *11*, 175. [CrossRef]
47. Seifert, M.E.; de Las Fuentes, L.; Ginsberg, C.; Rothstein, M.; Dietzen, D.J.; Cheng, S.C.; Ross, W.; Windus, D.; Dávila-Román, V.G.; Hruska, K.A. Left ventricular mass progression despite stable blood pressure and kidney function in stage 3 chronic kidney disease. *Am. J. Nephrol.* **2014**, *39*, 392–399. [CrossRef]
48. Memon, F.; El-Abbadi, M.; Nakatani, T.; Taguchi, T.; Lanske, B.; Razzaque, M.S. Does Fgf23-klotho activity influence vascular and soft tissue calcification through regulating mineral ion metabolism? *Kidney Int.* **2008**, *74*, 566–570. [CrossRef]
49. Yamada, S.; Giachelli, C.M. Vascular calcification in CKD-MBD: Roles for phosphate, FGF23, and Klotho. *Bone* **2017**, *100*, 87–93. [CrossRef]
50. Faul, C.; Amaral, A.P.; Oskouei, B.; Hu, M.-C.; Sloan, A.; Isakova, T.; Gutiérrez, O.M.; Aguillon-Prada, R.; Lincoln, J.; Hare, J.M.; et al. FGF23 induces left ventricular hypertrophy. *J. Clin. Invest.* **2011**, *121*, 4393–4408. [CrossRef]
51. Bergmann, M.W. WNT signaling in adult cardiac hypertrophy and remodeling: Lessons learned from cardiac development. *Circ. Res.* **2010**, *107*, 1198–1208. [CrossRef] [PubMed]
52. Yu, L.; Meng, W.; Ding, J.; Cheng, M. Klotho inhibits angiotensin II-induced cardiomyocyte hypertrophy through suppression of the AT1R/beta catenin pathway. *Biochem. Biophys. Res. Commun.* **2016**, *473*, 455–461. [CrossRef] [PubMed]
53. Milovanova, L.Y.; Dobrosmyslov, I.A.; Milovanov, Y.S.; Taranova, M.V.; Kozlov, V.V.; Milovanova, S.Y.; Kozevnikova, E.I. Fibroblast growth factor-23 (FGF-23) / soluble Klotho protein (sKlotho) / sclerostin glycoprotein ratio disturbance is a novel risk factor for cardiovascular complications in ESRD patients receiving treatment with regular hemodialysis or hemodiafiltration. *Ter. Arkh.* **2018**, *90*, 48–54. [CrossRef] [PubMed]
54. Li, L.; Zhao, Q.; Kong, W. Extracellular matrix remodeling and cardiac fibrosis. *Matrix Biol. J. Int. Soc. Matrix Biol.* **2018**, *68–69*, 490–506. [CrossRef]
55. Ye, B.; Ge, Y.; Perens, G.; Hong, L.; Xu, H.; Fishbein, M.C.; Li, F. Canonical Wnt/β-catenin signaling in epicardial fibrosis of failed pediatric heart allografts with diastolic dysfunction. *Cardiovasc. Pathol. Off. J. Soc. Cardiovasc. Pathol.* **2013**, *22*, 54–57. [CrossRef]
56. Działo, E.; Tkacz, K.; Błyszczuk, P. Crosstalk between the TGF-β and WNT signalling pathways during cardiac fibrogenesis. *Acta Biochim. Pol.* **2018**, *65*, 341–349. [CrossRef]
57. Akhmetshina, A.; Palumbo, K.; Dees, C.; Bergmann, C.; Venalis, P.; Zerr, P.; Horn, A.; Kireva, T.; Beyer, C.; Zwerina, J.; et al. Activation of canonical Wnt signalling is required for TGF-β-mediated fibrosis. *Nat. Commun.* **2012**, *3*, 735. [CrossRef]
58. Liu, Q.; Zhu, L.-J.; Waaga-Gasser, A.M.; Ding, Y.; Cao, M.; Jadhav, S.J.; Kirollos, S.; Shekar, P.S.; Padera, R.F.; Chang, Y.-C.; et al. The axis of local cardiac endogenous Klotho-TGF-β1-Wnt signaling mediates cardiac fibrosis in human. *J. Mol. Cell. Cardiol.* **2019**, *136*, 113–124. [CrossRef]

59. Doi, S.; Zou, Y.; Togao, O.; Pastor, J.V.; John, G.B.; Wang, L.; Shiizaki, K.; Gotschall, R.; Schiavi, S.; Yorioka, N.; et al. Klotho inhibits transforming growth factor-beta1 (TGF-beta1) signaling and suppresses renal fibrosis and cancer metastasis in mice. *J. Biol. Chem.* **2011**, *286*, 8655–8665. [CrossRef]
60. Hao, H.; Li, X.; Li, Q.; Lin, H.; Chen, Z.; Xie, J.; Xuan, W.; Liao, W.; Bin, J.; Huang, X.; et al. FGF23 promotes myocardial fibrosis in mice through activation of β-catenin. *Oncotarget* **2016**, *7*, 64649–64664. [CrossRef]
61. Schumacher, D.; Alampour-Rajabi, S.; Ponomariov, V.; Curaj, A.; Wu, Z.; Staudt, M.; Rusu, M.; Jankowski, V.; Marx, N.; Jankowski, J.; et al. Cardiac FGF23: New insights into the role and function of FGF23 after acute myocardial infarction. *Cardiovasc. Pathol. Off. J. Soc. Cardiovasc. Pathol.* **2019**, *40*, 47–54. [CrossRef] [PubMed]
62. Libby, P. Inflammation in atherosclerosis. *Nature* **2002**, *420*, 868–874. [CrossRef] [PubMed]
63. Christman, M.A.; Goetz, D.J.; Dickerson, E.; McCall, K.D.; Lewis, C.J.; Benencia, F.; Silver, M.J.; Kohn, L.D.; Malgor, R. Wnt5a is expressed in murine and human atherosclerotic lesions. *Am. J. Physiol. Heart Circ. Physiol.* **2008**, *294*, H2864–H2870. [CrossRef] [PubMed]
64. Moreno, J.A.; Izquierdo, M.C.; Sanchez-Niño, M.D.; Suárez-Alvarez, B.; Lopez-Larrea, C.; Jakubowski, A.; Blanco, J.; Ramirez, R.; Selgas, R.; Ruiz-Ortega, M.; et al. The inflammatory cytokines TWEAK and TNFα reduce renal klotho expression through NFκB. *J. Am. Soc. Nephrol. JASN* **2011**, *22*, 1315–1325. [CrossRef]
65. Yao, Y.; Wang, Y.; Zhang, Y.; Liu, C. Klotho ameliorates oxidized low density lipoprotein (ox-LDL)-induced oxidative stress via regulating LOX-1 and PI3K/Akt/eNOS pathways. *Lipids Health Dis.* **2017**, *16*, 77. [CrossRef]
66. Rodríguez-Ortiz, M.E.; Alcalá-Díaz, J.F.; Canalejo, A.; Torres-Peña, J.D.; Gómez-Delgado, F.; Muñoz-Castañeda, J.R.; Delgado-Lista, J.; Rodríguez, M.; López-Miranda, J.; Almadén, Y. Fibroblast growth factor 23 predicts carotid atherosclerosis in individuals without kidney disease. The CORDIOPREV study. *Eur. J. Intern. Med.* **2019**. [CrossRef]
67. Chen, A.; Sun, Y.; Cui, J.; Zhao, B.; Wang, H.; Chen, X.; Mao, Y. Associations of sclerostin with carotid artery atherosclerosis and all-cause mortality in Chinese patients undergoing maintenance hemodialysis. *BMC Nephrol.* **2018**, *19*, 264. [CrossRef]
68. London, G.M.; Marchais, S.J.; Guérin, A.P.; Métivier, F. Arteriosclerosis, vascular calcifications and cardiovascular disease in uremia. *Curr. Opin. Nephrol. Hypertens.* **2005**, *14*, 525–531. [CrossRef]
69. Shanahan, C.M.; Crouthamel, M.H.; Kapustin, A.; Giachelli, C.M. Arterial calcification in chronic kidney disease: Key roles for calcium and phosphate. *Circ. Res.* **2011**, *109*, 697–711. [CrossRef]
70. Cozzolino, M.; Dusso, A.S.; Slatopolsky, E. Role of calcium-phosphate product and bone-associated proteins on vascular calcification in renal failure. *J. Am. Soc. Nephrol.* **2001**, *12*, 2511–2516.
71. Montes de Oca, A.; Guerrero, F.; Martinez-Moreno, J.M.; Madueño, J.A.; Herencia, C.; Peralta, A.; Almaden, Y.; Lopez, I.; Aguilera-Tejero, E.; Gundlach, K.; et al. Magnesium inhibits Wnt/β-catenin activity and reverses the osteogenic transformation of vascular smooth muscle cells. *PLoS ONE* **2014**, *9*, e89525. [CrossRef] [PubMed]
72. Voelkl, J.; Lang, F.; Eckardt, K.-U.; Amann, K.; Kuro-O, M.; Pasch, A.; Pieske, B.; Alesutan, I. Signaling pathways involved in vascular smooth muscle cell calcification during hyperphosphatemia. *Cell. Mol. Life Sci. CMLS* **2019**, *76*, 2077–2091. [CrossRef] [PubMed]
73. Chen, T.; Mao, H.; Chen, C.; Wu, L.; Wang, N.; Zhao, X.; Qian, J.; Xing, C. The Role and Mechanism of α-Klotho in the Calcification of Rat Aortic Vascular Smooth Muscle Cells. Available online: https://www.hindawi.com/journals/bmri/2015/194362/abs/ (accessed on 2 January 2020).
74. Rodríguez-Ortiz, M.E.; Díaz-Tocados, J.M.; Muñoz-Castañeda, J.R.; Herencia, C.; Pineda, C.; Martínez-Moreno, J.M.; Montes de Oca, A.; López-Baltanás, R.; Alcalá-Díaz, J.; Ortiz, A.; et al. Inflammation both increases and causes resistance to FGF23 in normal and uremic rats. *Clin. Sci. Lond. Engl. 1979* **2020**, *134*, 15–32. [CrossRef] [PubMed]
75. Scialla, J.J.; Lau, W.L.; Reilly, M.P.; Isakova, T.; Yang, H.-Y.; Crouthamel, M.H.; Chavkin, N.W.; Rahman, M.; Wahl, P.; Amaral, A.P.; et al. Fibroblast growth factor 23 is not associated with and does not induce arterial calcification. *Kidney Int.* **2013**, *83*, 1159–1168. [CrossRef] [PubMed]
76. Zhu, D.; Mackenzie, N.C.W.; Millan, J.L.; Farquharson, C.; MacRae, V.E. A protective role for FGF-23 in local defence against disrupted arterial wall integrity? *Mol. Cell. Endocrinol.* **2013**, *372*, 1–11. [CrossRef]
77. Jimbo, R.; Kawakami-Mori, F.; Mu, S.; Hirohama, D.; Majtan, B.; Shimizu, Y.; Yatomi, Y.; Fukumoto, S.; Fujita, T.; Shimosawa, T. Fibroblast growth factor 23 accelerates phosphate-induced vascular calcification in the absence of Klotho deficiency. *Kidney Int.* **2014**, *85*, 1103–1111. [CrossRef]

78. Verkaik, M.; Juni, R.P.; van Loon, E.P.M.; van Poelgeest, E.M.; Kwekkeboom, R.F.J.; Gam, Z.; Richards, W.G.; Ter Wee, P.M.; Hoenderop, J.G.; Eringa, E.C.; et al. FGF23 impairs peripheral microvascular function in renal failure. *Am. J. Physiol. Heart Circ. Physiol.* **2018**, *315*, H1414–H1424. [CrossRef]
79. Evenepoel, P.; D'Haese, P.; Brandenburg, V. Sclerostin and DKK1: New players in renal bone and vascular disease. *Kidney Int.* **2015**, *88*, 235–240. [CrossRef]
80. Cejka, D.; Herberth, J.; Branscum, A.J.; Fardo, D.W.; Monier-Faugere, M.-C.; Diarra, D.; Haas, M.; Malluche, H.H. Sclerostin and Dickkopf-1 in renal osteodystrophy. *Clin. J. Am. Soc. Nephrol. CJASN* **2011**, *6*, 877–882. [CrossRef]
81. Behets, G.J.; Viaene, L.; Meijers, B.; Blocki, F.; Brandenburg, V.M.; Verhulst, A.; D'Haese, P.C.; Evenepoel, P. Circulating levels of sclerostin but not DKK1 associate with laboratory parameters of CKD-MBD. *PLoS ONE* **2017**, *12*, e0176411. [CrossRef]
82. Sabbagh, Y.; Graciolli, F.G.; O'Brien, S.; Tang, W.; dos Reis, L.M.; Ryan, S.; Phillips, L.; Boulanger, J.; Song, W.; Bracken, C.; et al. Repression of osteocyte Wnt/β-catenin signaling is an early event in the progression of renal osteodystrophy. *J. Bone Miner. Res. Off. J. Am. Soc. Bone Miner. Res.* **2012**, *27*, 1757–1772. [CrossRef] [PubMed]
83. Pelletier, S.; Dubourg, L.; Carlier, M.-C.; Hadj-Aissa, A.; Fouque, D. The relation between renal function and serum sclerostin in adult patients with CKD. *Clin. J. Am. Soc. Nephrol. CJASN* **2013**, *8*, 819–823. [CrossRef] [PubMed]
84. Cejka, D.; Jäger-Lansky, A.; Kieweg, H.; Weber, M.; Bieglmayer, C.; Haider, D.G.; Diarra, D.; Patsch, J.M.; Kainberger, F.; Bohle, B.; et al. Sclerostin serum levels correlate positively with bone mineral density and microarchitecture in haemodialysis patients. *Nephrol. Dial. Transplant. Off. Publ. Eur. Dial. Transpl. Assoc. Eur. Ren. Assoc.* **2012**, *27*, 226–230. [CrossRef] [PubMed]
85. Moe, S.M.; Chen, N.X.; Newman, C.L.; Organ, J.M.; Kneissel, M.; Kramer, I.; Gattone, V.H.; Allen, M.R. Anti-sclerostin antibody treatment in a rat model of progressive renal osteodystrophy. *J. Bone Miner. Res. Off. J. Am. Soc. Bone Miner. Res.* **2015**, *30*, 499–509. [CrossRef] [PubMed]
86. Carrillo-López, N.; Panizo, S.; Alonso-Montes, C.; Román-García, P.; Rodríguez, I.; Martínez-Salgado, C.; Dusso, A.S.; Naves, M.; Cannata-Andía, J.B. Direct inhibition of osteoblastic Wnt pathway by fibroblast growth factor 23 contributes to bone loss in chronic kidney disease. *Kidney Int* **2016**, *90*, 77–89. [CrossRef]
87. Fayed, A.; Elgohary, R.; Fawzy, M. Evaluating the role of serum sclerostin as an indicator of activity and damage in Egyptian patients with rheumatoid arthritis: University hospital experience. *Clin. Rheumatol.* **2019**. [CrossRef]
88. Raimann, A.; Ertl, D.A.; Helmreich, M.; Sagmeister, S.; Egerbacher, M.; Haeusler, G. Fibroblast growth factor 23 and Klotho are present in the growth plate. *Connect. Tissue Res.* **2013**, *54*, 108–117. [CrossRef]
89. Yuan, Q.; Sato, T.; Densmore, M.; Saito, H.; Schüler, C.; Erben, R.G.; Lanske, B. Deletion of PTH rescues skeletal abnormalities and high osteopontin levels in Klotho-/- mice. *PLoS Genet.* **2012**, *8*, e1002726. [CrossRef]
90. Ma, L.; Gao, M.; Wu, L.; Zhao, X.; Mao, H.; Xing, C. The suppressive effect of soluble Klotho on fibroblastic growth factor 23 synthesis in UMR-106 osteoblast-like cells. *Cell Biol. Int.* **2018**, *42*, 1270–1274. [CrossRef]
91. Zhang, W.; Xue, D.; Hu, D.; Xie, T.; Tao, Y.; Zhu, T.; Chen, E.; Pan, Z. Secreted klotho protein attenuates osteogenic differentiation of human bone marrow mesenchymal stem cells in vitro via inactivation of the FGFR1/ERK signaling pathway. *Growth Factors Chur Switz.* **2015**, *33*, 356–365. [CrossRef]
92. Shalhoub, V.; Ward, S.C.; Sun, B.; Stevens, J.; Renshaw, L.; Hawkins, N.; Richards, W.G. Fibroblast growth factor 23 (FGF23) and alpha-klotho stimulate osteoblastic MC3T3.E1 cell proliferation and inhibit mineralization. *Calcif. Tissue Int.* **2011**, *89*, 140–150. [CrossRef] [PubMed]
93. Haffner, D.; Leifheit-Nestler, M. Extrarenal effects of FGF23. *Pediatr. Nephrol.* **2017**, *32*, 753–765. [CrossRef] [PubMed]
94. Richter, B.; Faul, C. FGF23 Actions on Target Tissues—With and Without Klotho. *Front. Endocrinol.* **2018**, *9*, 189. [CrossRef] [PubMed]
95. Shardell, M.; Semba, R.D.; Rosano, C.; Kalyani, R.R.; Bandinelli, S.; Chia, C.W.; Ferrucci, L. Plasma Klotho and Cognitive Decline in Older Adults: Findings From the InCHIANTI Study. *J. Gerontol. A. Biol. Sci. Med. Sci.* **2016**, *71*, 677–682. [CrossRef]
96. Semba, R.D.; Moghekar, A.R.; Hu, J.; Sun, K.; Turner, R.; Ferrucci, L.; O'Brien, R. Klotho in the cerebrospinal fluid of adults with and without Alzheimer's disease. *Neurosci. Lett.* **2014**, *558*, 37–40. [CrossRef]

97. Ullah, M.; Sun, Z. Klotho Deficiency Accelerates Stem Cells Aging by Impairing Telomerase Activity. *J. Gerontol. Ser. A* **2019**, *74*, 1396–1407. [CrossRef]
98. Kuro-o, M. Klotho and aging. *Biochim. Biophys. Acta BBA Gen. Subj.* **2009**, *1790*, 1049–1058. [CrossRef]
99. Li, D.; Jing, D.; Liu, Z.; Chen, Y.; Huang, F.; Behnisch, T. Enhanced Expression of Secreted α-Klotho in the Hippocampus Alters Nesting Behavior and Memory Formation in Mice. *Front. Cell. Neurosci.* **2019**, *13*, 133. [CrossRef]
100. Massó, A.; Sánchez, A.; Bosch, A.; Giménez-Llort, L.; Chillón, M. Secreted αKlotho isoform protects against age-dependent memory deficits. *Mol. Psychiatry* **2018**, *23*, 1937–1947. [CrossRef]
101. Abraham, C.R.; Mullen, P.C.; Tucker-Zhou, T.; Chen, C.D.; Zeldich, E. Klotho Is a Neuroprotective and Cognition-Enhancing Protein. In *Vitamins & Hormones*; Elsevier: Amsterdam, The Netherlands, 2016; Volume 101, pp. 215–238. ISBN 978-0-12-804819-1.
102. Barnes, J.W.; Duncan, D.; Helton, S.; Hutcheson, S.; Kurundkar, D.; Logsdon, N.J.; Locy, M.; Garth, J.; Denson, R.; Farver, C.; et al. Role of fibroblast growth factor 23 and klotho cross talk in idiopathic pulmonary fibrosis. *Am. J. Physiol. Lung Cell. Mol. Physiol.* **2019**, *317*, L141–L154. [CrossRef]
103. Buendia-Roldan, I.; Machuca, N.; Mejía, M.; Maldonado, M.; Pardo, A.; Selman, M. Lower levels of α-Klotho in serum are associated with decreased lung function in individuals with interstitial lung abnormalities. *Sci. Rep.* **2019**, *9*, 10801. [CrossRef] [PubMed]
104. Gao, W.; Yuan, C.; Zhang, J.; Li, L.; Yu, L.; Wiegman, C.H.; Barnes, P.J.; Adcock, I.M.; Huang, M.; Yao, X. Klotho expression is reduced in COPD airway epithelial cells: Effects on inflammation and oxidant injury. *Clin. Sci. Lond. Engl. 1979* **2015**, *129*, 1011–1023. [CrossRef] [PubMed]
105. Krick, S.; Grabner, A.; Baumlin, N.; Yanucil, C.; Helton, S.; Grosche, A.; Sailland, J.; Geraghty, P.; Viera, L.; Russell, D.W.; et al. Fibroblast growth factor 23 and Klotho contribute to airway inflammation. *Eur. Respir. J.* **2018**, *52*. [CrossRef] [PubMed]
106. Baarsma, H.A.; Skronska-Wasek, W.; Mutze, K.; Ciolek, F.; Wagner, D.E.; John-Schuster, G.; Heinzelmann, K.; Günther, A.; Bracke, K.R.; Dagouassat, M.; et al. Noncanonical WNT-5A signaling impairs endogenous lung repair in COPD. *J. Exp. Med.* **2017**, *214*, 143–163. [CrossRef]
107. Kumawat, K.; Gosens, R. WNT-5A: Signaling and functions in health and disease. *Cell. Mol. Life Sci. CMLS* **2016**, *73*, 567–587. [CrossRef]
108. Singh, S.; Grabner, A.; Yanucil, C.; Schramm, K.; Czaya, B.; Krick, S.; Czaja, M.J.; Bartz, R.; Abraham, R.; Di Marco, G.S.; et al. Fibroblast growth factor 23 directly targets hepatocytes to promote inflammation in chronic kidney disease. *Kidney Int.* **2016**, *90*, 985–996. [CrossRef]
109. Perugorria, M.J.; Olaizola, P.; Labiano, I.; Esparza-Baquer, A.; Marzioni, M.; Marin, J.J.G.; Bujanda, L.; Banales, J.M. Wnt–β-catenin signalling in liver development, health and disease. *Nat. Rev. Gastroenterol. Hepatol.* **2019**, *16*, 121–136. [CrossRef]
110. Rao, Z.; Landry, T.; Li, P.; Bunner, W.; Laing, B.T.; Yuan, Y.; Huang, H. Administration of alpha klotho reduces liver and adipose lipid accumulation in obese mice. *Heliyon* **2019**, *5*, e01494. [CrossRef]
111. Somm, E.; Henry, H.; Bruce, S.J.; Bonnet, N.; Montandon, S.A.; Niederländer, N.J.; Messina, A.; Aeby, S.; Rosikiewicz, M.; Fajas, L.; et al. β-Klotho deficiency shifts the gut-liver bile acid axis and induces hepatic alterations in mice. *Am. J. Physiol. Endocrinol. Metab.* **2018**, *315*, E833–E847. [CrossRef]
112. Beljaars, L.; Daliri, S.; Dijkhuizen, C.; Poelstra, K.; Gosens, R. WNT-5A regulates TGF-β-related activities in liver fibrosis. *Am. J. Physiol. Gastrointest. Liver Physiol.* **2017**, *312*, G219–G227. [CrossRef]

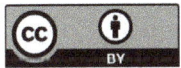

© 2020 by the authors. Licensee MDPI, Basel, Switzerland. This article is an open access article distributed under the terms and conditions of the Creative Commons Attribution (CC BY) license (http://creativecommons.org/licenses/by/4.0/).

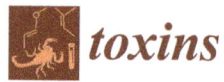

Review

Parathyroid Hormone: A Uremic Toxin

Eduardo J. Duque [1], Rosilene M. Elias [1,2] and Rosa M. A. Moysés [1,*]

1. LIM 16, Nephrology Department, Hospital das Clínicas HCFMUSP, Universidade de São Paulo, São Paulo 05403-000, Brazil; eduardojorgeduque@gmail.com (E.J.D.); rosilenemotta@hotmail.com (R.M.E.)
2. Post-Graduation, Universidade Nove de Julho (UNINOVE), São Paulo 01525-000, Brazil
* Correspondence: rosa.moyses@uol.com.br

Received: 31 January 2020; Accepted: 8 March 2020; Published: 17 March 2020

Abstract: Parathyroid hormone (PTH) has an important role in the maintenance of serum calcium levels. It activates renal 1α-hydroxylase and increases the synthesis of the active form of vitamin D (1,25[OH]$_2$D$_3$). PTH promotes calcium release from the bone and enhances tubular calcium resorption through direct action on these sites. Hallmarks of secondary hyperparathyroidism associated with chronic kidney disease (CKD) include increase in serum fibroblast growth factor 23 (FGF-23), reduction in renal 1,25[OH]$_2$D$_3$ production with a decline in its serum levels, decrease in intestinal calcium absorption, and, at later stages, hyperphosphatemia and high levels of PTH. In this paper, we aim to critically discuss severe CKD-related hyperparathyroidism, in which PTH, through calcium-dependent and -independent mechanisms, leads to harmful effects and manifestations of the uremic syndrome, such as bone loss, skin and soft tissue calcification, cardiomyopathy, immunodeficiency, impairment of erythropoiesis, increase of energy expenditure, and muscle weakness.

Keywords: parathyroid hormone; secondary hyperparathyroidism; uremic toxin

Key Contribution: Secondary hyperparathyroidism is a serious and common complication of CKD; with a negative impact on morbidity and mortality of patients on dialysis. Persistent high levels of PTH cause abnormalities in the cellular function of different target organs; contributing to several findings of the uremic syndrome.

---

1. Introduction

Parathyroid hormone (PTH) is a 9400 D molecular weight peptide, containing 84 amino acids that are secreted after cleavage from preproparathyroid hormone (115 amino acids) to proparathyroid hormone (90 amino acids). The active biological form is the intact PTH (1–84), whose half-life in the circulation is less than three minutes, and which clearance occurs mainly in the liver (60%–70%) and kidney (20%–30%) [1].

The secretion of PTH is regulated by changes of extracellular calcium through a feedback mainly mediated by the calcium-sensing receptor (CaSR). This receptor, a G protein-coupled receptor on parathyroid cells, regulates calcium-influenced PTH secretion [2]. A reduction of ionized calcium stimulates the PTH secretion, whereas high levels suppress the PTH release and enhance calcitonin secretion.

The effects of PTH are summarized in Figure 1. In renal proximal tubular cells, PTH inhibits phosphate reabsorption and upregulates the 1α-hydroxylase gene, responsible for conversion of 25-hydroxyvitamin D to the active metabolite 1,25-dihydroxyvitamin D (1,25[OH]$_2$D$_3$). It also increases calcium reabsorption by inserting calcium channels in the apical membrane of distal tubules and stimulating basolateral sodium-calcium transporters [3].

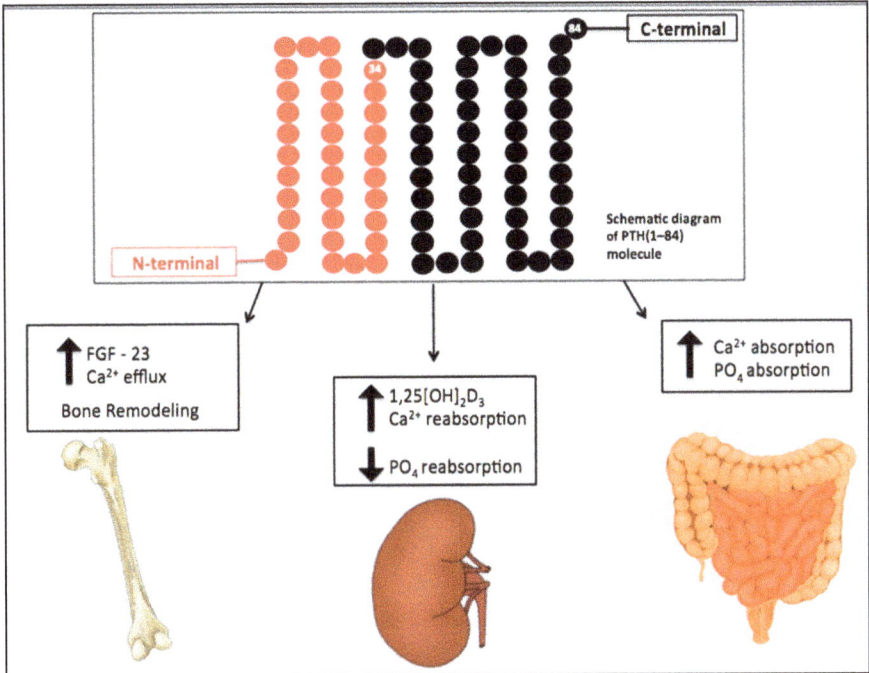

Figure 1. Physiological actions of parathyroid hormone (PTH). PTH plays a key role in the maintenance of calcium levels. It stimulates bone turnover and calcium release from the skeleton. In renal tubular cells, PTH increases calcium reabsorption, inhibits phosphate reabsorption, and upregulates the 1α-hydroxylase gene, responsible for conversion of 25-hydroxyvitamin D to the active metabolite, $1,25[OH]_2D_3$. It also enhances calcium and phosphate intestinal absorption by increasing the production of activated vitamin D. Down arrow = decrease, Up arrow = increase.

In bone tissue, PTH influences gene expression in osteoblasts, supporting the synthesis of proteins required for bone formation and osteoclast differentiation. Intermittent exposure to PTH is antiosteoporotic and osteoanabolic via stimulation of bone formation, which is mediated by Wnt signaling activation. Upon binding to the frizzled receptor and co-receptors, LRP5 and LRP6, Wnt activates a signaling pathway, leading to translocation of beta-catenin into the nucleus, specific gene expression, protein synthesis, and bone formation. Extracellular regulators of Wnt signaling include dickkopf 1 and sclerostin, a product of the *SOST* gene expressed by osteocytes that inhibits Wnt signaling [4,5]. PTH inhibits sclerostin and, therefore, stimulates bone formation.

Continuous exposure to PTH increases osteoclast activity, causing osteoporotic changes [6], mostly mediated by enhancing the production of RANKL (receptor activator of nuclear factor-κB ligand) and decreasing the production of osteoprotegerin (OPG), a natural decoy of RANKL, by osteoblasts and stromal cell. By binding to RANK (receptor activator of nuclear factor-κB), a member of the tumor necrosis factor family expressed by osteoclasts and their precursors, RANKL controls the differentiation, proliferation, and survival of osteoclasts [7]. As a result, continuous exposure to high levels of PTH causes bone loss, whereas intermittent exposure leads to bone mass gain.

2. CKD-Associated Secondary Hyperparathyroidism

Chronic kidney disease-mineral and bone disorder (CKD-MBD) involves a broad systemic disorder manifested in uremic patients by disturbances in mineral and bone metabolism and extraosseous calcification [8]. This syndrome comprises one or a combination of the following conditions: vascular or other soft tissue calcification, vitamin D deficiency, abnormalities in bone turnover, abnormal metabolism of calcium and phosphate, an increase of levels of fibroblast growth factor- 23 (FGF-23) and PTH.

The earliest abnormality that occurs with impaired kidney function is an increase in the level of FGF-23, a member of the family of the fibroblast growth factors which acts on phosphorus (P) metabolism. High FGF-23 results in increased phosphaturia, by inhibition of sodium-dependent P reabsorption (Na-P co-transporters IIa and IIc) [9], and deficiency of activated vitamin D, by inhibition of 1α hydroxylase [10]. For FGF-23 to exert its phosphaturic effect through FGF receptor, the klotho protein, expressed in the renal proximal tubules and parathyroid gland, is required as a cofactor. CKD progression is associated with a significant decrease in the expression of klotho, which causes high circulating levels of phosphate and vascular calcification in mice with CKD [11]. In addition, production of kidney calcitriol, the active form of vitamin D, decreases as CKD progresses. In normal conditions, calcitriol promotes intestinal absorption of calcium and phosphorus, and decreases the synthesis of PTH by binding to the vitamin D receptor (VDR) in the nucleus of the parathyroid cell. Therefore, calcitriol reduction allows an increase in the transcription of the PTH gene. Indirectly, it also stimulates PTH secretion due to a decrease in intestinal calcium absorption. Since parathyroid glands express FGF receptors and klotho [12], another mechanism regulating PTH secretion involves FGF-23, by reducing PTH mRNA through Klotho-dependent and Klotho-independent pathways [13]. However, as FGF-23 also inhibits the activity of 1α-hydroxylase, sustained high levels of FGF-23 are associated with an increase in PTH [10]. Calcitriol deficiency also influences the parathyroid set point for calcium-regulated PTH secretion and, possibly, decreases the expression of vitamin D and calcium receptors. Higher concentrations of calcium are needed to reduce PTH release in vitro from the parathyroid of uremic patients compared with healthy controls. Thus, renal klotho loss, hyperphosphatemia, vitamin D deficiency, and an increase in FGF-23 [12] are pathogenic mechanisms of hyperparathyroidism progression (Figure 2).

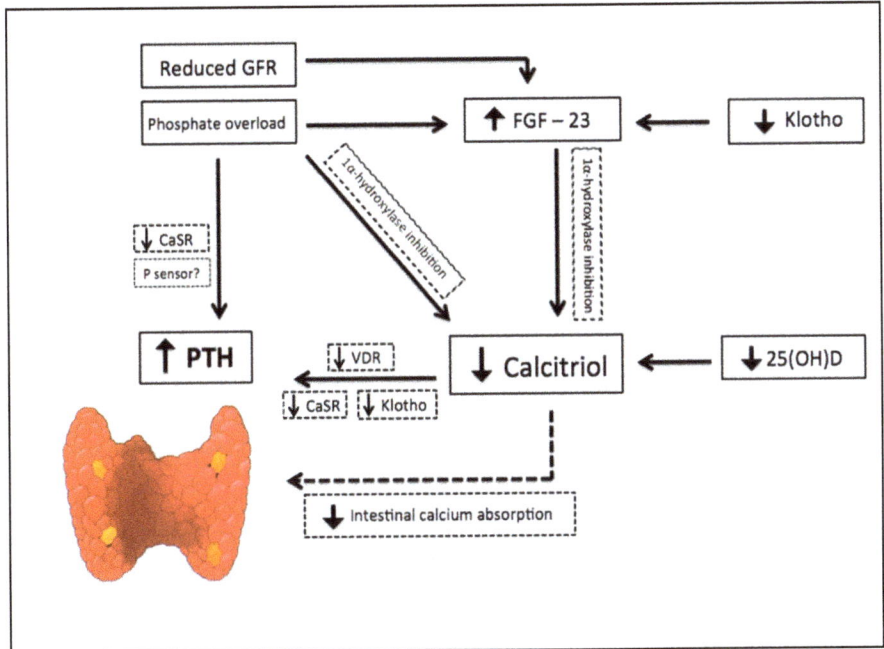

Figure 2. Pathogenic mechanisms of hyperparathyroidism progression in Chronic Kidney Disease (CKD). CKD progression is associated with phosphate overload, high levels of fibroblast growth factor- 23 (FGF-23), significant decrease in the expression of klotho, and a reduction of renal calcitriol production. Calcitriol deficiency influences parathyroid set point for calcium-regulated PTH secretion and decreases the expression of vitamin D and calcium receptors. Indirectly, calcitriol deficiency also stimulates PTH secretion due to a decrease in intestinal calcium absorption. Down arrow = decrease, Up arrow = increase.

Secondary hyperparathyroidism (sHPT) is often observed in patients with CKD, mainly in those requiring dialysis therapy. PTH starts to rise when the estimated glomerular filtration rate (eGFR) drops to approximately 50 mL/min/1.73 m^2. Further decline of renal function results in skeletal resistance to PTH, abnormal parathyroid growth and function. Persistent high levels of PTH generate an increase in FGF-23 expression and CKD osteodystrophy, favoring high bone turnover. This condition increases bone fragility, which may explain, at least in part, the association between sHPT and increased fracture risk. Furthermore, sHPT causes hyperphosphatemia, vascular and tissue calcification, anemia (by erythropoiesis impairment), and worse quality of life. The Dialysis Outcomes and Practice Patterns Study (DOPPS) has denoted that serum PTH higher than 600 pg/mL (63 pmol/L) is associated with a 21% increase in all-cause mortality risk [14].

Increased levels of FGF-23 and sHPT are closely related in the CKD setting. Whereas PTH acts directly on osteocytes to increase the FGF-23 expression, the FGF-23-receptor complex is downregulated in parathyroid glands, resulting in a loss of the ability of FGF-23 to decrease PTH expression. Moreover, as mentioned before, FGF-23 acts in the kidney by decreasing 1,25[OH]$_2$D$_3$ synthesis, and therefore contributing to enhance PTH levels.

Hyperphosphatemia has been recognized as an important player in the pathogenesis of sHPT [15]. Phosphate retention directly impairs renal 1α-hydroxylase activity, decreases 1,25[OH]$_2$D$_3$ synthesis, and affects posttranscriptional events that ultimately influence PTH mRNA stability and hormone synthesis. As CKD progresses, high phosphate levels influence the expression of factors involved in cell cycle regulation and parathyroid cell proliferation [16], and promote resistance to the actions of calcitriol in the parathyroid glands. High phosphate levels induce progression of sHPT and resistance to the effects of PTH in the bone. Moreover, it has been recently shown that phosphate at high concentrations acts as a noncompetitive antagonist of the CaSR, resulting in an increase of PTH secretion [17]. However, we should keep in mind that not only phosphate but other uremic toxins, such as indoxyl sulfate, are known to interfere with vitamin D metabolism and promote sHPT progression [18], as well as bone resistance to PTH.

Therapeutic arsenal for the treatment of sHPT includes calcitriol and vitamin D analogs, calcimimetics, and phosphate binders. Parathyroidectomy (PTX) is the surgical treatment indicated for cases with refractory hypercalcemia/hyperphosphatemia and severe symptoms such as extra skeletal calcification/calciphylaxis, intractable pruritus, and bone pain.

3. Effects of sHPT on BONE

Chronic PTH excess and bone resorption markers are associated with abnormal cortical and trabecular density, and fractures [19]. Cortical bone contributes to the mechanical strength of the skeleton, and this compartment is more adversely affected by hyperparathyroidism than the trabecular bone [20,21]. A histomorphometric evaluation in primary hyperparathyroidism has depicted that PTH promotes periosteal resorption and intracortical porosity [22].

A longitudinal study of 53 patients with stages 2 to 5 CKD, including those on dialysis, has shown that hyperparathyroidism and high serum concentration of bone turnover markers were associated with significant cortical loss, detected by dual-energy X-ray absorptiometry and high-resolution peripheral quantitative computed tomography [23]. The association of high levels of PTH and cortical porosity was also shown in dialysis patients [20]. In a post hoc analysis of the BRIC study, we observed an increased cortical porosity, evaluated through bone histomorphometry, which was associated with PTH levels, but not with the trabecular bone turnover [20].

In contrast to this effect in the cortical compartment, chronic excess of PTH might act as an anabolic agent for trabecular bone, increasing trabecular number and thickness [24]. Mice with prenatal conditional ablation of the PTH receptor (PTHR) by homologous recombination exhibit decreased trabecular bone compartment and increased thickness of cortical bone during fetal development [25].

Beyond consequences of PTH excess, the association between low levels of PTH and fractures is also a matter of debate. A U-shaped relationship between PTH and vertebral fractures has been shown in dialysis patients [26]. Moreover, Coco et al. [27] demonstrated a higher risk of hip fracture in patients on dialysis with lower PTH (around 195 pg/mL), and Iimori et al. [28] confirmed a high risk of fracture in patients with PTH levels below 150 pg/mL. However, according to Danese et al. [29], the risks for hip and vertebral fracture are weakly associated with PTH levels among patients on dialysis, with the lowest risk observed around a PTH concentration of 300 pg/mL.

Skeletal resistance to the PTH calcemic regulation further compromises the ability to maintain calcium levels in patients with advanced renal disease [30]. This resistance is not restricted to the effects of PTH on calcium release from the skeleton, but also involves the action of the hormone on the response of the bone cells [31]. We and others have shown increased bone expression of sclerostin in CKD patients [32,33], suggesting that this Wnt pathway inhibitor is related to the bone resistance to PTH. As a consequence, high serum PTH levels are needed to induce equivalent biologic responses in patients with CKD. Albeit some studies have described a down-regulation of PTHR in the context of CKD [34], we showed higher expression of PTHR1 in the osteocytes, mostly in earlier CKD stages [32]. However, this receptor activity was not evaluated in the mentioned study, and the current belief is that the PTHR activity might be compromised.

Some studies suggest that the transforming growth factor β (TGF-β) has a role in bone remodeling, regulating the recruitment of osteoclasts and osteoblasts. Downregulation of hormones and cytokines, such as IGF-1, IL-11, and TGF-β1, may be associated with age-related bone loss [35]. In vitro studies have shown that TGF-β increases the synthesis of bone proteins by osteoblastic cells [36], and local injection of TGF-β under the periosteum stimulates bone formation [37]. In contrast, transgenic mice overexpressing osteoblast-specific truncated TGF-β receptor present an increase in trabecular bone mass and a decrease in bone remodeling [38]. Furthermore, mice with knockout of the osteoblast TGF-β receptor develop a decrease in cortical bone and an increase in trabecular compartment, which is similar to the phenotype of animals expressing an active PTHR [39]. Thus, due to its dual effect, a fine balance of TGF-β production is required to prevent bone loss.

Pieces of evidence indicate that PTH and TGF-β operate together to exert their biological activities in the bone. Higher expression of TGF-β protein has been noted in high-turnover bones of patients with end-stage renal disease. In uremic animals, renal FGF-23 expression correlates with local TGF-β expression [40]. Patients with renal osteodystrophy have significantly higher levels of TGF-β than those without this condition [41]. Indeed, Santos et al. [42] demonstrated a significant high TGF-β expression in bone of patients with sHPT, which has improved after PTX.

PTH receptors are present in tissues unrelated to calcium homeostasis [43], but little is known about PTHR downregulation in the CKD context. Therefore, it is unknown whether PTH excessive levels, required to keep trabecular bone remodeling, might contribute to deleterious actions on nonclassical target organs.

4. Effects of sHPT on Cardiovascular System

sHPT promotes cardiovascular disease, regardless of calcium or phosphate levels [44]. There is some evidence of a correlation between serum levels of PTH and hypertension [45]. A study with 1784 individuals with mild renal dysfunction or normal eGFR followed for seven years revealed that PTH levels were able to predict hypertension in men, even after adjustments for age, smoking, and body mass index [46]. In addition, a meta-analysis with six prospective cohort studies, involving a total of 18,994 participants, showed that increased levels of PTH may be associated with a higher risk of hypertension [47]. Despite the evidence linking PTH with hypertension, the unanswered question is whether this relationship is causal. In particular, changes in systemic calcium metabolism are thought to play an important role in the regulation of blood pressure. Leiba et al. [48] have described some cases of hypertensive end-stage renal disease patients, who had a sudden drop in blood pressure after PTX. Heyliger et al. [49] documented a significant decrease in both systolic and diastolic blood pressure in 147 patients with hypertension undergoing PTX.

Parathyroid hyperfunction is associated with endothelial dysfunction and myocardial hypertrophy. In experimental studies using a rat model of CKD (5/6 nephrectomy) submitted to PTX, the continuous infusion of supraphysiological rates of 1–34 PTH was associated with myocardial hypertrophy and fibrosis along with a high myocardial expression of oxidative stress and inflammation markers [50]. There is an association between PTH levels, myocardial hypertrophy, and mortality, in patients with sHPT and in individuals from the general population [51]. An analysis with 2040 individuals has found that in women under 60 years and men over 59 years, PTH was a significant predictor of left ventricular hypertrophy [51].

PTH stimulation on cardiomyocytes promotes an increase in synthesis and expression of fetal-type proteins via activation of protein kinase C and affects contractile function by inhibiting β-adrenoceptor-mediated effects through the same pathway [52]. Therefore, this effect of PTH might suppress cardiomyocyte contractility.

Besides the aforementioned effect on cardiomyocytes, PTH acts on cardiac fibroblasts, inducing cardiac fibrosis in uremia [53]. As a promoter of fibroblast proliferation, TGF-β also generates cardiac fibrosis, as well as cardiomyocyte apoptosis and cardiac hypertrophy [54]. Beyond its role in bone turnover, PTH may mediate cardiovascular fibrosis and apoptosis through the TGF-β signaling pathway.

PTH might indirectly induce myocardial hypertrophy by increasing FGF-23 synthesis. High levels of FGF-23 have also been linked to left ventricular hypertrophy and mortality in patients with CKD. According to Gutierrez et al. [55], high levels of FGF-23 were independently associated with left ventricular hypertrophy in a group of 162 patients with CKD, not on dialysis. Furthermore, an experimental study has shown a direct effect of FGF-23 on myocardial hypertrophy [56].

CKD is associated with a high prevalence of arteriosclerosis or stiffening of the arteries independently of the presence of significant atherosclerosis. Calcification of the intimal and medial layers of vessels has an important role for arterial stiffening, and it is a key feature of the arterial disease in the kidney disease setting. Elevations in serum phosphate, calcium, and calcium-phosphate product, among other factors, are intimately involved in promoting calcification. Vascular calcification has been frequently documented in primary hyperparathyroidism and sHPT, although its pathophysiology is still a matter of debate. The question is whether there is a direct deleterious effect of PTH on vessels. An experimental study has shown that exposure of vascular endothelial cells to PTH led to decreased expression of the mRNA of OPG, a known protection factor of endothelial tissue [57]. However, the administration of 1–34 PTH to young mice has attenuated the progression of aortic valve calcification in a model of CKD [58]. Therefore, the association of long-term exposure of high PTH levels with vascular and valvular calcification [59] is probably explained by the large supply of calcium and phosphate from high bone turnover [60]. Indeed, sHPT is associated with an increased risk of calcific uremic arteriolopathy, also known as calciphylaxis. Elevations in phosphate and calcium levels compromise the vasculature, resulting in ischemic changes and plaque-like lesions that progress to painful skin lesions [61]. The prognosis of this condition is poor, and patients' survival generally reaches one year, in the best scenario [62].

In summary, although the role of PTH in mediating the RANK/RANKL/OPG axis in skeletal and extraskeletal calcification [63] has not yet been elucidated, this hormone should be included in the list of mediators of the bone–vascular interaction.

5. Effects of sHPT on CKD Progression

A recent meta-analysis suggests an independent association between serum phosphate levels, kidney failure, and mortality among patients with CKD not requiring dialysis [64]. Increased levels of phosphate may lead to tubular injury, interstitial fibrosis, endothelial dysfunction, and vascular calcification via phosphate or calcium-phosphate crystals [65].

A retrospective cohort study with 13,772 incident patients on hemodialysis has revealed an association between the decline of residual kidney function and abnormalities of MBD, such as high levels of phosphate, intact PTH, alkaline phosphatase, and low levels of calcium [66]. It has also been shown that diabetic predialysis CKD patients with sHPT usually require greater healthcare resource utilization and experience a faster kidney disease progression with a higher risk of dialysis initiation or death when compared with predialysis diabetic patients with CKD but without sHPT [67].

6. Effects of sHPT on CKD-Related Caquexia and Energy Expenditure

Muscle weakness is another condition possibly associated with hyperparathyroidism in patients with CKD, whose physiologic basis is not completely understood. Some studies using muscle biopsies of patients with CKD have revealed a decrease in muscle mitochondrial oxidative enzymes, such as citrate synthase and cytochrome c oxidase, and a decrease in the synthesis of contractile muscle proteins, myosin heavy chain, and mitochondrial proteins [68].

The diagnosis of uremic myopathy is based on clinical features and a multifactorial origin, caused by physical inactivity, reduced protein intake, immunological and myocellular alterations, inflammation, metabolic acidosis, abnormalities in insulin-like growth factor, and myostatin expression. Most of these mechanisms stimulate the ATP-dependent ubiquitin-proteosome system (UPS), one of the most important intracellular proteolysis pathways [69]. In addition, vitamin D deficiency is also recognized as a risk factor for CKD-related myopathy [70].

Experimental evidence supports the toxic effect of PTH on muscles. Animals exposed to high doses of PTH for four days showed muscle dysfunction, including a reduction of mitochondrial activity and a decrease in high-energy phosphate [71]. Gomez-Fernandez et al. [72] have described the weakness of the respiratory muscles in correlation with PTH levels.

Weight loss, a common feature of advanced CKD, might be related to the excess of PTH levels. CKD patients with sHPT who undergo PTX present, in general, a significant magnitude of weight gain (more than 5% above the baseline) [73]. Interestingly, patients undergoing dialysis with sHPT present an increase of resting energy expenditure that reduces significantly six months after PTX [74].

Kir et al. [75] uncovered evidence that PTH and PTH-related protein (PTHrP) signal, through the same receptor, work as potential mediators of body weight loss, in association with browning of adipose tissue and loss of muscle mass. They observed that injection of cancer cells into mice was responsible for increased concentration of PTHrP, with capacity to activate the uncoupling protein-1, inducing "browning" of white adipose tissue and energy generation. The pathway to browning includes PTH/PTHrP activation of protein kinase A and loss of muscle mass via the UPS. Deletion of PTHR abrogates the muscle atrophy and changes the regulation of thermogenic genes in mice with 5/6 nephrectomy.

This finding revealed that the deletion of PTHR in animal models acts as a critical factor for resistance to the development of sarcopenia. A higher concentration of brown adipose tissue might be an important factor associated with muscle wasting in CKD by increasing energy expenditure.

7. Effect of sHPT on Glucose Metabolism

Glucose intolerance is another condition associated with uremia, possibly due to decreased insulin secretion. Some evidence suggests that PTH has a role in this event since insulin resistance has been noted in patients with primary hyperparathyroidism [76]. There is, however, no convincing evidence of such effect in uremia.

Experimental studies in uremic animals have demonstrated an action of PTH on protein kinase C promoting an increase of cytosolic calcium in pancreatic islets. Excess PTH may interfere with the ability of the beta-cells to augment insulin secretion appropriately, affecting insulin secretion by calcium-dependent mechanisms [77]. Ahamed et al. [78] have documented a negative correlation between PTH and fasting insulin in uremic patients. Patients with severe hyperparathyroidism had relatively more impairment of pancreatic beta-cell function in comparison with those with mild hyperparathyroidism, and an intravenous dose of 1-cholecalciferol has been associated with an improvement of beta-cell function.

Mak et al. [79] have shown that patients on dialysis with 1,25-$(OH)_2D_3$ deficiency and sHPT were glucose-intolerant and insulin-resistant. After intravenous administration of 1,25-$(OH)_2D_3$, there was an increase of insulin secretion and an improvement of glucose tolerance. These events occurred without any change in serum PTH concentration. An improvement of glucose tolerance and insulin secretion has been described in children with uremia after handling sHPT markers, by phosphate restriction and oral phosphate binders [80]. Therefore, changes in metabolism could be explained by a reduction of PTH, phosphate and/or FGF-23 levels, as well as by normalization of serum calcitriol.

However, some studies have shown that the undercarboxylated form of osteocalcin, an osteoblast-specific protein, is associated with energy metabolism regulation [81]. Infusion of undercarboxylated osteocalcin improves glucose tolerance and insulin resistance in mice with insulin receptor deletion [82]. In sHPT, there is a PTH-mediated increase of carboxylated and undercarboxylated osteocalcin, which might lead to an increase in insulin sensitivity and energy expenditure [83]. Thus, these conflicting actions of PTH on glucose metabolism should be addressed in future studies.

8. Effect of sHPT on Central Nervous System

Toxic effects of PTH on the central nervous system have been suggested. The mechanism might involve an increase of levels of cytosolic calcium in brain synaptic terminals since the removal of parathyroid is capable to prevent an excess of calcium in uremic brains [84]. Guisado et al. [85] have shown a correlation between changes in the electroencephalogram (EEG), similar to those presented in the chronic uremia context, with the increase of brain calcium content. Furthermore, PTX before uremia induction prevented EEG abnormalities, whereas the administration of parathyroid extracts to healthy animals induced EEG changes similar to those observed in uremic animals.

It has also been suggested a harmful effect of PTH on cognitive function in CKD patients. However, there is still weak support due to the lack of research in this area [86].

9. Effect of sHPT on Hematopoietic and Immunological System

Hyperparathyroidism aggravates hematopoietic dysfunction [87], inhibiting erythropoiesis, accelerating erythrocyte sedimentation rate, and increasing osmotic fragility of erythrocytes through Ca-ATPase stimulation [88]. Elevated levels of PTH cause fibrosis of bone marrow [89], related to the synergism between FGF and TGF-β action on myofibroblast transdifferentiation. A regression of medullary fibrosis was demonstrated one year after PTX in uremic patients, accompanied by a reduction in IL-1, TNF-a, TGF-β, and FGF [42].

Cell-mediated immunity, involving lymphocyte function, is abnormal in uremia [90]. Chronic exposure to PTH is associated with a reduction of T lymphocyte proliferation, cytokine production, and impairment of immunoglobulins production. There are some beneficial effects of PTX on the immunologic parameters in the sHPT context. In this regard, patients with CKD on maintenance dialysis followed prospectively for one year after PTX presented an improvement in serum immunoglobulins and complement titles. This improvement in humoral immunity after PTX occurs probably due to the remarkable reduction of PTH, which directly affects B-cells, and partially improved nutritional state [91]. Thus, abnormalities of the "uremic immunodeficiency" may be related to the degree of sHPT.

Interestingly, T lymphocytes are essential to the PTH-mediated bone homeostasis. Some authors have shown the role of T lymphocytes in PTH–mediated skeleton homeostasis, suggesting that the immune system is essential to the bone actions of PTH. Hory et al. [92] have reported that transplantation of human parathyroid into athymic mice did not promote bone resorption. A subsequent study by Pettway et al. [93] has suggested an involvement between T cells and bone response to PTH. Intermittent PTH treatment could induce a faint anabolic response in the trabecular bone compartment of T cell-deficient mice.

10. Conclusions

sHPT has significant clinical implications not restricted to the pathophysiology of some mineral and bone metabolism disorder. There is a substantial body of evidence that supports the role of PTH in the pathogenesis of abnormalities in cell function, contributing to several uremic findings in patients with CKD by increasing intracellular calcium. The presence of PTH receptors in different tissues unrelated to calcium homeostasis may be the reason for such a number of nonclassical effects of severe sHPT.

The diversity of toxic effects involves myocardial dysfunction, cardiac hypertrophy, muscle weakness, osmotic fragility of erythrocytes, glucose intolerance, and abnormalities of the immune system (Figure 3). Moreover, there is evidence that PTX restores some of these organ dysfunctions, as shown in Table 1.

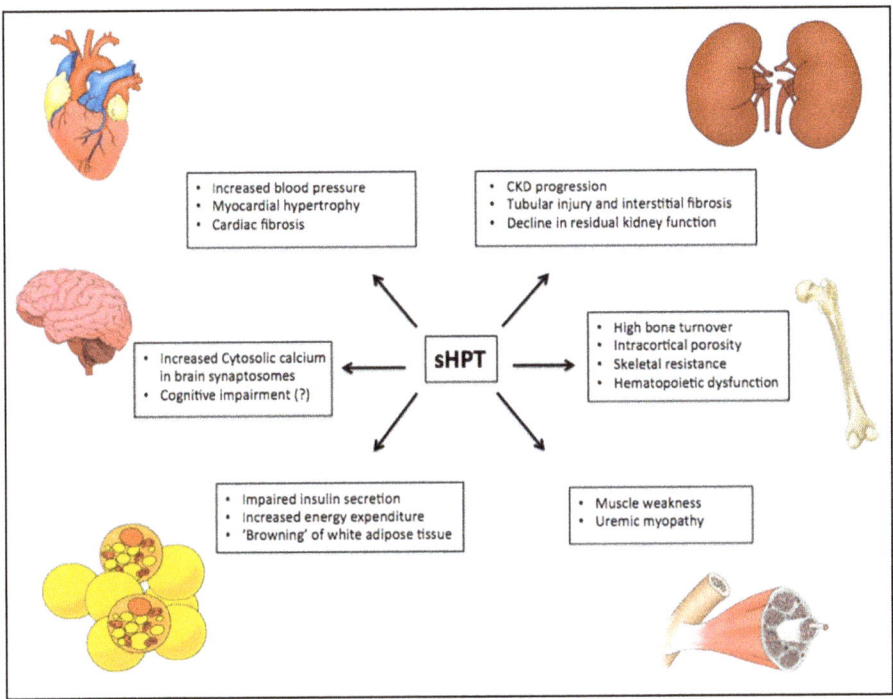

Figure 3. PTH-related manifestations on different target organs in uremic syndrome. Some studies have suggested the role of PTH in uremic syndrome through calcium-dependent and independent mechanisms. Among several toxic actions, it has been shown an association of high levels of PTH with myocardial hypertrophy and cardiovascular disease, nervous system disorders, development of sarcopenia, progression of chronic kidney disease, hematopoietic dysfunction, reduced insulin secretion by pancreatic beta-cells, increase of energy expenditure, "browning" of white adipose tissue, and high bone turnover with significant cortical compartment loss. CKD: chronic kidney disease.

Table 1. PTH-related manifestations and beneficial effects of Parathyroidectomy.

PTH-Related Manifestations	Parathyroidectomy Effects	Ref.
Hypertension Myocardial hypertrophy	Blood pressure reduction Beneficial effect on cardiovascular mortality	[44,46]
Abnormal bone density (mainly in cortical compartment)	Improvement of bone mineral density at lumbar spine and femoral neck	[19,94]
Increase of levels of cytosolic calcium in brain synaptic terminals	Improvement of cognitive function Prevention of electroencephalogram abnormalities in uremic animals	[85,95]
Hematopoietic dysfunction Accelerate erythrocyte sedimentation rate Increase of osmotic fragility of erythrocytes	Improvement of anemia Regression of medullar fibrosis	[87,96]
Reduction of T lymphocyte proliferation and cytokine production Impairment of immunoglobulins production	Improvement on serum immunoglobulins and complement titles	[90,91]
Increase in all-cause mortality risk	Improve of survival in patients with severe secondary Hyperparathyroidism Improvement of quality of life	[14,97]

Therefore, in view of the several adverse effects of high levels of PTH, a true uremic toxin, there is a need for closer monitoring for its levels in patients with CKD, in order to achieve more rigorous and early control of sHPT.

Funding: Drs Moyses and Elias are supported by CNPq (Conselho Nacional de Desenvolvimento Científico e Tecnológico). This financial support had no role in writing this review.

Conflicts of Interest: The authors declare no conflict of interest.

References

1. Goodman, W.G.; Salusky, I.B.; Juppner, H. New lessons from old assays: Parathyroid hormone (PTH), its receptors, and the potential biological relevance of PTH fragments. *Nephrol. Dial. Transplant.* **2002**, *17*, 1731–1736. [CrossRef] [PubMed]
2. Conigrave, A.D. The calcium-sensing receptor and the parathyroid: Past, present, future. *Front. Physiol.* **2016**, *7*, 563. [CrossRef] [PubMed]
3. Blaine, J.; Chonchol, M.; Levi, M. Renal control of calcium, phosphate, and magnesium homeostasis. *Clin. J. Am. Soc. Nephrol. CJASN* **2015**, *10*, 1257–1272. [CrossRef] [PubMed]
4. Baron, R.; Kneissel, M. WNT signaling in bone homeostasis and disease: From human mutations to treatments. *Nat. Med.* **2013**, *19*, 179–192. [CrossRef]
5. Baron, R.; Rawadi, G. Targeting the Wnt/beta-catenin pathway to regulate bone formation in the adult skeleton. *Endocrinology* **2007**, *148*, 2635–2643. [CrossRef]
6. Jilka, R.L. Molecular and cellular mechanisms of the anabolic effect of intermittent PTH. *Bone* **2007**, *40*, 1434–1446. [CrossRef]
7. Hofbauer, L.C.; Khosla, S.; Dunstan, C.R.; Lacey, D.L.; Boyle, W.J.; Riggs, B.L. The roles of osteoprotegerin and osteoprotegerin ligand in the paracrine regulation of bone resorption. *J. Bone Miner. Res.* **2000**, *15*, 2–12. [CrossRef]
8. National Kidney, F. K/DOQI clinical practice guidelines for bone metabolism and disease in chronic kidney disease. *Am. J. Kidney Dis.* **2003**, *42*, S1–S201.
9. Murer, H.; Hernando, N.; Forster, I.; Biber, J. Regulation of Na/Pi transporter in the proximal tubule. *Annu. Rev. Physiol.* **2003**, *65*, 531–542. [CrossRef]
10. Silver, J.; Naveh-Many, T. FGF-23 and secondary hyperparathyroidism in chronic kidney disease. *Nat. Rev. Nephrol.* **2013**, *9*, 641–649. [CrossRef]
11. Hu, M.C.; Shi, M.; Zhang, J.; Quinones, H.; Griffith, C.; Kuro-o, M.; Moe, O.W. Klotho deficiency causes vascular calcification in chronic kidney disease. *J. Am. Soc. Nephrol. JASN* **2011**, *22*, 124–136. [CrossRef] [PubMed]
12. Martin, A.; David, V.; Quarles, L.D. Regulation and function of the FGF23/klotho endocrine pathways. *Physiol. Rev.* **2012**, *92*, 131–155. [CrossRef] [PubMed]
13. Olauson, H.; Lindberg, K.; Amin, R.; Sato, T.; Jia, T.; Goetz, R.; Mohammadi, M.; Andersson, G.; Lanske, B.; Larsson, T.E. Parathyroid-specific deletion of Klotho unravels a novel calcineurin-dependent FGF23 signaling pathway that regulates PTH secretion. *PLoS Genet.* **2013**, *9*, e1003975. [CrossRef]
14. Tentori, F.; Blayney, M.J.; Albert, J.M.; Gillespie, B.W.; Kerr, P.G.; Bommer, J.; Young, E.W.; Akizawa, T.; Akiba, T.; Pisoni, R.L.; et al. Mortality risk for dialysis patients with different levels of serum calcium, phosphorus, and PTH: The Dialysis Outcomes and Practice Patterns Study (DOPPS). *Am. J. Kidney Dis.* **2008**, *52*, 519–530. [CrossRef] [PubMed]
15. Naveh-Many, T.; Rahamimov, R.; Livni, N.; Silver, J. Parathyroid cell proliferation in normal and chronic renal failure rats. The effects of calcium, phosphate, and vitamin D. *J. Clin. Investig.* **1995**, *96*, 1786–1793. [CrossRef] [PubMed]
16. Denda, M.; Finch, J.; Slatopolsky, E. Phosphorus accelerates the development of parathyroid hyperplasia and secondary hyperparathyroidism in rats with renal failure. *Am. J. Kidney Dis.* **1996**, *28*, 596–602. [CrossRef]
17. Centeno, P.P.; Herberger, A.; Mun, H.C.; Tu, C.; Nemeth, E.F.; Chang, W.; Conigrave, A.D.; Ward, D.T. Phosphate acts directly on the calcium-sensing receptor to stimulate parathyroid hormone secretion. *Nat. Commun.* **2019**, *10*, 4693. [CrossRef]

18. Goto, S.; Fujii, H.; Hamada, Y.; Yoshiya, K.; Fukagawa, M. Association between indoxyl sulfate and skeletal resistance in hemodialysis patients. *Ther. Apher. Dial.* **2010**, *14*, 417–423. [CrossRef]
19. Nickolas, T.L.; Cremers, S.; Zhang, A.; Thomas, V.; Stein, E.; Cohen, A.; Chauncey, R.; Nikkel, L.; Yin, M.T.; Liu, X.S.; et al. Discriminants of prevalent fractures in chronic kidney disease. *J. Am. Soc. Nephrol. JASN* **2011**, *22*, 1560–1572. [CrossRef]
20. Araujo, M.J.; Karohl, C.; Elias, R.M.; Barreto, F.C.; Barreto, D.V.; Canziani, M.E.; Carvalho, A.B.; Jorgetti, V.; Moyses, R.M. The pitfall of treating low bone turnover: Effects on cortical porosity. *Bone* **2016**, *91*, 75–80. [CrossRef]
21. Moe, S.M.; Chen, N.X.; Newman, C.L.; Gattone, V.H., 2nd; Organ, J.M.; Chen, X.; Allen, M.R. A comparison of calcium to zoledronic acid for improvement of cortical bone in an animal model of CKD. *J. Bone Miner. Res.* **2014**, *29*, 902–910. [CrossRef] [PubMed]
22. Duan, Y.; De Luca, V.; Seeman, E. Parathyroid hormone deficiency and excess: Similar effects on trabecular bone but differing effects on cortical bone. *J. Clin. Endocrinol. Metab.* **1999**, *84*, 718–722. [CrossRef] [PubMed]
23. Nickolas, T.L.; Stein, E.M.; Dworakowski, E.; Nishiyama, K.K.; Komandah-Kosseh, M.; Zhang, C.A.; McMahon, D.J.; Liu, X.S.; Boutroy, S.; Cremers, S.; et al. Rapid cortical bone loss in patients with chronic kidney disease. *J. Bone Miner. Res.* **2013**, *28*, 1811–1820. [CrossRef] [PubMed]
24. Parfitt, A.M. Hormonal influences on bone remodeling and bone loss: Application to the management of primary hyperparathyroidism. *Ann. Intern. Med.* **1996**, *125*, 413–415. [CrossRef]
25. Lanske, B.; Amling, M.; Neff, L.; Guiducci, J.; Baron, R.; Kronenberg, H.M. Ablation of the PTHrP gene or the PTH/PTHrP receptor gene leads to distinct abnormalities in bone development. *J. Clin. Investig.* **1999**, *104*, 399–407. [CrossRef]
26. Jansz, T.T.; Goto, N.A.; van Ballegooijen, A.J.; Willems, H.C.; Verhaar, M.C.; van Jaarsveld, B.C. The prevalence and incidence of vertebral fractures in end-stage renal disease and the role of parathyroid hormone. *Osteoporos. Int.* **2019**, 1–10. [CrossRef]
27. Coco, M.; Rush, H. Increased incidence of hip fractures in dialysis patients with low serum parathyroid hormone. *Am. J. Kidney Dis.* **2000**, *36*, 1115–1121. [CrossRef]
28. Iimori, S.; Mori, Y.; Akita, W.; Kuyama, T.; Takada, S.; Asai, T.; Kuwahara, M.; Sasaki, S.; Tsukamoto, Y. Diagnostic usefulness of bone mineral density and biochemical markers of bone turnover in predicting fracture in CKD stage 5D patients–a single-center cohort study. *Nephrol. Dial. Transplant.* **2012**, *27*, 345–351. [CrossRef]
29. Danese, M.D.; Kim, J.; Doan, Q.V.; Dylan, M.; Griffiths, R.; Chertow, G.M. PTH and the risks for hip, vertebral, and pelvic fractures among patients on dialysis. *Am. J. Kidney Dis.* **2006**, *47*, 149–156. [CrossRef]
30. Fukagawa, M.; Kazama, J.J.; Shigematsu, T. Skeletal resistance to pth as a basic abnormality underlying uremic bone diseases. *Am. J. Kidney Dis.* **2001**, *38*, S152–S155. [CrossRef]
31. Iwasaki-Ishizuka, Y.; Yamato, H.; Nii-Kono, T.; Kurokawa, K.; Fukagawa, M. Downregulation of parathyroid hormone receptor gene expression and osteoblastic dysfunction associated with skeletal resistance to parathyroid hormone in a rat model of renal failure with low turnover bone. *Nephrol. Dial. Transplant.* **2005**, *20*, 1904–1911. [CrossRef] [PubMed]
32. Graciolli, F.G.; Neves, K.R.; Barreto, F.; Barreto, D.V.; Dos Reis, L.M.; Canziani, M.E.; Sabbagh, Y.; Carvalho, A.B.; Jorgetti, V.; Elias, R.M.; et al. The complexity of chronic kidney disease-mineral and bone disorder across stages of chronic kidney disease. *Kidney Int.* **2017**, *91*, 1436–1446. [CrossRef] [PubMed]
33. Boltenstal, H.; Qureshi, A.R.; Behets, G.J.; Lindholm, B.; Stenvinkel, P.; D'Haese, P.C.; Haarhaus, M. Association of serum sclerostin with bone sclerostin in chronic kidney disease is lost in glucocorticoid treated patients. *Calcif. Tissue Int.* **2019**, *104*, 214–223. [CrossRef] [PubMed]
34. Picton, M.L.; Moore, P.R.; Mawer, E.B.; Houghton, D.; Freemont, A.J.; Hutchison, A.J.; Gokal, R.; Hoyland, J.A. Down-regulation of human osteoblast PTH/PTHrP receptor mRNA in end-stage renal failure. *Kidney Int.* **2000**, *58*, 1440–1449. [CrossRef] [PubMed]
35. Manolagas, S.C. Birth and death of bone cells: Basic regulatory mechanisms and implications for the pathogenesis and treatment of osteoporosis. *Endocr. Rev.* **2000**, *21*, 115–137. [CrossRef] [PubMed]
36. Bonewald, L.F.; Dallas, S.L. Role of active and latent transforming growth factor beta in bone formation. *J. Cell. Biochem.* **1994**, *55*, 350–357. [CrossRef] [PubMed]
37. Noda, M.; Camilliere, J.J. In vivo stimulation of bone formation by transforming growth factor-beta. *Endocrinology* **1989**, *124*, 2991–2994. [CrossRef]

38. Filvaroff, E.; Erlebacher, A.; Ye, J.; Gitelman, S.E.; Lotz, J.; Heillman, M.; Derynck, R. Inhibition of TGF-beta receptor signaling in osteoblasts leads to decreased bone remodeling and increased trabecular bone mass. *Development* **1999**, *126*, 4267–4279.
39. Qiu, T.; Wu, X.; Zhang, F.; Clemens, T.L.; Wan, M.; Cao, X. TGF-beta type II receptor phosphorylates PTH receptor to integrate bone remodelling signalling. *Nat. Cell Biol.* **2010**, *12*, 224–234. [CrossRef]
40. Mace, M.L.; Gravesen, E.; Nordholm, A.; Hofman-Bang, J.; Secher, T.; Olgaard, K.; Lewin, E. Kidney fibroblast growth factor 23 does not contribute to elevation of its circulating levels in uremia. *Kidney Int.* **2017**, *92*, 165–178. [CrossRef]
41. Jiang, X.; Kanai, H.; Shigehara, T.; Maezawa, A.; Yano, S.; Naruse, T. Metabolism of transforming growth factor-beta in patients receiving hemodialysis especially those with renal osteodystrophy. *Ren. Fail.* **1998**, *20*, 135–145. [CrossRef] [PubMed]
42. Santos, F.R.; Moyses, R.M.; Montenegro, F.L.; Jorgetti, V.; Noronha, I.L. IL-1beta, TNF-alpha, TGF-beta, and bFGF expression in bone biopsies before and after parathyroidectomy. *Kidney Int.* **2003**, *63*, 899–907. [CrossRef] [PubMed]
43. Ritz, E.; Stefanski, A.; Rambausek, M. The role of the parathyroid glands in the uremic syndrome. *Am. J. Kidney Dis.* **1995**, *26*, 808–813. [CrossRef]
44. Lishmanov, A.; Dorairajan, S.; Pak, Y.; Chaudhary, K.; Chockalingam, A. Elevated serum parathyroid hormone is a cardiovascular risk factor in moderate chronic kidney disease. *Int. Urol. Nephrol.* **2012**, *44*, 541–547. [CrossRef]
45. Jorde, R.; Sundsfjord, J.; Haug, E.; Bonaa, K.H. Relation between low calcium intake, parathyroid hormone, and blood pressure. *Hypertension* **2000**, *35*, 1154–1159. [CrossRef]
46. Jorde, R.; Svartberg, J.; Sundsfjord, J. Serum parathyroid hormone as a predictor of increase in systolic blood pressure in men. *J Hypertens* **2005**, *23*, 1639–1644. [CrossRef]
47. Zhang, Y.; Zhang, D.Z. Circulating parathyroid hormone and risk of hypertension: A meta-analysis. *Clin. Chim. Acta* **2018**, *482*, 40–45. [CrossRef]
48. Leiba, A.; Cohen, M.S.; Dinour, D.; Holtzman, E.J. Severe and long-lasting hypotension occuring immediately after parathyroidectomy in hypertensive hemodialysis patients: A case series. *J. Hum. Hypertens.* **2013**, *27*, 399–401. [CrossRef]
49. Heyliger, A.; Tangpricha, V.; Weber, C.; Sharma, J. Parathyroidectomy decreases systolic and diastolic blood pressure in hypertensive patients with primary hyperparathyroidism. *Surgery* **2009**, *146*, 1042–1047. [CrossRef]
50. Custodio, M.R.; Koike, M.K.; Neves, K.R.; dos Reis, L.M.; Graciolli, F.G.; Neves, C.L.; Batista, D.G.; Magalhaes, A.O.; Hawlitschek, P.; Oliveira, I.B.; et al. Parathyroid hormone and phosphorus overload in uremia: Impact on cardiovascular system. *Nephrol. Dial. Transplant.* **2012**, *27*, 1437–1445. [CrossRef]
51. Saleh, F.N.; Schirmer, H.; Sundsfjord, J.; Jorde, R. Parathyroid hormone and left ventricular hypertrophy. *Eur. Heart J.* **2003**, *24*, 2054–2060. [CrossRef]
52. Schlüter, K.-D.; Piper, H.M. Cardiovascular actions of parathyroid hormone and parathyroid hormone-related peptide. *Cardiovasc. Res.* **1998**, *37*, 34–41. [CrossRef]
53. Amann, K.; Ritz, E.; Wiest, G.; Klaus, G.; Mall, G. A role of parathyroid hormone for the activation of cardiac fibroblasts in uremia. *J. Am. Soc. Nephrol. JASN* **1994**, *4*, 1814–1819. [PubMed]
54. Huntgeburth, M.; Tiemann, K.; Shahverdyan, R.; Schluter, K.D.; Schreckenberg, R.; Gross, M.L.; Modersheim, S.; Caglayan, E.; Muller-Ehmsen, J.; Ghanem, A.; et al. Transforming growth factor beta(1) oppositely regulates the hypertrophic and contractile response to beta-adrenergic stimulation in the heart. *PLoS ONE* **2011**, *6*, e26628. [CrossRef] [PubMed]
55. Gutierrez, O.M.; Januzzi, J.L.; Isakova, T.; Laliberte, K.; Smith, K.; Collerone, G.; Sarwar, A.; Hoffmann, U.; Coglianese, E.; Christenson, R.; et al. Fibroblast growth factor 23 and left ventricular hypertrophy in chronic kidney disease. *Circulation* **2009**, *119*, 2545–2552. [CrossRef]
56. Faul, C.; Amaral, A.P.; Oskouei, B.; Hu, M.C.; Sloan, A.; Isakova, T.; Gutierrez, O.M.; Aguillon-Prada, R.; Lincoln, J.; Hare, J.M.; et al. FGF23 induces left ventricular hypertrophy. *J. Clin. Investig.* **2011**, *121*, 4393–4408. [CrossRef]
57. Rashid, G.; Plotkin, E.; Klein, O.; Green, J.; Bernheim, J.; Benchetrit, S. Parathyroid hormone decreases endothelial osteoprotegerin secretion: Role of protein kinase A and C. *Am. J. Physiol. Ren. Physiol.* **2009**, *296*, F60–F66. [CrossRef]

58. Shao, J.S.; Cheng, S.L.; Charlton-Kachigian, N.; Loewy, A.P.; Towler, D.A. Teriparatide (human parathyroid hormone (1–34)) inhibits osteogenic vascular calcification in diabetic low density lipoprotein receptor-deficient mice. *J. Biol. Chem.* **2003**, *278*, 50195–50202. [CrossRef]
59. Linefsky, J.P.; O'Brien, K.D.; Katz, R.; de Boer, I.H.; Barasch, E.; Jenny, N.S.; Siscovick, D.S.; Kestenbaum, B. Association of serum phosphate levels with aortic valve sclerosis and annular calcification: The cardiovascular health study. *J. Am. Coll. Cardiol.* **2011**, *58*, 291–297. [CrossRef]
60. Neves, K.R.; Graciolli, F.G.; dos Reis, L.M.; Graciolli, R.G.; Neves, C.L.; Magalhaes, A.O.; Custodio, M.R.; Batista, D.G.; Jorgetti, V.; Moyses, R.M. Vascular calcification: Contribution of parathyroid hormone in renal failure. *Kidney Int.* **2007**, *71*, 1262–1270. [CrossRef]
61. McCarthy, J.T.; El-Azhary, R.A.; Patzelt, M.T.; Weaver, A.L.; Albright, R.C.; Bridges, A.D.; Claus, P.L.; Davis, M.D.; Dillon, J.J.; El-Zoghby, Z.M.; et al. Survival, risk factors, and effect of treatment in 101 patients with calciphylaxis. *Mayo Clin. Proc.* **2016**, *91*, 1384–1394. [CrossRef] [PubMed]
62. Nigwekar, S.U.; Zhao, S.; Wenger, J.; Hymes, J.L.; Maddux, F.W.; Thadhani, R.I.; Chan, K.E. A nationally representative study of calcific uremic arteriolopathy risk factors. *J. Am. Soc. Nephrol. JASN* **2016**, *27*, 3421–3429. [CrossRef] [PubMed]
63. Hofbauer, L.C.; Brueck, C.C.; Shanahan, C.M.; Schoppet, M.; Dobnig, H. Vascular calcification and osteoporosis–from clinical observation towards molecular understanding. *Osteoporos. Int.* **2007**, *18*, 251–259. [CrossRef] [PubMed]
64. Da, J.; Xie, X.; Wolf, M.; Disthabanchong, S.; Wang, J.; Zha, Y.; Lv, J.; Zhang, L.; Wang, H. Serum phosphorus and progression of CKD and mortality: A meta-analysis of cohort studies. *Am. J. Kidney Dis.* **2015**, *66*, 258–265. [CrossRef]
65. Neves, K.R.; Graciolli, F.G.; dos Reis, L.M.; Pasqualucci, C.A.; Moyses, R.M.; Jorgetti, V. Adverse effects of hyperphosphatemia on myocardial hypertrophy, renal function, and bone in rats with renal failure. *Kidney Int.* **2004**, *66*, 2237–2244. [CrossRef]
66. Lee, Y.J.; Okuda, Y.; Sy, J.; Obi, Y.; Kang, D.H.; Nguyen, S.; Hsiung, J.T.; Park, C.; Rhee, C.M.; Kovesdy, C.P.; et al. Association of mineral bone disorder with decline in residual kidney function in incident hemodialysis patients. *J. Bone Miner. Res.* **2019**, *35*, 317–325. [CrossRef]
67. Schumock, G.T.; Andress, D.L.; Marx, S.E.; Sterz, R.; Joyce, A.T.; Kalantar-Zadeh, K. Association of secondary hyperparathyroidism with CKD progression, health care costs and survival in diabetic predialysis CKD patients. *Nephron. Clin. Pract.* **2009**, *113*, c54–c61. [CrossRef]
68. Adey, D.; Kumar, R.; McCarthy, J.T.; Nair, K.S. Reduced synthesis of muscle proteins in chronic renal failure. *Am. J. Physiol. Endocrinol. Metab.* **2000**, *278*, E219–E225. [CrossRef]
69. Workeneh, B.T.; Mitch, W.E. Review of muscle wasting associated with chronic kidney disease. *Am. J. Clin. Nutr.* **2010**, *91*, 1128S–1132S. [CrossRef]
70. Molina, P.; Carrero, J.J.; Bover, J.; Chauveau, P.; Mazzaferro, S.; Torres, P.U.; European Renal, N.; Chronic Kidney, D.-M.; Bone Disorder Working Groups of the European Renal Association-European Dialysis Transplant Association. Vitamin D, a modulator of musculoskeletal health in chronic kidney disease. *J. Cachexia Sarcopenia Muscle* **2017**, *8*, 686–701. [CrossRef]
71. Baczynski, R.; Massry, S.G.; Magott, M.; el-Belbessi, S.; Kohan, R.; Brautbar, N. Effect of parathyroid hormone on energy metabolism of skeletal muscle. *Kidney Int.* **1985**, *28*, 722–727. [CrossRef] [PubMed]
72. Gomez-Fernandez, P.; Sanchez Agudo, L.; Calatrava, J.M.; Martinez, M.E.; Escuin Sancho, F.; Selgas, R.; Sanchez Sicilia, L. Parathormone as a uremic toxin. Possible effect on respiratory muscle function in uremia. *Med. Clin.* **1984**, *82*, 395–397.
73. Khajehdehi, P.; Ali, M.; Al-Gebory, F.; Henry, G.; Bastani, B. The effects of parathyroidectomy on nutritional and biochemical status of hemodialysis patients with severe secondary hyperparathyroidism. *J. Ren. Nutr.* **1999**, *9*, 186–191. [CrossRef]
74. Cuppari, L.; de Carvalho, A.B.; Avesani, C.M.; Kamimura, M.A.; Dos Santos Lobao, R.R.; Draibe, S.A. Increased resting energy expenditure in hemodialysis patients with severe hyperparathyroidism. *J. Am. Soc. Nephrol. JASN* **2004**, *15*, 2933–2939. [CrossRef] [PubMed]
75. Kir, S.; Komaba, H.; Garcia, A.P.; Economopoulos, K.P.; Liu, W.; Lanske, B.; Hodin, R.A.; Spiegelman, B.M. PTH/PTHrP receptor mediates cachexia in models of kidney failure and cancer. *Cell Metab.* **2016**, *23*, 315–323. [CrossRef] [PubMed]

76. Fadda, G.Z.; Akmal, M.; Premdas, F.H.; Lipson, L.G.; Massry, S.G. Insulin release from pancreatic islets: Effects of CRF and excess PTH. *Kidney Int.* **1988**, *33*, 1066–1072. [CrossRef]
77. Amend, W.J., Jr.; Steinberg, S.M.; Lowrie, E.G.; Lazarus, J.M.; Soeldner, J.S.; Hampers, C.L.; Merrill, J.P. The influence of serum calcium and parathyroid hormone upon glucose metabolism in uremia. *J. Lab. Clin. Med.* **1975**, *86*, 435–444.
78. Ahamed, N.A.; Abdul-Aziz, M.Y.; El-Bauomy, A.; Salem, T.S. Parathyroid hormone: eFfects on glucose homeostasis and insulin sensitivity in chronic renal failure patients on regular hemodialysis. *J. Taibah Univ. Med. Sci.* **2008**, *3*, 44–54. [CrossRef]
79. Mak, R.H. Intravenous 1,25 dihydroxycholecalciferol corrects glucose intolerance in hemodialysis patients. *Kidney Int.* **1992**, *41*, 1049–1054. [CrossRef]
80. Mak, R.H.; Turner, C.; Haycock, G.B.; Chantler, C. Secondary hyperparathyroidism and glucose intolerance in children with uremia. *Kidney Int. Suppl.* **1983**, *16*, S128–S133.
81. Wolf, G. Energy regulation by the skeleton. *Nutr. Rev.* **2008**, *66*, 229–233. [CrossRef]
82. Fulzele, K.; Riddle, R.C.; DiGirolamo, D.J.; Cao, X.; Wan, C.; Chen, D.; Faugere, M.C.; Aja, S.; Hussain, M.A.; Bruning, J.C.; et al. Insulin receptor signaling in osteoblasts regulates postnatal bone acquisition and body composition. *Cell* **2010**, *142*, 309–319. [CrossRef] [PubMed]
83. Goldenstein, P.T.; Graciolli, F.G.; Antunes, G.L.; Dominguez, W.V.; Dos Reis, L.M.; Moe, S.; Elias, R.M.; Jorgetti, V.; Moyses, R.M.A. A prospective study of the influence of the skeleton on calcium mass transfer during hemodialysis. *PLoS ONE* **2018**, *13*, e0198946. [CrossRef]
84. Fraser, C.L.; Sarnacki, P.; Arieff, A.I. Calcium transport abnormality in uremic rat brain synaptosomes. *J. Clin. Investig.* **1985**, *76*, 1789–1795. [CrossRef] [PubMed]
85. Guisado, R.; Arieff, A.I.; Massry, S.G.; Lazarowitz, V.; Kerian, A. Changes in the electroencephalogram in acute uremia. Effects of parathyroid hormone and brain electrolytes. *J. Clin. Investig.* **1975**, *55*, 738–745. [CrossRef] [PubMed]
86. Lourida, I.; Thompson-Coon, J.; Dickens, C.M.; Soni, M.; Kuzma, E.; Kos, K.; Llewellyn, D.J. Parathyroid hormone, cognitive function and dementia: A systematic review. *PLoS ONE* **2015**, *10*, e0127574. [CrossRef] [PubMed]
87. Meytes, D.; Bogin, E.; Ma, A.; Dukes, P.P.; Massry, S.G. Effect of parathyroid hormone on erythropoiesis. *J. Clin. Investig.* **1981**, *67*, 1263–1269. [CrossRef]
88. Levi, J.; Malachi, T.; Djaldetti, M.; Bogin, E. Biochemical changes associated with the osmotic fragility of young and mature erythrocytes caused by parathyroid hormone in relation to the uremic syndrome. *Clin. Biochem.* **1987**, *20*, 121–125. [CrossRef]
89. Brickman, A.S.; Sherrard, D.J.; Jowsey, J.; Singer, F.R.; Baylink, D.J.; Maloney, N.; Massry, S.G.; Norman, A.W.; Coburn, J.W. 1,25-dihydroxycholecalciferol. Effect on skeletal lesions and plasma parathyroid hormone levels in uremic osteodystrophy. *Arch. Intern. Med.* **1974**, *134*, 883–888. [CrossRef]
90. Klinger, M.; Alexiewicz, J.M.; Linker-Israeli, M.; Pitts, T.O.; Gaciong, Z.; Fadda, G.Z.; Massry, S.G. Effect of parathyroid hormone on human T cell activation. *Kidney Int.* **1990**, *37*, 1543–1551. [CrossRef]
91. Yasunaga, C.; Nakamoto, M.; Matsuo, K.; Nishihara, G.; Yoshida, T.; Goya, T. Effects of a parathyroidectomy on the immune system and nutritional condition in chronic dialysis patients with secondary hyperparathyroidism. *Am. J. Surg.* **1999**, *178*, 332–336. [CrossRef]
92. Hory, B.G.; Roussanne, M.C.; Rostand, S.; Bourdeau, A.; Drueke, T.B.; Gogusev, J. Absence of response to human parathyroid hormone in athymic mice grafted with human parathyroid adenoma, hyperplasia or parathyroid cells maintained in culture. *J. Endocrinol. Investig.* **2000**, *23*, 273–279. [CrossRef] [PubMed]
93. Pettway, G.J.; Schneider, A.; Koh, A.J.; Widjaja, E.; Morris, M.D.; Meganck, J.A.; Goldstein, S.A.; McCauley, L.K. Anabolic actions of PTH (1-34): Use of a novel tissue engineering model to investigate temporal effects on bone. *Bone* **2005**, *36*, 959–970. [CrossRef] [PubMed]
94. Chou, F.F.; Chen, J.B.; Lee, C.H.; Chen, S.H.; Sheen-Chen, S.M. Parathyroidectomy can improve bone mineral density in patients with symptomatic secondary hyperparathyroidism. *Arch. Surg.* **2001**, *136*, 1064–1068. [CrossRef]
95. Chou, F.F.; Chen, J.B.; Hsieh, K.C.; Liou, C.W. Cognitive changes after parathyroidectomy in patients with secondary hyperparathyroidism. *Surgery* **2008**, *143*, 526–532. [CrossRef]

96. Mandolfo, S.; Malberti, F.; Farina, M.; Villa, G.; Scanziani, R.; Surian, M.; Imbasciati, E. Parathyroidectomy and response to erythropoietin therapy in anaemic patients with chronic renal failure. *Nephrol. Dial. Transplant.* **1998**, *13*, 2708–2709. [CrossRef]
97. Goldenstein, P.T.; Elias, R.M.; Pires de Freitas do Carmo, L.; Coelho, F.O.; Magalhaes, L.P.; Antunes, G.L.; Custodio, M.R.; Montenegro, F.L.; Titan, S.M.; Jorgetti, V.; et al. Parathyroidectomy improves survival in patients with severe hyperparathyroidism: A comparative study. *PLoS ONE* **2013**, *8*, e68870. [CrossRef]

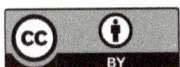 © 2020 by the authors. Licensee MDPI, Basel, Switzerland. This article is an open access article distributed under the terms and conditions of the Creative Commons Attribution (CC BY) license (http://creativecommons.org/licenses/by/4.0/).

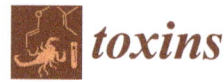

Review

The Role of Gut Dysbiosis in the Bone–Vascular Axis in Chronic Kidney Disease

Pieter Evenepoel [1,2,*], Sander Dejongh [1,2], Kristin Verbeke [3] and Bjorn Meijers [1,2]

[1] Laboratory of Nephrology, Department of Immunology and Microbiology, KU Leuven—University of Leuven, B-3000 Leuven, Belgium; sander.dejongh@kuleuven.be (S.D.); Bjorn.meijers@uzleuven.be (B.M.)
[2] Department of Nephrology and Renal Transplantation, University Hospitals Leuven, B-3000 Leuven, Belgium
[3] Translational Research Center for Gastrointestinal Disorders (TARGID), KU Leuven—University of Leuven, B-3000 Leuven, Belgium; kristin.verbeke@kuleuven.be
* Correspondence: pieter.evenepoel@uzleuven.be; Tel.: +32-16-344591; Fax: +32-16-344599

Received: 30 March 2020; Accepted: 16 April 2020; Published: 29 April 2020

Abstract: Patients with chronic kidney disease (CKD) are at increased risk of bone mineral density loss and vascular calcification. Bone demineralization and vascular mineralization often concur in CKD, similar to what observed in the general population. This contradictory association is commonly referred to as the 'calcification paradox' or the bone–vascular axis. Mounting evidence indicates that CKD-associated gut dysbiosis may be involved in the pathogenesis of the bone–vascular axis. A disrupted intestinal barrier function, a metabolic shift from a predominant saccharolytic to a proteolytic fermentation pattern, and a decreased generation of vitamin K may, alone or in concert, drive a vascular and skeletal pathobiology in CKD patients. A better understanding of the role of gut dysbiosis in the bone–vascular axis may open avenues for novel therapeutics, including nutriceuticals.

Keywords: bone; vascular calcification; gut; CKD

Key Contribution: Gut dysbiosis is common in patients with CKD and is increasingly recognized to be involved in the pathogenesis of the bone-vascular axis.

1. Introduction

Chronic kidney disease (CKD) is recognized as a major noncommunicable disease of growing epidemic dimensions worldwide. CDK–mineral and bone disorder (CKD–MBD) is one of the many complications associated with CKD. It represents a systemic disorder of mineral and bone metabolism due to CKD, manifested with either one or a combination of the following: (1) abnormalities of calcium, phosphorus (phosphate), parathyroid hormone, or vitamin D metabolism; (2) abnormalities in bone turnover, mineralization, volume, linear growth, or strength; and (3) vascular or other soft-tissue calcification. CKD–MBD explains, at least in part, the high morbidity and mortality of CKD patients [1].

Bone demineralization and vascular mineralization often concur in CKD, as in the general population. This contradictory association is often referred to as the 'calcification paradox' or the bone–vascular axis [2]. Mounting evidence indicates that CKD-associated gut dysbiosis may be involved in the pathogenesis of the bone–vascular axis. The present review aims to update the current evidence on the role of gut dysbiosis in the bone–vascular axis.

2. Bone–Vascular Axis

Mounting evidence indicates that CKD is a state of impaired bone quantity [3–9]. In clinical practice, bone quantity is most commonly assessed by dual-energy X-ray absorptiometry (DXA). A decreased bone quantity [6,10], along with an impaired bone quality [11], contributes to an excessively high fracture risk in CKD patients. Epidemiological evidence demonstrates that the fracture risk increases along with the progression of CKD, with CKD stage-5D patients showing a non-vertebral fracture risk that is up to six times higher than the fracture risk of age- and gender-matched controls [12,13]. Fractures are a major cause of morbidity and, compared to CKD patients without fractures, those with fractures experience a several-fold increased risk of mortality [14,15]. Fractures also impose a large financial burden on healthcare systems.

Vascular calcification is a condition characterized by calcium phosphate crystal deposition in the intima, media, or cardiac valves [16]. Media calcification is most common among patients with CKD, with prevalence and severity paralleling the progression of renal failure [17]. Vascular calcification is observed in more than 60% of patients with CKD stage 5D [16]. Vascular calcification is an active, cell-regulated process. Its pathophysiology varies across vascular beds and remains incompletely understood, despite major progress in the last decade [18–21]. Vascular calcification is an established independent risk factor for cardiovascular disease (CVD), the leading cause of morbidity and mortality in patients with CKD [22,23].

Many clinical studies have demonstrated an association between low bone mass and vascular calcification in patients with CKD [24–29]. The association between osteoporosis and vascular calcification is not specific to CKD. It also is commonly observed in the elderly and in patients with diabetes mellitus or chronic obstructive pulmonary disease [30–35]. Importantly, the association remains significant after adjustment for age, which suggests an age-independent relationship [26,27,29–33,36,37]. Vascular calcification and bone mineralization are both actively regulated processes showing many similarities. The co-existence of bone loss with vascular calcification should therefore be considered a paradoxical phenomenon. It is commonly referred to as the 'calcification paradox'. It most likely reflects direct bone–vascular cross-talk and/or the involvement of common pathogenic factors [2,35].

3. Gut Microbial Ecosystem in Health and CKD

The human gut harbors a complex and dynamic microbial ecosystem that is shaped by diet and host factors [38]. The human microbiome project has shown that the composition of the microbial ecosystem is quite different from one individual to the other. This variability in composition is not continuous and random, but stratified. Nutrient intake patterns are associated with both the degree of diversity and certain clusters of microbial species that are often found to act in concert. The microbial ecosystem thrives on the nutritional leftovers brought to them via the digestive tract. This requires substantial metabolic flexibility, as nutrient availability is dependent on host nutrient intake and digestion. A complex web of overlapping metabolic pathways allows access to nutritional sources inaccessible to mammalian metabolism, thereby supplementing the host metabolism.

The gut microbiota provides the host with a variety of functions including the digestion of complex dietary components, production of vitamins, maturation of the immune system, protection against pathogens, and regulation of host metabolism [39]. A compelling set of bidirectional links between the gut microbiota and the host (patho) physiology has emerged, and metabolites produced by the microbiota are increasingly implicated as crucial executors of the microbial influence on the host. Of note, microbial metabolites do account for about 10% of circulating metabolites [40].

CKD is associated with a disturbed gut microbiota composition and metabolism [41–43]. These disturbances reflect the aggregate consequences of CKD, more specifically, the effects of kidney dysfunction combined with the effects of therapeutic interventions and dietary modifications. Kidney dysfunction has a major impact on a number of physiological systems, including the gastrointestinal tract. More specifically, gastrointestinal assimilation and motility, both known to modify the colonic microenvironment, may be disturbed in CKD [44,45]. CKD, furthermore, causes an increased influx of urea, uric acid, and oxalate into the colon. Urea is converted to ammonia and subsequently to ammonium hydroxide, which can raise the colonic pH and result in mucosal damage. Patients with CKD, furthermore, often consume a diet low in dietary fiber to avoid hyperkaliemia. These and other dietary measures may importantly impact on gut microbiota composition and metabolism. Finally, not only antibiotics, but also non-antibiotic drugs are increasingly recognized to extensively affect human gut bacteria [46]. This is especially relevant in the setting of CKD, as pill burden in these patients is huge.

Using bacterial DNA isolated from fecal samples, Vaziri et al. showed highly significant differences in the abundance of over 200 bacterial operational taxonomic units between hemodialysis patients and healthy controls [41]. Additional studies demonstrated that patients with End Stage Kidney Disease (ESKD) had an increased number of bacteria that possess urease, uricase, and p-cresol- and indole-forming enzymes, and a contraction of families or genera possessing butyrate-forming enzymes (e.g., *Roseburiae*, *Lactobacillaceae*, and *Prevotellaceae*) [47,48]. Metabolomics studies showed clear differences in the levels of fecal metabolites (including phenols, indoles, and aldehydes) between patients with CKD and healthy controls. Of interest, the differences in fecal metabolite profiles were greater between patients on hemodialysis and unrelated healthy individuals than between patients on hemodialysis and household members exposed to the same diet [43]. Gryp et al., conversely, failed to observe increasing levels of p-cresyl sulfate, p-cresyl glucuronide, indoxyl sulfate, indole-3-acetic acid levels, and their precursors in stool and urine samples of patients along with the progression of CKD. In addition, anaerobic culture of fecal samples showed no difference in ex vivo p-cresol, indole, and indole-3-acetic acid generation (https://doi.org/10.1016/j.kint.2020.01.028). The use of animal models enables the effects of CKD to be separated from those of therapeutic interventions and diet. Studies with uremic rats confirm that renal dysfunction itself induces profound changes in the gut microbiota composition [41] and metabolism [43]. Taken together, current evidence indicates that CKD causes a microbial metabolism shift away from saccharolytic fermentation and towards proteolytic fermentation. Given some contradictory findings, additional prospective studies are required to confirm this shift.

CKD-induced changes to the composition and function of the intestinal microbiota also impair the intestinal barrier function, a condition commonly referred to as leaky gut [38]. A leaky gut in CKD is evidenced by the observation of increased concentrations of bacterial components, such as endotoxin or DNA, in the circulation of patients with increasing CKD stage. The levels of bacterial components are the highest in patients with ESKD treated with dialysis [49,50]. Although circulating bacterial components in patients on dialysis might derive from external sources such as dialysate fluids, the intestinal microbiota is by far the most likely source of these components in patients with CKD not on dialysis [50]. One study showed that after a few days of feeding uremic rodents with a non-pathogenic but green fluorescent *Escherichia coli* strain, green fluorescent bacterial colonies could be cultured from mouse livers, demonstrating that CKD facilitates the translocation across the intestinal barrier not only of bacterial components but also of entire living bacteria [51,52]. Our current understanding of the effects of CKD on the intestinal barrier function is in line with studies from the 1990s that demonstrated that orally ingested high-molecular-mass polyethylene glycols cross the intestinal barrier and enter the circulation and urine of uremic animals and patients [53]. Some but not all studies in animal models of CKD have demonstrated superficial mucosal erosions or disrupted tight junctions between intestinal epithelial cells in several parts of the gastrointestinal tract [52,54,55], in line with autopsy findings of patients on maintenance hemodialysis, which frequently show subtle pathologies indicative of diffuse gastrointestinal wall inflammation. Both an increased exposure to urea-derived ammonia and ammonium hydroxide [56] and a decreased generation of butyrate may contribute to a leaky gut [57]. Butyrate maintains the barrier function by at least two not mutually exclusive mechanisms. Butyrate is the primary energy source for colonic epithelial cells and undergoes fatty-acid oxidation to such an extent that these cells are slightly hypoxic. This leads to hypoxia-inducible factor-1-mediated upregulation of tight junction genes [58]. In addition, butyrate functions as a histone deacetylase (HDAC) inhibitor, and this has been shown to upregulate tight junction genes as well as the major intestinal mucin *MUC2* [59,60] gene and to downregulate the expression of pro-inflammatory cytokines [61]. Treatment of uremic rats with the symbiont *Bifidobacterium animalis* subsp. lactis Bi-07 attenuated epithelial erosion and decreased intestinal inflammation [52].

4. Gut–Bone–Vascular Axis in CKD

Acknowledging that the gut microbiome is a key regulator of bone [62–64] and cardiovascular [65–67] health, gut dysbiosis may be hypothesized to be involved in the pathogenesis of the bone–vascular axis. The present review discusses mechanisms by which gut dysbiosis may contribute to vascular calcification and bone demineralization in the setting of CKD. We herein will separately discuss the role of increased protein fermentation, decreased carbohydrate fermentation, vitamin K deficiency, and gut-derived inflammation (Figure 1).

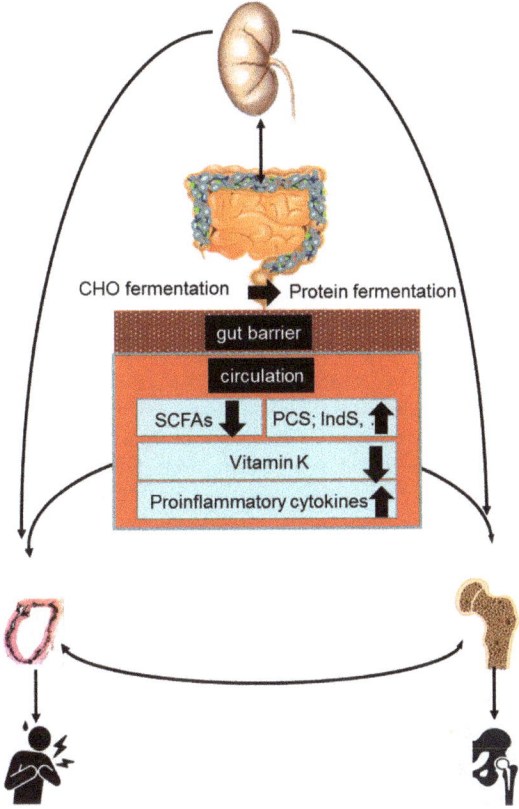

Figure 1. The kidney–gut–bone–vascular axis. Chronic kidney disease is associated with gut dysbiosis, characterized by a metabolic shift towards a predominantly proteolytic fermentation pattern and a leaky gut. Gut dysbiosis may induce bone loss and vascular calcification and as such may play a pathogenic role in the bone–vascular axis in CKD. Underlying pathophysiological mechanisms include increased exposure to protein fermentation metabolites (such as p-cresyl sulfate (PCS) and indoxyl sulfate (IndS)), a leaky gut contributing to inflammation, and deficiency of vitamin K and short-chain fatty acids (SCFAs).

5. Role of Increased Protein Fermentation in the Bone–Vascular Axis

End products of protein fermentation such as phenols and indoles are largely [68] transported across the colonic epithelium via active and passive transport mechanisms [57,69] and subsequently metabolized by phase 1 and 2 reactions (e.g., towards *p*-cresyl sulfate (PCS) and indoxyl sulfate (IndS)) in the colonic epithelium and liver before entering the systemic circulation 70. Whether CKD affects transport kinetics and metabolism of protein fermentation metabolites remains to be investigated.

Protein fermentation metabolites are cleared from the circulation by the kidneys, mainly by tubular secretion, since most are strongly protein-bound [70]. Plasma concentrations of PCS and IndS increase along the progression of CKD to reach levels in patients with ESKD being 10- to 50-fold higher than in healthy controls. These high levels reflect both an increased intestinal production and absorption and a decreased renal clearance [71]. At uremic concentrations, PCS and IndS may disturb several biological processes and confer direct and indirect toxicity in various cells and tissues, at least partly by generating intracellular oxidative stress [72].

Experimental studies revealed that IndS and PCS may promote vascular calcification through various mechanisms [73–75]. These mechanisms include (a) increased shedding of endothelial microparticles [76,77], (b) impaired autophagic flux in endothelial cells [78], (c) downregulation of MiR-29b [79], and (d) suppression of the nuclear factor erythroid 2-related factor 2 (NRF2), a master regulator of cellular antioxidant activity [80]. Dahl salt-sensitive hypertensive IndS-administered rats presented aortic calcification and upregulation of osteogenic genes when compared to control rats, indicating a pro-calcifying role of IndS in an in vivo animal model [81]. In a subsequent experiment by the same group, Dahl salt-sensitive hypertensive IndS-administered rats presented markers of senescence in the area of aortic calcification [82]. Recently, Opdebeeck et al. reported that both IndS and PCS independently promote vascular calcification in the adenine-induced CKD rat model. This was demonstrated in the aorta, as well as in peripheral arteries. Uremic toxin-induced vascular calcification was associated with the activation of inflammation and coagulation pathways [83].

In line with these experimental data, the circulating levels of PCS and IndS have been repeatedly associated with cardiovascular morbidity (including arterial stiffness, vascular calcification, ischemic and thrombotic events, and atrial fibrillation) and mortality in patients with CKD across stages of the disease [84–86] Also in the general population, clear associations between PCS and IndS concentrations and cardiovascular endpoints have been reported. For example, in a population-based study in Belgium, the prevalence of hypertension increased along with PCS and IndS quartiles [87].

Evidence of the skeletal toxicity of protein fermentation metabolites is much more limited. Protein fermentation metabolites may confer direct toxicity to bone cells and disrupt bone matrix characteristics, thereby compromising bone quality and strength [88,89]. IndS promotes osteoblast apoptosis [90] and inhibits osteoclast differentiation [91]. The latter may occur through aryl hydrocarbon receptor signaling-dependent suppression of receptor activator of nuclear factor kappa-B ligand (RANKL) production [92]. IndS also causes the deterioration of bone mechanical properties [93,94] and bone architecture. Finally, IndS may induce skeletal resistance to parathyroid hormone (PTH) [95]. Increased protein fermentation may contribute to the high prevalence of a dynamic bone disease in patients with CKD, despite these patients often presenting with PTH levels exceeding the normal upper limit severalfold [96].

Protein fermentation metabolites may also affect bone and vascular health indirectly, e.g., by promoting inflammation (vide infra) and epigenetic silencing of Klotho, an anti-aging protein [97–99]. Emerging evidence indicate that Klotho deficiency is involved in the pathogenesis of vascular calcification and bone loss in CKD. *Klotho*-null mice [100,101] show extensive vascular calcification and a low-turnover osteopenia phenotype. The bone phenotype, most probably, results from systemic disturbances in mineral metabolism associated with disrupted FGF23–Klotho signaling rather than from a functional defect of Klotho in osteocytes [102,103].

6. Role of Decreased Carbohydrate Fermentation in the Bone–Vascular Axis

Fermentation of complex carbohydrates results in the generation of short-chain fatty acids (SCFAs) [104]. The main SCFAs are butyrate, propionate, and acetate, which are found in the intestine in a molar ratio of 60:20:20. SCFAs are efficiently absorbed by the gut mucosa by poorly selective anion-transporting proteins [105]. SCFAs, not used by the colonocytes as a source of energy, enter the portal circulation and subsequently either are metabolized by the liver or enter the systemic circulation. SCFAs entering the systemic circulation have important impacts on host physiology as sources of energy, regulators of gene expression (e.g., via inhibition of HDAC), and signaling molecules that are recognized by specific receptors. Especially butyrate is a pleiotropic molecule, functioning as a ligand for certain G protein-coupled receptor (GPCR, e.g., GPCR41 and 43, also known as free-fatty acid receptor 3 and 2) and as a peroxisome proliferator-activated receptor agonist [57].

Production of both propionate and butyrate is reduced in animal CKD models [106]. Human studies, so far, yielded inconsistent findings with regard to both the overall capacity of microbiota to produce butyrate [107] and the circulating levels of SCFAs [108,109]. Chinese patients with CKD stage 5 showed a reduction in the most abundant butyrate-producing microbial species 48 and almost threefold lower plasma butyrate levels than healthy controls [108]. A comparable study in the Netherlands, however, failed to confirm these findings [107].

An increasing body of evidence implicates SCFAs in the pathogenesis of bone disease [64]. SCFAs may promote a positive bone balance by suppressing osteoclastogenesis and stimulating osteoblastogenesis. Mechanistically, propionate and butyrate induce metabolic reprogramming of osteoclasts, resulting in enhanced glycolysis at the expense of oxidative phosphorylation, thereby downregulating essential osteoclast genes [110]. Butyrate, furthermore, suppresses osteoclast differentiation, most probably by increasing the production of osteoprotegerin (OPG) by human osteoblasts [111,112]. Butyrate is also capable of stimulating bone formation [111,113]. The underlying mechanisms remain poorly defined. Butyrate promotes the differentiation of naïve $CD4^+$ cells into regulatory T cells (Tregs). The expansion of Tregs in the bone marrow leads to increased production of Wnt10b. This Wnt ligand subsequently activates Wnt signaling in osteoblastic cells, leading to osteoblast proliferation, differentiation, and survival [113]. Remarkably, this anabolic effect is only seen in trabecular bone. It is unclear whether, and if so, to what extent, the weak inhibition of HDACs accounts for the bone anabolic effects of butyrate [114].

SCFAs may also protect bone indirectly, e.g., by suppressing inflammation (vide infra) and by increasing insulin-like growth factor 1 (IGF-1), a distinct bone anabolic factor [115]. Finally, the CKD-induced microbial metabolism shift away from saccharolytic fermentation and towards proteolytic fermentation creates a colonic microenvironment (e.g., a higher luminal pH) that may hamper calcium absorption [62]. The contribution of calcium absorption in the colon to the overall calcium influx is probably limited. Nevertheless impaired colonic calcium absorption may contribute to a tight, if not negative, calcium balance, commonly observed in CKD patients free of calcium supplements [116].

Studies exploring the role of SCFAs in vascular (patho)biology are limited. Butyrate activates NRF2 at the transcription level [117–120]. This effect is mediated by HDAC inhibition. One of the downstream effects of NRF2 activation is the upregulation of the glutathione/glutathione S-transferase (GST) antioxidant system resulting in a beneficial smooth muscle cell (VSMC) redox state [121]. Activation of NRF2 signaling has been shown to alleviate high phosphate-induced calcification of VSMCs [122]. SCFAs also have anti-inflammatory properties and thus may indirectly protect against vascular calcification (vide infra).

7. Role of Vitamin K Deficiency in the Bone–Vascular Axis

Microbiota are capable of producing menaquinones (vitamin K2). To what extent the microbial production of menaquinones (vitamin K2) contributes to the overall vitamin K status of the host remains a matter of ongoing debate [123]. Experimental studies on the effect of oral and colorectal administration of vitamin K on circulating prothrombin concentration in vitamin K-deficient rats demonstrated that the bioavailability of colonic vitamin K is more than 50-fold lower than the bioavailability of oral vitamin K [123]. Conversely, data from germ-free rodents [124] and experimental and clinical studies with broad-spectrum antibiotics indicate that gut microbial metabolism may be important to maintain adequate vitamin K stores in the mammalian host [125–127].

Recent data indicate that a large majority of patients with CKD are vitamin K-deficient [128–133]. Besides dietary restrictions, therapy with vitamin K antagonists and phosphate chelators, and impaired vitamin K recycling, a decreased microbial production related to gut dysbiosis may account for the high prevalence of functional vitamin K deficiency in CKD [129,130,134,135].

Vitamin K deficiency is a well-recognized risk factor of vascular calcification and arterial stiffness, both in the general population and in CKD patients [136,137]. Accelerated vascular calcification in individuals with functional vitamin K deficiency is explained by incomplete γ-carboxylation and reduced function of matrix Gla protein (MGP) in the vasculature [138]. MGP is a 14 kDa secretory protein synthesized by chondrocytes, VSMCs, endothelial cells (ECs), and fibroblasts. γ-Carboxylated MGP inhibits vascular mineralization both directly, as a part of a complex with fetuin-A (also known as α-2-HS-glycoprotein), and indirectly, by interfering with the binding of bone morphogenetic protein-2 (BMP-2) to its receptor and thereby inhibiting BMP-2-induced osteogenic differentiation.

Low dietary intake of vitamin K, therapy with vitamin K antagonists, and functional vitamin K deficiency, as determined by circulating biomarkers (such as dephosphorylated–uncarboxylated MGP), are associated with low bone mineral density (BMD) and increased risk of fractures, both in the general population [90–92] and in patients with CKD [133,139]. Vitamin K-dependent γ-carboxylation of Gla-containing bone proteins such as MGP and osteocalcin (also referred to as bone Gla protein) may positively impact mineralization and bone quality. However, much remains to be learned on the role of MGP and osteocalcin in bone biology [140–142]. Vitamin K may affect bone health also directly by targeting the steroid and xenobiotic-sensing nuclear receptor (SXR), expressed in osteoblasts [141,143]. Finally, vitamin K deficiency may trigger micro-inflammation and thus contribute to the calcification paradox (vide infra) [133,144].

8. Role of Inflammation in the Bone–Vascular Axis

CKD is well-recognized as a state of micro-inflammation [25,145]. Several factors contribute to the inflammatory status in CKD. Only in recent years, gut dysbiosis has been recognized as another important culprit [54,146]. The pathways linking gut dysbiosis to inflammation are manifold.

First, gut dysbiosis is associated with a dysfunctional epithelial barrier [69,147]. The disruption of the gut epithelial barrier enables the entry of endotoxin and other microbial components into the systemic circulation, which in turn may elicit an inflammatory response [148]. Several studies in animal models of CKD have documented superficial mucosal erosions, mucin loss, or disrupted tight junctions between intestinal epithelial cells in several parts of the gastrointestinal tract [54,55,149,150], in line with autopsy findings in patients on chronic hemodialysis, which who show subtle pathologies indicative of diffuse gastrointestinal wall inflammation [151]. Besides gut dysbiosis, sympathetic overactivity and intestinal congestion due to hypervolemia as a result of heart failure are hypothesized to contribute to increased intestinal permeability in CKD [38].

Second, both an increased exposure to protein fermentation metabolites and a decreased exposure to SCFAs have been hypothesized to contribute to micro-inflammation in CKD. PCS was shown to activate leucocyte free-radical production [152] and IndS-induced proinflammatory cytokines in human primary macrophages, by a mechanism involving the activation of Delta-like 4 (Dll4)–Notch signaling [153]. Other studies, conversely, failed to confirm the proinflammatory properties of PCS and IndS [154]. Moreover, clinical studies investigating the relationship between serum levels of gut-derived uremic toxins, markers of inflammation, yielded inconsistent findings [155]. The anti-inflammatory immune-regulatory properties of circulating SCFAs are well established and best characterized for butyrate. Butyrate stimulates the production of ketone bodies, including β-hydroxybutyrate, known to suppress the activation of the NACHT leucine-rich repeat and pyd domains-containing 3 (NLRP3) inflammasome [156] and suppresses nuclear factor kappa-B (NF- kappa-B) signaling in immune cells [157,158]. Butyrate may also mediate systemic anti-inflammatory effects by inhibition of HDACs [57,159]. However, the clinical relevance of the latter mechanism is questionable, as butyrate circulates only at micromolar levels, which is far below the IC50 for HDAC inhibition.

Finally, vitamin K deficiency is associated with inflammation [133,144]. Both causality of the relationship and its underlying molecular mechanisms remain to be defined.

Inflammation may be a common soil for bone loss and vascular calcification [24,25,160–166]. The pathophysiological mechanisms linking inflammation to vascular calcification are complex and multifaceted. Inflammatory cytokines and C-reactive protein may (a) promote endothelial-to-mesenchymal transition [161], (b) augment osteo–chondrogenic differentiation of vascular smooth muscle cells through activation of Msx2–Wnt/β-catenin signaling [167] and induction of oxidative stress [168], and (c) repress the production of fetuin-A, an important calcification inhibitor [169]. Vascular calcification, in turn, may elicit an inflammatory response and as such trigger a self-perpetuating vicious circle.

Experimental data indicate that inflammatory cytokines, either circulating or locally produced in the bone, such as TNF-α, IL-6, and IL-1β, may induce increased bone resorption [170–173]. These effects are mediated, in part, via cytokine-induced increases in RANKL, a key stimulator of bone resorption, expressed by osteoblasts and T cells [174]. TNF-α is also an inhibitor of bone formation [175], further tilting the balance towards bone loss [161]. In disagreement with these data, Barreto et al., reported a positive correlation between TNF-α levels and bone area [176]. These authors speculate that elevated TNF-α expression may represent a homeostatic feedback mechanism to counteract excessive bone mass gain.

9. Therapeutic Options

Targeting gut microbiota composition and metabolism may be appealing to tackle the immense burden of cardiovascular disease and fractures simultaneously. Human trials and experimental murine models have shown that nutrition (e.g., diets high in dietary fiber), probiotics, prebiotics, or supplementation of SCFAs may have beneficial effects on the skeleton [64,177,178] and cardiovascular system [179]. The potential of food as a medicine in the setting of CKD is huge, but many questions remain with regard to the optimal use of nutriceuticals. A 'one-size-fits-all' approach is unlikely to be successful. Omics, undoubtedly, will prove useful in personalizing nutritional therapy [180,181].

Author Contributions: Writing—original draft preparation, P.E.; writing—review and editing, P.E., S.D., K.V., B.M. All authors have read and agreed to the published version of the manuscript.

Funding: This research received no external funding.

Conflicts of Interest: The authors declare no conflict of interest.

References

1. Moe, S.; Drueke, T.; Cunningham, J.; Goodman, W.; Martin, K.; Olgaard, K.; Ott, S.; Sprague, S.; Lameire, N.; Eknoyan, G. Definition, evaluation, and classification of renal osteodystrophy: A position statement from Kidney Disease: Improving Global Outcomes (KDIGO). *Kidney Int.* **2006**, *69*, 1945–1953. [CrossRef]
2. Evenepoel, P.; Opdebeeck, B.; David, K.; D'Haese, P.C. Bone-Vascular Axis in Chronic Kidney Disease. *Adv. Chronic. Kidney Dis.* **2019**, *26*, 472–483. [CrossRef]
3. Stein, M.S.; Packham, D.K.; Ebeling, P.R.; Wark, J.D.; Becker, G.J. Prevalence and risk factors for osteopenia in dialysis patients. *Am. J. Kidney Dis.* **1996**, *28*, 515–522. [CrossRef]
4. Rix, M.; Andreassen, H.; Eskildsen, P.; Langdahl, B.; Olgaard, K. Bone mineral density and biochemical markers of bone turnover in patients with predialysis chronic renal failure. *Kidney Int.* **1999**, *56*, 1084–1093. [CrossRef]
5. Urena, P.; Bernard-Poenaru, O.; Ostertag, A.; Baudoin, C.; Cohen-Solal, M.; Cantor, T.; de Vernejoul, M.C. Bone mineral density, biochemical markers and skeletal fractures in haemodialysis patients. *Nephrol. Dial. Transplant.* **2003**, *18*, 2325–2331. [CrossRef]
6. Evenepoel, P.; Claes, K.; Meijers, B.; Laurent, M.R.; Bammens, B.; Naesens, M.; Sprangers, B.; Pottel, H.; Cavalier, E.; Kuypers, D. Bone mineral density, bone turnover markers, and incident fractures in de novo kidney transplant recipients. *Kidney Int.* **2019**, *95*, 1461–1470. [CrossRef]
7. Chen, H.; Lips, P.; Vervloet, M.G.; van Schoor, N.M.; de Jongh, R.T. Association of renal function with bone mineral density and fracture risk in the Longitudinal Aging Study Amsterdam. *Osteoporos. Int* **2018**, *29*, 2129–2138. [CrossRef]

8. Klawansky, S.; Komaroff, E.; Cavanaugh, P.F., Jr.; Mitchell, D.Y.; Gordon, M.J.; Connelly, J.E.; Ross, S.D. Relationship between age, renal function and bone mineral density in the US population. *Osteoporos. Int.* **2003**, *14*, 570–576. [CrossRef]
9. Ishani, A.; Blackwell, T.; Jamal, S.A.; Cummings, S.R.; Ensrud, K.E. The effect of raloxifene treatment in postmenopausal women with CKD. *J. Am. Soc. Nephrol.* **2008**, *19*, 1430–1438. [CrossRef]
10. Ketteler, M.; Block, G.A.; Evenepoel, P.; Fukagawa, M.; Herzog, C.A.; McCann, L.; Moe, S.M.; Shroff, R.; Tonelli, M.A.; Toussaint, N.D.; et al. Executive summary of the 2017 KDIGO Chronic Kidney Disease-Mineral and Bone Disorder (CKD-MBD) Guideline Update: What's changed and why it matters. *Kidney Int.* **2017**, *92*, 26–36. [CrossRef]
11. Malluche, H.H.; Porter, D.S.; Monier-Faugere, M.C.; Mawad, H.; Pienkowski, D. Differences in bone quality in low- and high-turnover renal osteodystrophy. *J. Am. Soc. Nephrol.* **2012**, *23*, 525–532. [CrossRef]
12. Jadoul, M.; Albert, J.M.; Akiba, T.; Akizawa, T.; Arab, L.; Bragg-Gresham, J.L.; Mason, N.; Prutz, K.G.; Young, E.W.; Pisoni, R.L. Incidence and risk factors for hip or other bone fractures among hemodialysis patients in the Dialysis Outcomes and Practice Patterns Study. *Kidney Int.* **2006**, *70*, 1358–1366. [CrossRef]
13. Rodriguez, G.M.; Naves, D.M.; Cannata Andia, J.B. Bone metabolism, vascular calcifications and mortality: Associations beyond mere coincidence. *J. Nephrol.* **2005**, *18*, 458–463.
14. Tentori, F.; McCullough, K.; Kilpatrick, R.D.; Bradbury, B.D.; Robinson, B.M.; Kerr, P.G.; Pisoni, R.L. High rates of death and hospitalization follow bone fracture among hemodialysis patients. *Kidney Int.* **2014**, *85*, 166–173. [CrossRef]
15. Naves, M.; Diaz-Lopez, J.B.; Gomez, C.; Rodriguez-Rebollar, A.; Rodriguez-Garcia, M.; Cannata-Andia, J.B. The effect of vertebral fracture as a risk factor for osteoporotic fracture and mortality in a Spanish population. *Osteoporos. Int.* **2003**, *14*, 520–524. [CrossRef]
16. Vervloet, M.; Cozzolino, M. Vascular calcification in chronic kidney disease: Different bricks in the wall? *Kidney Int.* **2017**, *91*, 808–817. [CrossRef]
17. Budoff, M.J.; Rader, D.J.; Reilly, M.P.; Mohler III, E.R.; Lash, J.; Yang, W.; Rosen, L.; Glenn, M.; Teal, V.; Feldman, H.I. Relationship of estimated GFR and coronary artery calcification in the CRIC (Chronic Renal Insufficiency Cohort) Study. *Am. J. Kidney Dis.* **2011**, *58*, 519–526. [CrossRef]
18. Neven, E.; De Schutter, T.M.; De Broe, M.E.; D'Haese, P.C. Cell biological and physicochemical aspects of arterial calcification. *Kidney Int.* **2011**, *79*, 1166–1177. [CrossRef]
19. Schlieper, G. Vascular calcification in chronic kidney disease: Not all arteries are created equal. *Kidney Int.* **2014**, *85*, 501–503. [CrossRef]
20. Shanahan, C.M.; Crouthamel, M.H.; Kapustin, A.; Giachelli, C.M. Arterial calcification in chronic kidney disease: Key roles for calcium and phosphate. *Circ. Res.* **2011**, *109*, 697–711. [CrossRef]
21. O'Neill, W.C.; Adams, A.L. Breast arterial calcification in chronic kidney disease: Absence of smooth muscle apoptosis and osteogenic transdifferentiation. *Kidney Int.* **2014**, *85*, 668–676. [CrossRef]
22. Okuno, S.; Ishimura, E.; Kitatani, K.; Fujino, Y.; Kohno, K.; Maeno, Y.; Maekawa, K.; Yamakawa, T.; Imanishi, Y.; Inaba, M.; et al. Presence of abdominal aortic calcification is significantly associated with all-cause and cardiovascular mortality in maintenance hemodialysis patients. *Am. J. Kidney Dis.* **2007**, *49*, 417–425. [CrossRef]
23. Claes, K.J.; Heye, S.; Bammens, B.; Kuypers, D.R.; Meijers, B.; Naesens, M.; Vanrenterghem, Y.; Evenepoel, P. Aortic calcifications and arterial stiffness as predictors of cardiovascular events in incident renal transplant recipients. *Transpl. Int* **2013**, *26*, 973–981. [CrossRef]
24. Chen, Z.; Qureshi, A.R.; Ripsweden, J.; Wennberg, L.; Heimburger, O.; Lindholm, B.; Barany, P.; Haarhaus, M.; Brismar, T.B.; Stenvinkel, P. Vertebral bone density associates with coronary artery calcification and is an independent predictor of poor outcome in end-stage renal disease patients. *Bone* **2016**, *92*, 50–57. [CrossRef]
25. Viaene, L.; Behets, G.J.; Heye, S.; Claes, K.; Monbaliu, D.; Pirenne, J.; D'Haese, P.C.; Evenepoel, P. Inflammation and the bone-vascular axis in end-stage renal disease. *Osteoporos. Int.* **2016**, *27*, 489–497. [CrossRef]
26. Naves, M.; Rodriguez-Garcia, M.; Diaz-Lopez, J.B.; Gomez-Alonso, C.; Cannata-Andia, J.B. Progression of vascular calcifications is associated with greater bone loss and increased bone fractures. *Osteoporos. Int.* **2008**, *19*, 1161–1166. [CrossRef]
27. Adragao, T.; Herberth, J.; Monier-Faugere, M.C.; Branscum, A.J.; Ferreira, A.; Frazao, J.M.; Dias, C.J.; Malluche, H.H. Low bone volume–a risk factor for coronary calcifications in hemodialysis patients. *Clin. J. Am. Soc. Nephrol.* **2009**, *4*, 450–455. [CrossRef]

28. Cejka, D.; Weber, M.; Diarra, D.; Reiter, T.; Kainberger, F.; Haas, M. Inverse association between bone microarchitecture assessed by HR-pQCT and coronary artery calcification in patients with end-stage renal disease. *Bone* **2014**, *64*, 33–38. [CrossRef]
29. Barreto, D.V.; Barreto, F.C.; Carvalho, A.B.; Cuppari, L.; Cendoroglo, M.; Draibe, S.A.; Moyses, R.M.; Neves, K.R.; Jorgetti, V.; Blair, A.; et al. Coronary calcification in hemodialysis patients: The contribution of traditional and uremia-related risk factors. *Kidney Int.* **2005**, *67*, 1576–1582. [CrossRef]
30. Schulz, E.; Arfai, K.; Liu, X.; Sayre, J.; Gilsanz, V. Aortic calcification and the risk of osteoporosis and fractures. *J. Clin. Endocrinol. Metab.* **2004**, *89*, 4246–4253. [CrossRef]
31. Tanko, L.B.; Christiansen, C.; Cox, D.A.; Geiger, M.J.; McNabb, M.A.; Cummings, S.R. Relationship between osteoporosis and cardiovascular disease in postmenopausal women. *J. Bone Miner. Res.* **2005**, *20*, 1912–1920. [CrossRef]
32. Hyder, J.A.; Allison, M.A.; Wong, N.; Papa, A.; Lang, T.F.; Sirlin, C.; Gapstur, S.M.; Ouyang, P.; Carr, J.J.; Criqui, M.H. Association of coronary artery and aortic calcium with lumbar bone density: The MESA Abdominal Aortic Calcium Study. *Am. J. Epidemiol.* **2009**, *169*, 186–194. [CrossRef]
33. Lampropoulos, C.E.; Papaioannou, I.; D'Cruz, D.P. Osteoporosis—A risk factor for cardiovascular disease? *Nat. Rev. Rheumatol.* **2012**, *8*, 587–598. [CrossRef]
34. Flipon, E.; Liabeuf, S.; Fardellone, P.; Mentaverri, R.; Ryckelynck, T.; Grados, F.; Kamel, S.; Massy, Z.A.; Dargent-Molina, P.; Brazier, M. Is vascular calcification associated with bone mineral density and osteoporotic fractures in ambulatory, elderly women? *Osteoporos. Int.* **2011**. [CrossRef]
35. Persy, V.; D'Haese, P. Vascular calcification and bone disease: The calcification paradox. *Trends Mol. Med.* **2009**, *15*, 405–416. [CrossRef]
36. London, G.M.; Marty, C.; Marchais, S.J.; Guerin, A.P.; Metivier, F.; de Vernejoul, M.C. Arterial Calcifications and Bone Histomorphometry in End-Stage Renal Disease. *J. Am. Soc. Nephrol.* **2004**, *15*, 1943–1951. [CrossRef]
37. Rodriguez-Garcia, M.; Gomez-Alonso, C.; Naves-Diaz, M.; Diaz-Lopez, J.B.; Diaz-Corte, C.; Cannata-Andia, J.B. Vascular calcifications, vertebral fractures and mortality in haemodialysis patients. *Nephrol. Dial. Transplant.* **2009**, *24*, 239–246. [CrossRef]
38. Meijers, B.; Evenepoel, P.; Anders, H.J. Intestinal microbiome and fitness in kidney disease. *Nat. Rev. Nephrol.* **2019**, *15*, 531–545. [CrossRef]
39. Kau, A.L.; Ahern, P.P.; Griffin, N.W.; Goodman, A.L.; Gordon, J.I. Human nutrition, the gut microbiome and the immune system. *Nature* **2011**, *474*, 327–336. [CrossRef]
40. Wikoff, W.R.; Anfora, A.T.; Liu, J.; Schultz, P.G.; Lesley, S.A.; Peters, E.C.; Siuzdak, G. Metabolomics analysis reveals large effects of gut microflora on mammalian blood metabolites. *Proc. Natl. Acad. Sci. USA* **2009**, *106*, 3698–3703. [CrossRef]
41. Vaziri, N.D.; Wong, J.; Pahl, M.; Piceno, Y.M.; Yuan, J.; Desantis, T.Z.; Ni, Z.; Nguyen, T.H.; Andersen, G.L. Chronic kidney disease alters intestinal microbial flora. *Kidney Int.* **2012**. [CrossRef] [PubMed]
42. Jiang, S.; Xie, S.; Lv, D.; Wang, P.; He, H.; Zhang, T.; Zhou, Y.; Lin, Q.; Zhou, H.; Jiang, J.; et al. Alteration of the gut microbiota in Chinese population with chronic kidney disease. *Sci. Rep.* **2017**, *7*, 2870. [CrossRef] [PubMed]
43. Poesen, R.; Windey, K.; Neven, E.; Kuypers, D.; De Preter, V.; Augustijns, P.; D'Haese, P.; Evenepoel, P.; Verbeke, K.; Meijers, B. The Influence of CKD on Colonic Microbial Metabolism. *J. Am. Soc. Nephrol.* **2016**, *27*, 1389–1399. [CrossRef] [PubMed]
44. Bammens, B.; Verbeke, K.; Vanrenterghem, Y.; Evenepoel, P. Evidence for impaired assimilation of protein in chronic renal failure. *Kidney Int.* **2003**, *64*, 2196–2203. [CrossRef] [PubMed]
45. Evenepoel, P.; Meijers, B.K.I.; Bammens, B.R.M.; Verbeke, K. Uremic toxins originating from colonic microbial metabolism. *Kidney Int.* **2009**, *76*, S12–S19. [CrossRef] [PubMed]
46. Maier, L.; Pruteanu, M.; Kuhn, M.; Zeller, G.; Telzerow, A.; Anderson, E.E.; Brochado, A.R.; Fernandez, K.C.; Dose, H.; Mori, H.; et al. Extensive impact of non-antibiotic drugs on human gut bacteria. *Nature* **2018**, *555*, 623–628. [CrossRef] [PubMed]
47. Wong, J.; Piceno, Y.M.; Desantis, T.Z.; Pahl, M.; Andersen, G.L.; Vaziri, N.D. Expansion of urease- and uricase-containing, indole- and p-cresol-forming and contraction of short-chain fatty acid-producing intestinal microbiota in ESRD. *Am. J. Nephrol.* **2014**, *39*, 230–237. [CrossRef] [PubMed]

48. Jiang, S.; Xie, S.; Lv, D.; Zhang, Y.; Deng, J.; Zeng, L.; Chen, Y. A reduction in the butyrate producing species Roseburia spp. and Faecalibacterium prausnitzii is associated with chronic kidney disease progression. *Antonie Leeuwenhoek* **2016**, *109*, 1389–1396. [CrossRef]
49. Poesen, R.; Ramezani, A.; Claes, K.; Augustijns, P.; Kuypers, D.; Barrows, I.R.; Muralidharan, J.; Evenepoel, P.; Meijers, B.; Raj, D.S. Associations of Soluble CD14 and Endotoxin with Mortality, Cardiovascular Disease, and Progression of Kidney Disease among Patients with CKD. *Clin. J. Am. Soc. Nephrol.* **2015**, *10*, 1525–1533. [CrossRef]
50. McIntyre, C.W.; Harrison, L.E.; Eldehni, M.T.; Jefferies, H.J.; Szeto, C.C.; John, S.G.; Sigrist, M.K.; Burton, J.O.; Hothi, D.; Korsheed, S.; et al. Circulating endotoxemia: A novel factor in systemic inflammation and cardiovascular disease in chronic kidney disease. *Clin. J. Am. Soc. Nephrol.* **2011**, *6*, 133–141. [CrossRef]
51. Andersen, K.; Kesper, M.S.; Marschner, J.A.; Konrad, L.; Ryu, M.; Kumar, V.S.; Kulkarni, O.P.; Mulay, S.R.; Romoli, S.; Demleitner, J.; et al. Intestinal Dysbiosis, Barrier Dysfunction, and Bacterial Translocation Account for CKD-Related Systemic Inflammation. *J. Am. Soc. Nephrol.* **2017**, *28*, 76–83. [CrossRef] [PubMed]
52. Wei, M.; Wang, Z.; Liu, H.; Jiang, H.; Wang, M.; Liang, S.; Shi, K.; Feng, J. Probiotic Bifidobacterium animalis subsp. lactis Bi-07 alleviates bacterial translocation and ameliorates microinflammation in experimental uraemia. *Nephrology (Carlton.)* **2014**, *19*, 500–506. [CrossRef] [PubMed]
53. Magnusson, M.; Magnusson, K.E.; Sundqvist, T.; Denneberg, T. Impaired intestinal barrier function measured by differently sized polyethylene glycols in patients with chronic renal failure. *Gut* **1991**, *32*, 754–759. [CrossRef]
54. Anders, H.J.; Andersen, K.; Stecher, B. The intestinal microbiota, a leaky gut, and abnormal immunity in kidney disease. *Kidney Int.* **2013**, *83*, 1010–1016. [CrossRef] [PubMed]
55. Vaziri, N.D.; Yuan, J.; Nazertehrani, S.; Ni, Z.; Liu, S. Chronic kidney disease causes disruption of gastric and small intestinal epithelial tight junction. *Am. J. Nephrol.* **2013**, *38*, 99–103. [CrossRef] [PubMed]
56. Vaziri, N.D.; Yuan, J.; Norris, K. Role of urea in intestinal barrier dysfunction and disruption of epithelial tight junction in chronic kidney disease. *Am. J. Nephrol.* **2013**, *37*, 1–6. [CrossRef] [PubMed]
57. Bach Knudsen, K.E.; Laerke, H.N.; Hedemann, M.S.; Nielsen, T.S.; Ingerslev, A.K.; Gundelund Nielsen, D.S.; Theil, P.K.; Purup, S.; Hald, S.; Schioldan, A.G.; et al. Impact of Diet-Modulated Butyrate Production on Intestinal Barrier Function and Inflammation. *Nutrients* **2018**, *10*, 499. [CrossRef]
58. Kelly, C.J.; Zheng, L.; Campbell, E.L.; Saeedi, B.; Scholz, C.C.; Bayless, A.J.; Wilson, K.E.; Glover, L.E.; Kominsky, D.J.; Magnuson, A.; et al. Crosstalk between Microbiota-Derived Short-Chain Fatty Acids and Intestinal Epithelial HIF Augments Tissue Barrier Function. *Cell Host. Microbe* **2015**, *17*, 662–671. [CrossRef]
59. Hatayama, H.; Iwashita, J.; Kuwajima, A.; Abe, T. The short chain fatty acid, butyrate, stimulates MUC2 mucin production in the human colon cancer cell line, LS174T. *Biochem. Biophys. Res. Commun.* **2007**, *356*, 599–603. [CrossRef]
60. Schilderink, R.; Verseijden, C.; Seppen, J.; Muncan, V.; van den Brink, G.R.; Lambers, T.T.; van Tol, E.A.; de Jonge, W.J. The SCFA butyrate stimulates the epithelial production of retinoic acid via inhibition of epithelial HDAC. *Am. J. Physiol. Gastrointest. Liver Physiol.* **2016**, *310*, G1138–G1146. [CrossRef]
61. Chang, P.V.; Hao, L.; Offermanns, S.; Medzhitov, R. The microbial metabolite butyrate regulates intestinal macrophage function via histone deacetylase inhibition. *Proc. Natl. Acad. Sci. USA* **2014**, *111*, 2247–2252. [CrossRef] [PubMed]
62. Weaver, C.M. Diet, gut microbiome, and bone health. *Curr. Osteoporos. Rep.* **2015**, *13*, 125–130. [CrossRef] [PubMed]
63. Hernandez, C.J.; Guss, J.D.; Luna, M.; Goldring, S.R. Links Between the Microbiome and Bone. *J. Bone Miner. Res.* **2016**, *31*, 1638–1646. [CrossRef] [PubMed]
64. Zaiss, M.M.; Jones, R.M.; Schett, G.; Pacifici, R. The gut-bone axis: How bacterial metabolites bridge the distance. *J. Clin. Investig.* **2019**, *129*, 3018–3028. [CrossRef] [PubMed]
65. Karlsson, F.H.; Fak, F.; Nookaew, I.; Tremaroli, V.; Fagerberg, B.; Petranovic, D.; Backhed, F.; Nielsen, J. Symptomatic atherosclerosis is associated with an altered gut metagenome. *Nat. Commun.* **2012**, *3*, 1245. [CrossRef] [PubMed]
66. Jie, Z.; Xia, H.; Zhong, S.L.; Feng, Q.; Li, S.; Liang, S.; Zhong, H.; Liu, Z.; Gao, Y.; Zhao, H.; et al. The gut microbiome in atherosclerotic cardiovascular disease. *Nat. Commun.* **2017**, *8*, 845. [CrossRef]
67. Jovanovich, A.; Isakova, T.; Stubbs, J. Microbiome and Cardiovascular Disease in CKD. *Clin. J. Am. Soc. Nephrol.* **2018**, *13*, 1598–1604. [CrossRef]

68. Evenepoel, P.; Claus, D.; Geypens, B.; Hiele, M.; Geboes, K.; Rutgeerts, P.; Ghoos, Y. Amount and fate of egg protein escaping assimilation in the small intestine of humans. *AJP-Gastrointest. Liver Physiol.* **1999**, *277*, G935–G943. [CrossRef]
69. Meijers, B.; Farre, R.; Dejongh, S.; Vicario, M.; Evenepoel, P. Intestinal Barrier Function in Chronic Kidney Disease. *Toxins (Basel)* **2018**, *10*, 298. [CrossRef]
70. Poesen, R.; Evenepoel, P.; de Loor, H.; Kuypers, D.; Augustijns, P.; Meijers, B. Metabolism, Protein Binding, and Renal Clearance of Microbiota-Derived p-Cresol in Patients with CKD. *Clin. J. Am. Soc. Nephrol.* **2016**, *11*, 1136–1144. [CrossRef]
71. Poesen, R.; Viaene, L.; Verbeke, K.; Claes, K.; Bammens, B.; Sprangers, B.; Naesens, M.; Vanrenterghem, Y.; Kuypers, D.; Evenepoel, P.; et al. Renal clearance and intestinal generation of p-cresyl sulfate and indoxyl sulfate in CKD. *Clin. J. Am. Soc. Nephrol.* **2013**, *8*, 1508–1514. [CrossRef] [PubMed]
72. Vanholder, R.; Schepers, E.; Pletinck, A.; Nagler, E.V.; Glorieux, G. The uremic toxicity of indoxyl sulfate and p-cresyl sulfate: A systematic review. *J. Am. Soc. Nephrol.* **2014**, *25*, 1897–1907. [CrossRef] [PubMed]
73. Gryp, T.; Vanholder, R.; Vaneechoutte, M.; Glorieux, G. p-Cresyl Sulfate. *Toxins (Basel)* **2017**, *9*, 52. [CrossRef] [PubMed]
74. Tumur, Z.; Shimizu, H.; Enomoto, A.; Miyazaki, H.; Niwa, T. Indoxyl sulfate upregulates expression of ICAM-1 and MCP-1 by oxidative stress-induced NF-kappaB activation. *Am. J. Nephrol.* **2010**, *31*, 435–441. [CrossRef] [PubMed]
75. Muteliefu, G.; Enomoto, A.; Jiang, P.; Takahashi, M.; Niwa, T. Indoxyl sulphate induces oxidative stress and the expression of osteoblast-specific proteins in vascular smooth muscle cells. *Nephrol. Dial. Transplant.* **2009**, *24*, 2051–2058. [CrossRef]
76. Meijers, B.K.; Van, K.S.; Verbeke, K.; Dehaen, W.; Vanrenterghem, Y.; Hoylaerts, M.F.; Evenepoel, P. The uremic retention solute p-cresyl sulfate and markers of endothelial damage. *Am. J. Kidney Dis.* **2009**, *54*, 891–901. [CrossRef]
77. Buendia, P.; Montes de Oca, A.; Madueno, J.A.; Merino, A.; Martin-Malo, A.; Aljama, P.; Ramirez, R.; Rodriguez, M.; Carracedo, J. Endothelial microparticles mediate inflammation-induced vascular calcification. *FASEB J.* **2015**, *29*, 173–181. [CrossRef]
78. Rodrigues, S.D.; Santos, S.S.; Meireles, T.; Romero, N.; Glorieux, G.; Pecoits-Filho, R.; Zhang, D.D.; Nakao, L.S. Uremic toxins promote accumulation of oxidized protein and increased sensitivity to hydrogen peroxide in endothelial cells by impairing the autophagic flux. *Biochem. Biophys. Res. Commun.* **2019**. [CrossRef]
79. Zhang, H.; Chen, J.; Shen, Z.; Gu, Y.; Xu, L.; Hu, J.; Zhang, X.; Ding, X. Indoxyl sulfate accelerates vascular smooth muscle cell calcification via microRNA-29b dependent regulation of Wnt/beta-catenin signaling. *Toxicol. Lett.* **2018**, *284*, 29–36. [CrossRef]
80. Stockler-Pinto, M.B.; Soulage, C.O.; Borges, N.A.; Cardozo, L.F.M.F.; Dolenga, C.J.; Nakao, L.S.; Pecoits-Filho, R.; Fouque, D.; Mafra, D. From bench to the hemodialysis clinic: Protein-bound uremic toxins modulate NF-kappaB/Nrf2 expression. *Int Urol. Nephrol.* **2018**, *50*, 347–354. [CrossRef]
81. Adijiang, A.; Goto, S.; Uramoto, S.; Nishijima, F.; Niwa, T. Indoxyl sulphate promotes aortic calcification with expression of osteoblast-specific proteins in hypertensive rats. *Nephrol. Dial. Transplant.* **2008**, *23*, 1892–1901. [CrossRef] [PubMed]
82. Adijiang, A.; Higuchi, Y.; Nishijima, F.; Shimizu, H.; Niwa, T. Indoxyl sulfate, a uremic toxin, promotes cell senescence in aorta of hypertensive rats. *Biochem. Biophys. Res. Commun.* **2010**, *399*, 637–641. [CrossRef] [PubMed]
83. Opdebeeck, B.; Maudsley, S.; Azmi, A.; De, M.A.; De, L.W.; Meijers, B.; Verhulst, A.; Evenepoel, P.; D'Haese, P.C.; Neven, E. Indoxyl Sulfate and p-Cresyl Sulfate Promote Vascular Calcification and Associate with Glucose Intolerance. *J. Am. Soc. Nephrol.* **2019**, *30*, 751–766. [CrossRef] [PubMed]
84. Meijers, B.K.I.; Claes, K.; Bammens, B.; de Loor, H.; Viaene, L.; Verbeke, K.; Kuypers, D.; Vanrenterghem, Y.; Evenepoel, P. p-Cresol and Cardiovascular Risk in Mild-to-Moderate Kidney Disease. *Clin. J. Am. Soc. Nephrol.* **2010**, *5*, 1182–1189. [CrossRef] [PubMed]
85. Barreto, F.C.; Barreto, D.V.; Liabeuf, S.; Meert, N.; Glorieux, G.; Temmar, M.; Choukroun, G.; Vanholder, R.; Massy, Z.A. Serum indoxyl sulfate is associated with vascular disease and mortality in chronic kidney disease patients. *Clin. J. Am. Soc. Nephrol.* **2009**, *4*, 1551–1558. [CrossRef]

86. Liabeuf, S.; Barreto, D.V.; Barreto, F.C.; Meert, N.; Glorieux, G.; Schepers, E.; Temmar, M.; Choukroun, G.; Vanholder, R.; Massy, Z.A.; et al. Free p-cresylsulphate is a predictor of mortality in patients at different stages of chronic kidney disease. *Nephrol. Dial. Transplant.* **2010**, *25*, 1183–1191. [CrossRef]
87. Viaene, L.; Thijs, L.; Jin, Y.; Liu, Y.; Gu, Y.; Meijers, B.; Claes, K.; Staessen, J.; Evenepoel, P. Heritability and Clinical Determinants of Serum Indoxyl Sulfate and p-Cresyl Sulfate, Candidate Biomarkers of the Human Microbiome Enterotype. *PLoS ONE* **2014**, *9*, e79682. [CrossRef]
88. Kazama, J.J.; Iwasaki, Y.; Fukagawa, M. Uremic osteoporosis. *Kidney Int. Suppl. (2011)* **2013**, *3*, 446–450. [CrossRef]
89. Tanaka, H.; Iwasaki, Y.; Yamato, H.; Mori, Y.; Komaba, H.; Watanabe, H.; Maruyama, T.; Fukagawa, M. p-Cresyl sulfate induces osteoblast dysfunction through activating JNK and p38 MAPK pathways. *Bone* **2013**, *56*, 347–354. [CrossRef]
90. Kim, Y.H.; Kwak, K.A.; Gil, H.W.; Song, H.Y.; Hong, S.Y. Indoxyl sulfate promotes apoptosis in cultured osteoblast cells. *BMC Pharmacol. Toxicol.* **2013**, *14*, 60. [CrossRef]
91. Mozar, A.; Louvet, L.; Godin, C.; Mentaverri, R.; Brazier, M.; Kamel, S.; Massy, Z.A. Indoxyl sulphate inhibits osteoclast differentiation and function. *Nephrol. Dial. Transplant.* **2012**, *27*, 2176–2181. [CrossRef] [PubMed]
92. Lanza, D.; Perna, A.F.; Oliva, A.; Vanholder, R.; Pletinck, A.; Guastaferro, S.; Di, N.A.; Vigorito, C.; Capasso, G.; Jankowski, V.; et al. Impact of the uremic milieu on the osteogenic potential of mesenchymal stem cells. *PLoS ONE* **2015**, *10*, e0116468. [CrossRef] [PubMed]
93. Iwasaki, Y.; Kazama, J.J.; Yamato, H.; Fukagawa, M. Changes in chemical composition of cortical bone associated with bone fragility in rat model with chronic kidney disease. *Bone* **2011**, *48*, 1260–1267. [CrossRef] [PubMed]
94. Iwasaki, Y.; Kazama, J.J.; Yamato, H.; Shimoda, H.; Fukagawa, M. Accumulated uremic toxins attenuate bone mechanical properties in rats with chronic kidney disease. *Bone* **2013**, *57*, 477–483. [CrossRef] [PubMed]
95. Nii-Kono, T.; Iwasaki, Y.; Uchida, M.; Fujieda, A.; Hosokawa, A.; Motojima, M.; Yamato, H.; Kurokawa, K.; Fukagawa, M. Indoxyl sulfate induces skeletal resistance to parathyroid hormone in cultured osteoblastic cells. *Kidney Int.* **2007**. [CrossRef]
96. Evenepoel, P.; Bover, J.; Urena, T.P. Parathyroid hormone metabolism and signaling in health and chronic kidney disease. *Kidney Int.* **2016**, *90*, 1184–1190. [CrossRef]
97. Sun, C.Y.; Chang, S.C.; Wu, M.S. Suppression of Klotho expression by protein-bound uremic toxins is associated with increased DNA methyltransferase expression and DNA hypermethylation. *Kidney Int.* **2012**, *81*, 640–650. [CrossRef]
98. Chen, J.; Zhang, X.; Zhang, H.; Liu, T.; Zhang, H.; Teng, J.; Ji, J.; Ding, X. Indoxyl Sulfate Enhance the Hypermethylation of Klotho and Promote the Process of Vascular Calcification in Chronic Kidney Disease. *Int. J. Biol. Sci.* **2016**, *12*, 1236–1246. [CrossRef]
99. Mencke, R.; Hillebrands, J.L. The role of the anti-ageing protein Klotho in vascular physiology and pathophysiology. *Ageing Res. Rev.* **2017**, *35*, 124–146. [CrossRef]
100. Kawaguchi, H.; Manabe, N.; Miyaura, C.; Chikuda, H.; Nakamura, K.; Kuro-o, M. Independent impairment of osteoblast and osteoclast differentiation in klotho mouse exhibiting low-turnover osteopenia. *J. Clin. Investig.* **1999**, *104*, 229–237. [CrossRef]
101. Lindberg, K.; Olauson, H.; Amin, R.; Ponnusamy, A.; Goetz, R.; Taylor, R.F.; Mohammadi, M.; Canfield, A.; Kublickiene, K.; Larsson, T.E. Arterial klotho expression and FGF23 effects on vascular calcification and function. *PLoS ONE* **2013**, *8*, e60658. [CrossRef] [PubMed]
102. Rhee, Y.; Bivi, N.; Farrow, E.; Lezcano, V.; Plotkin, L.I.; White, K.E.; Bellido, T. Parathyroid hormone receptor signaling in osteocytes increases the expression of fibroblast growth factor-23 in vitro and in vivo. *Bone* **2011**, *49*, 636–643. [CrossRef] [PubMed]
103. Komaba, H.; Kaludjerovic, J.; Hu, D.Z.; Nagano, K.; Amano, K.; Ide, N.; Sato, T.; Densmore, M.J.; Hanai, J.I.; Olauson, H.; et al. Klotho expression in osteocytes regulates bone metabolism and controls bone formation. *Kidney Int.* **2017**, *92*, 599–611. [CrossRef] [PubMed]
104. Louis, P.; Flint, H.J. Formation of propionate and butyrate by the human colonic microbiota. *Environ. Microbiol.* **2017**, *19*, 29–41. [CrossRef]
105. Stumpff, F. A look at the smelly side of physiology: Transport of short chain fatty acids. *Pflugers Arch.* **2018**, *470*, 571–598. [CrossRef]

106. Mishima, E.; Fukuda, S.; Mukawa, C.; Yuri, A.; Kanemitsu, Y.; Matsumoto, Y.; Akiyama, Y.; Fukuda, N.N.; Tsukamoto, H.; Asaji, K.; et al. Evaluation of the impact of gut microbiota on uremic solute accumulation by a CE-TOFMS-based metabolomics approach. *Kidney Int.* **2017**, *92*, 634–645. [CrossRef]
107. Terpstra, M.L.; Sinnige, M.J.; Hugenholtz, F.; Peters-Sengers, H.; Remmerswaal, E.B.; Geerlings, S.E.; Bemelman, F.J. Butyrate production in patients with end-stage renal disease. *Int. J. Nephrol. Renovasc. Dis.* **2019**, *12*, 87–101. [CrossRef]
108. Wang, S.; Lv, D.; Jiang, S.; Jiang, J.; Liang, M.; Hou, F.; Chen, Y. Quantitative reduction in short-chain fatty acids, especially butyrate, contributes to the progression of chronic kidney disease. *Clin. Sci. (Lond.)* **2019**, *133*, 1857–1870. [CrossRef]
109. Jadoon, A.; Mathew, A.V.; Byun, J.; Gadegbeku, C.A.; Gipson, D.S.; Afshinnia, F.; Pennathur, S. Gut Microbial Product Predicts Cardiovascular Risk in Chronic Kidney Disease Patients. *Am. J. Nephrol.* **2018**, *48*, 269–277. [CrossRef]
110. Lucas, S.; Omata, Y.; Hofmann, J.; Bottcher, M.; Iljazovic, A.; Sarter, K.; Albrecht, O.; Schulz, O.; Krishnacoumar, B.; Kronke, G.; et al. Short-chain fatty acids regulate systemic bone mass and protect from pathological bone loss. *Nat. Commun.* **2018**, *9*, 55. [CrossRef]
111. Katono, T.; Kawato, T.; Tanabe, N.; Suzuki, N.; Iida, T.; Morozumi, A.; Ochiai, K.; Maeno, M. Sodium butyrate stimulates mineralized nodule formation and osteoprotegerin expression by human osteoblasts. *Arch. Oral Biol.* **2008**, *53*, 903–909. [CrossRef] [PubMed]
112. Montalvany-Antonucci, C.C.; Duffles, L.F.; de Arruda, J.A.A.; Zicker, M.C.; de Oliveira, S.; Macari, S.; Garlet, G.P.; Madeira, M.F.M.; Fukada, S.Y.; Andrade, I.; et al. Short-chain fatty acids and FFAR2 as suppressors of bone resorption. *Bone* **2019**, *125*, 112–121. [CrossRef] [PubMed]
113. Tyagi, A.M.; Yu, M.; Darby, T.M.; Vaccaro, C.; Li, J.Y.; Owens, J.A.; Hsu, E.; Adams, J.; Weitzmann, M.N.; Jones, R.M.; et al. The Microbial Metabolite Butyrate Stimulates Bone Formation via T Regulatory Cell-Mediated Regulation of WNT10B Expression. *Immunity* **2018**, *49*, 1116–1131. [CrossRef] [PubMed]
114. Schroeder, T.M.; Westendorf, J.J. Histone deacetylase inhibitors promote osteoblast maturation. *J. Bone Miner. Res.* **2005**, *20*, 2254–2263. [CrossRef]
115. Yan, J.; Herzog, J.W.; Tsang, K.; Brennan, C.A.; Bower, M.A.; Garrett, W.S.; Sartor, B.R.; Aliprantis, A.O.; Charles, J.F. Gut microbiota induce IGF-1 and promote bone formation and growth. *Proc. Natl. Acad. Sci. USA* **2016**, *113*, E7554–E7563. [CrossRef]
116. Evenepoel, P.; Viaene, L.; Meijers, B. Calcium balance in chronic kidney disease: Walking the tightrope. *Kidney Int.* **2012**, *81*, 1057–1059. [CrossRef]
117. Sun, B.; Jia, Y.; Yang, S.; Zhao, N.; Hu, Y.; Hong, J.; Gao, S.; Zhao, R. Sodium butyrate protects against high-fat diet-induced oxidative stress in rat liver by promoting expression of nuclear factor E2-related factor 2. *Br. J. Nutr.* **2019**, *122*, 400–410. [CrossRef]
118. Wu, J.; Jiang, Z.; Zhang, H.; Liang, W.; Huang, W.; Zhang, H.; Li, Y.; Wang, Z.; Wang, J.; Jia, Y.; et al. Sodium butyrate attenuates diabetes-induced aortic endothelial dysfunction via P300-mediated transcriptional activation of Nrf2. *Free Radic. Biol. Med.* **2018**, *124*, 454–465. [CrossRef]
119. Yaku, K.; Enami, Y.; Kurajyo, C.; Matsui-Yuasa, I.; Konishi, Y.; Kojima-Yuasa, A. The enhancement of phase 2 enzyme activities by sodium butyrate in normal intestinal epithelial cells is associated with Nrf2 and p53. *Mol. Cell Biochem.* **2012**, *370*, 7–14. [CrossRef]
120. Guo, W.; Liu, J.; Sun, J.; Gong, Q.; Ma, H.; Kan, X.; Cao, Y.; Wang, J.; Fu, S. Butyrate alleviates oxidative stress by regulating NRF2 nuclear accumulation and H3K9/14 acetylation via GPR109A in bovine mammary epithelial cells and mammary glands. *Free Radic. Biol. Med.* **2020**. [CrossRef]
121. Ranganna, K.; Mathew, O.P.; Yatsu, F.M.; Yousefipour, Z.; Hayes, B.E.; Milton, S.G. Involvement of glutathione/glutathione S-transferase antioxidant system in butyrate-inhibited vascular smooth muscle cell proliferation. *FEBS J.* **2007**, *274*, 5962–5978. [CrossRef] [PubMed]
122. Wei, R.; Enaka, M.; Muragaki, Y. Activation of KEAP1/NRF2/P62 signaling alleviates high phosphate-induced calcification of vascular smooth muscle cells by suppressing reactive oxygen species production. *Sci. Rep.* **2019**, *9*, 10366. [CrossRef] [PubMed]
123. Groenen-van Dooren, M.M.; Ronden, J.E.; Soute, B.A.; Vermeer, C. Bioavailability of phylloquinone and menaquinones after oral and colorectal administration in vitamin K-deficient rats. *Biochem. Pharmacol.* **1995**, *50*, 797–801. [CrossRef]

124. Komai, M.; Shirakawa, H.; Kimura, S. Newly developed model for vitamin K deficiency in germfree mice. *Int, J. Vitam. Nutr. Res.* **1988**, *58*, 55–59.
125. Allison, P.M.; Mummah-Schendel, L.L.; Kindberg, C.G.; Harms, C.S.; Bang, N.U.; Suttie, J.W. Effects of a vitamin K-deficient diet and antibiotics in normal human volunteers. *J. Lab. Clin. Med.* **1987**, *110*, 180–188. [PubMed]
126. Frick, P.G.; Riedler, G.; Brogli, H. Dose response and minimal daily requirement for vitamin K in man. *J. Appl. Physiol* **1967**, *23*, 387–389. [CrossRef]
127. Guss, J.D.; Taylor, E.; Rouse, Z.; Roubert, S.; Higgins, C.H.; Thomas, C.J.; Baker, S.P.; Vashishth, D.; Donnelly, E.; Shea, M.K.; et al. The microbial metagenome and bone tissue composition in mice with microbiome-induced reductions in bone strength. *Bone* **2019**, *127*, 146–154. [CrossRef]
128. Krueger, T.; Westenfeld, R.; Ketteler, M.; Schurgers, L.J.; Floege, J. Vitamin K deficiency in CKD patients: A modifiable risk factor for vascular calcification? *Kidney Int.* **2009**, *76*, 18–22. [CrossRef]
129. Holden, R.M.; Morton, A.R.; Garland, J.S.; Pavlov, A.; Day, A.G.; Booth, S.L. Vitamins K and D status in stages 3-5 chronic kidney disease. *Clin. J. Am. Soc. Nephrol.* **2010**, *5*, 590–597. [CrossRef]
130. Cranenburg, E.C.; Schurgers, L.J.; Uiterwijk, H.H.; Beulens, J.W.; Dalmeijer, G.W.; Westerhuis, R.; Magdeleyns, E.J.; Herfs, M.; Vermeer, C.; Laverman, G.D. Vitamin K intake and status are low in hemodialysis patients. *Kidney Int.* **2012**, *82*, 605–610. [CrossRef]
131. Schlieper, G.; Westenfeld, R.; Kruger, T.; Cranenburg, E.C.; Magdeleyns, E.J.; Brandenburg, V.M.; Djuric, Z.; Damjanovic, T.; Ketteler, M.; Vermeer, C.; et al. Circulating nonphosphorylated carboxylated matrix gla protein predicts survival in ESRD. *J. Am. Soc. Nephrol.* **2011**, *22*, 387–395. [CrossRef] [PubMed]
132. Boxma, P.Y.; van den Berg, E.; Geleijnse, J.M.; Laverman, G.D.; Schurgers, L.J.; Vermeer, C.; Kema, I.P.; Muskiet, F.A.; Navis, G.; Bakker, S.J.; et al. Vitamin k intake and plasma desphospho-uncarboxylated matrix Gla-protein levels in kidney transplant recipients. *PLoS ONE* **2012**, *7*, e47991. [CrossRef] [PubMed]
133. Evenepoel, P.; Claes, K.; Meijers, B.; Laurent, M.; Bammens, B.; Naesens, M.; Sprangers, B.; Pottel, H.; Cavalier, E.; Kuypers, D. Poor Vitamin K Status Is Associated With Low Bone Mineral Density and Increased Fracture Risk in End-Stage Renal Disease. *J. Bone Miner. Res.* **2019**, *34*, 262–269. [CrossRef] [PubMed]
134. Jansz, T.T.; Neradova, A.; van Ballegooijen, A.J.; Verhaar, M.C.; Vervloet, M.G.; Schurgers, L.J.; van Jaarsveld, B.C. The role of kidney transplantation and phosphate binder use in vitamin K status. *PLoS ONE* **2018**, *13*, e0203157. [CrossRef] [PubMed]
135. Kaesler, N.; Magdeleyns, E.; Herfs, M.; Schettgen, T.; Brandenburg, V.; Fliser, D.; Vermeer, C.; Floege, J.; Schlieper, G.; Kruger, T. Impaired vitamin K recycling in uremia is rescued by vitamin K supplementation. *Kidney Int.* **2014**, *86*, 286–293. [CrossRef]
136. Delanaye, P.; Krzesinski, J.M.; Warling, X.; Moonen, M.; Smelten, N.; Medart, L.; Pottel, H.; Cavalier, E. Dephosphorylated-uncarboxylated Matrix Gla protein concentration is predictive of vitamin K status and is correlated with vascular calcification in a cohort of hemodialysis patients. *BMC. Nephrol.* **2014**, *15*, 145. [CrossRef]
137. Fain, M.E.; Kapuku, G.K.; Paulson, W.D.; Williams, C.F.; Raed, A.; Dong, Y.; Knapen, M.H.J.; Vermeer, C.; Pollock, N.K. Inactive Matrix Gla Protein, Arterial Stiffness, and Endothelial Function in African American Hemodialysis Patients. *Am. J. Hypertens.* **2018**, *31*, 735–741. [CrossRef]
138. Schurgers, L.J.; Barreto, D.V.; Barreto, F.C.; Liabeuf, S.; Renard, C.; Magdeleyns, E.J.; Vermeer, C.; Choukroun, G.; Massy, Z.A. The circulating inactive form of matrix gla protein is a surrogate marker for vascular calcification in chronic kidney disease: A preliminary report. *Clin. J. Am. Soc. Nephrol.* **2010**, *5*, 568–575. [CrossRef]
139. Fusaro, M.; Noale, M.; Viola, V.; Galli, F.; Tripepi, G.; Vajente, N.; Plebani, M.; Zaninotto, M.; Guglielmi, G.; Miotto, D.; et al. Vitamin K, vertebral fractures, vascular calcifications, and mortality: VItamin K Italian (VIKI) dialysis study. *J. Bone Miner. Res.* **2012**, *27*, 2271–2278. [CrossRef]
140. Zoch, M.L.; Clemens, T.L.; Riddle, R.C. New insights into the biology of osteocalcin. *Bone* **2016**, *82*, 42–49. [CrossRef]
141. Azuma, K.; Shiba, S.; Hasegawa, T.; Ikeda, K.; Urano, T.; Horie-Inoue, K.; Ouchi, Y.; Amizuka, N.; Inoue, S. Osteoblast-Specific gamma-Glutamyl Carboxylase-Deficient Mice Display Enhanced Bone Formation with Aberrant Mineralization. *J. Bone Miner. Res.* **2015**, *30*, 1245–1254. [CrossRef] [PubMed]

142. Suzuki, Y.; Maruyama-Nagao, A.; Sakuraba, K.; Kawai, S. Level of serum undercarboxylated osteocalcin correlates with bone quality assessed by calcaneal quantitative ultrasound sonometry in young Japanese females. *Exp. Ther. Med.* **2017**, *13*, 1937–1943. [CrossRef] [PubMed]
143. Tabb, M.M.; Sun, A.; Zhou, C.; Grun, F.; Errandi, J.; Romero, K.; Pham, H.; Inoue, S.; Mallick, S.; Lin, M.; et al. Vitamin K2 regulation of bone homeostasis is mediated by the steroid and xenobiotic receptor SXR. *J. Biol. Chem.* **2003**, *278*, 43919–43927. [CrossRef] [PubMed]
144. Shea, M.K.; Booth, S.L.; Massaro, J.M.; Jacques, P.F.; D'Agostino, R.B., Sr.; Dawson-Hughes, B.; Ordovas, J.M.; O'Donnell, C.J.; Kathiresan, S.; Keaney, J.F.; et al. Vitamin K and vitamin D status: Associations with inflammatory markers in the Framingham Offspring Study. *Am. J. Epidemiol.* **2008**, *167*, 313–320. [CrossRef]
145. Stenvinkel, P.; Wanner, C.; Metzger, T.; Heimburger, O.; Mallamaci, F.; Tripepi, G.; Malatino, L.; Zoccali, C. Inflammation and outcome in end-stage renal failure: Does female gender constitute a survival advantage? *Kidney Int.* **2002**, *62*, 1791–1798. [CrossRef]
146. Kotanko, P.; Carter, M.; Levin, N.W. Intestinal bacterial microflora–a potential source of chronic inflammation in patients with chronic kidney disease. *Nephrol. Dial. Transplant.* **2006**, *21*, 2057–2060. [CrossRef] [PubMed]
147. Vaziri, N.D. CKD impairs barrier function and alters microbial flora of the intestine: A major link to inflammation and uremic toxicity. *Curr. Opin. Nephrol. Hypertens.* **2012**, *21*, 587–592. [CrossRef]
148. Lau, W.L.; Kalantar-Zadeh, K.; Vaziri, N.D. The Gut as a Source of Inflammation in Chronic Kidney Disease. *Nephron* **2015**, *130*, 92–98. [CrossRef]
149. Gonzalez, A.; Krieg, R.; Massey, H.D.; Carl, D.; Ghosh, S.; Gehr, T.W.B.; Ghosh, S.S. Sodium butyrate ameliorates insulin resistance and renal failure in CKD rats by modulating intestinal permeability and mucin expression. *Nephrol. Dial. Transplant.* **2019**, *34*, 783–794. [CrossRef]
150. Yang, J.; Lim, S.Y.; Ko, Y.S.; Lee, H.Y.; Oh, S.W.; Kim, M.G.; Cho, W.Y.; Jo, S.K. Intestinal barrier disruption and dysregulated mucosal immunity contribute to kidney fibrosis in chronic kidney disease. *Nephrol. Dial. Transplant.* **2019**, *34*, 419–428. [CrossRef]
151. Vaziri, N.D.; Dure-Smith, B.; Miller, R.; Mirahmadi, M.K. Pathology of gastrointestinal tract in chronic hemodialysis patients: An autopsy study of 78 cases. *Am. J. Gastroenterol.* **1985**, *80*, 608–611. [PubMed]
152. Schepers, E.; Meert, N.; Glorieux, G.; Goeman, J.; Van der Eycken, J.; Vanholder, R. P-cresylsulphate, the main in vivo metabolite of p-cresol, activates leucocyte free radical production. *Nephrol. Dial. Transplant.* **2007**, *22*, 592–596. [CrossRef] [PubMed]
153. Nakano, T.; Katsuki, S.; Chen, M.; Decano, J.L.; Halu, A.; Lee, L.H.; Pestana, D.V.S.; Kum, A.S.T.; Kuromoto, R.K.; Golden, W.S.; et al. Uremic Toxin Indoxyl Sulfate Promotes Proinflammatory Macrophage Activation Via the Interplay of OATP2B1 and Dll4-Notch Signaling. *Circulation* **2019**, *139*, 78–96. [CrossRef] [PubMed]
154. Viaene, L.; Evenepoel, P.; Meijers, B.; Vanderschueren, D.; Overbergh, L.; Mathieu, C. Uremia Suppresses Immune Signal-Induced CYP27B1 Expression in Human Monocytes. *Am. J. Nephrol.* **2012**, *36*, 497–508. [CrossRef]
155. Hsu, H.J.; Yen, C.H.; Wu, I.W.; Hsu, K.H.; Chen, C.K.; Sun, C.Y.; Chou, C.C.; Chen, C.Y.; Tsai, C.J.; Wu, M.S.; et al. The association of uremic toxins and inflammation in hemodialysis patients. *PLoS ONE* **2014**, *9*, e102691. [CrossRef]
156. Youm, Y.H.; Nguyen, K.Y.; Grant, R.W.; Goldberg, E.L.; Bodogai, M.; Kim, D.; D'Agostino, D.; Planavsky, N.; Lupfer, C.; Kanneganti, T.D.; et al. The ketone metabolite beta-hydroxybutyrate blocks NLRP3 inflammasome-mediated inflammatory disease. *Nat. Med.* **2015**, *21*, 263–269. [CrossRef]
157. Tedelind, S.; Westberg, F.; Kjerrulf, M.; Vidal, A. Anti-inflammatory properties of the short-chain fatty acids acetate and propionate: A study with relevance to inflammatory bowel disease. *World, J. Gastroenterol.* **2007**, *13*, 2826–2832. [CrossRef]
158. Meijer, K.; de Vos, P.; Priebe, M.G. Butyrate and other short-chain fatty acids as modulators of immunity: What relevance for health? *Curr. Opin. Clin. Nutr. Metab. Care* **2010**, *13*, 715–721. [CrossRef]
159. Koh, A.; De, V.F.; Kovatcheva-Datchary, P.; Backhed, F. From Dietary Fiber to Host Physiology: Short-Chain Fatty Acids as Key Bacterial Metabolites. *Cell* **2016**, *165*, 1332–1345. [CrossRef]
160. Hjortnaes, J.; Butcher, J.; Figueiredo, J.L.; Riccio, M.; Kohler, R.H.; Kozloff, K.M.; Weissleder, R.; Aikawa, E. Arterial and aortic valve calcification inversely correlates with osteoporotic bone remodelling: A role for inflammation. *Eur. Heart, J.* **2010**, *31*, 1975–1984. [CrossRef]
161. Khosla, S. The bone and beyond: A shift in calcium. *Nat. Med.* **2011**, *17*, 430–431. [CrossRef] [PubMed]

162. New, S.E.; Aikawa, E. Molecular imaging insights into early inflammatory stages of arterial and aortic valve calcification. *Circ. Res.* **2011**, *108*, 1381–1391. [CrossRef] [PubMed]
163. Panuccio, V.; Enia, G.; Tripepi, R.; Aliotta, R.; Mallamaci, F.; Tripepi, G.; Zoccali, C. Pro-inflammatory cytokines and bone fractures in CKD patients. An exploratory single centre study. *BMC. Nephrol.* **2012**, *13*, 134. [CrossRef]
164. Oh, J.; Wunsch, R.; Turzer, M.; Bahner, M.; Raggi, P.; Querfeld, U.; Mehls, O.; Schaefer, F. Advanced coronary and carotid arteriopathy in young adults with childhood-onset chronic renal failure. *Circulation* **2002**, *106*, 100–105. [CrossRef] [PubMed]
165. Guerin, A.P.; London, G.M.; Marchais, S.J.; Metivier, F. Arterial stiffening and vascular calcifications in end-stage renal disease. *Nephrol. Dial. Transplant.* **2000**, *15*, 1014–1021. [CrossRef] [PubMed]
166. Cauley, J.A.; Barbour, K.E.; Harrison, S.L.; Cloonan, Y.K.; Danielson, M.E.; Ensrud, K.E.; Fink, H.A.; Orwoll, E.S.; Boudreau, R. Inflammatory Markers and the Risk of Hip and Vertebral Fractures in Men: The Osteoporotic Fractures in Men (MrOS). *J. Bone Miner. Res.* **2016**, *31*, 2129–2138. [CrossRef]
167. Al-Aly, Z.; Shao, J.S.; Lai, C.F.; Huang, E.; Cai, J.; Behrmann, A.; Cheng, S.L.; Towler, D.A. Aortic Msx2-Wnt Calcification Cascade Is Regulated by TNF-+¦GÇôDependent Signals in Diabetic LdlrGêÆ/GêÆ Mice. *Arterioscler. Thromb. Vasc. Biol.* **2007**, *27*, 2589–2596. [CrossRef]
168. Henze, L.A.; Luong, T.T.D.; Boehme, B.; Masyout, J.; Schneider, M.P.; Brachs, S.; Lang, F.; Pieske, B.; Pasch, A.; Eckardt, K.U.; et al. Impact of C-reactive protein on osteo-/chondrogenic transdifferentiation and calcification of vascular smooth muscle cells. *Aging (Albany. NY)* **2019**, *11*, 5445–5462. [CrossRef]
169. Ketteler, M.; Bongartz, P.; Westenfeld, R.; Wildberger, J.E.; Mahnken, A.H.; Böhm, R.; Metzger, T.; Wanner, C.; Jahnen-Dechent, W.; Floege, J. Association of low fetuin-A (AHSG) concentrations in serum with cardiovascular mortality in patients on dialysis: A cross-sectional study. *Lancet* **2003**, *361*, 827–833. [CrossRef]
170. Feyen, J.H.; Elford, P.; Di Padova, F.E.; Trechsel, U. Interleukin-6 is produced by bone and modulated by parathyroid hormone. *J. Bone Miner. Res.* **1989**, *4*, 633–638. [CrossRef]
171. Pfeilschifter, J.; Chenu, C.; Bird, A.; Mundy, G.R.; Roodman, G.D. Interleukin-1 and tumor necrosis factor stimulate the formation of human osteoclastlike cells in vitro. *J. Bone Miner. Res.* **1989**, *4*, 113–118. [CrossRef] [PubMed]
172. Ferreira, A.; Saraiva, M.; Behets, G.; Macedo, A.; Galvao, M.; D'Haese, P.; Drueke, T.B. Evaluation of bone remodeling in hemodialysis patients: Serum biochemistry, circulating cytokines and bone histomorphometry. *J. Nephrol.* **2009**, *22*, 783–793. [PubMed]
173. Cafiero, C.; Gigante, M.; Brunetti, G.; Simone, S.; Chaoul, N.; Oranger, A.; Ranieri, E.; Colucci, S.; Pertosa, G.B.; Grano, M.; et al. Inflammation induces osteoclast differentiation from peripheral mononuclear cells in chronic kidney disease patients: Crosstalk between the immune and bone systems. *Nephrol. Dial. Transplant.* **2018**, *33*, 65–75. [CrossRef] [PubMed]
174. Hofbauer, L.C.; Lacey, D.L.; Dunstan, C.R.; Spelsberg, T.C.; Riggs, B.L.; Khosla, S. Interleukin-1beta and tumor necrosis factor-alpha, but not interleukin-6, stimulate osteoprotegerin ligand gene expression in human osteoblastic cells. *Bone* **1999**, *25*, 255–259. [CrossRef]
175. Kobayashi, K.; Takahashi, N.; Jimi, E.; Udagawa, N.; Takami, M.; Kotake, S.; Nakagawa, N.; Kinosaki, M.; Yamaguchi, K.; Shima, N.; et al. Tumor necrosis factor alpha stimulates osteoclast differentiation by a mechanism independent of the ODF/RANKL-RANK interaction. *J. Exp. Med.* **2000**, *191*, 275–286. [CrossRef]
176. Barreto, F.C.; Barreto, D.V.; Moyses, R.M.; Neves, C.L.; Jorgetti, V.; Draibe, S.A.; Canziani, M.E.; Carvalho, A.B. Osteoporosis in hemodialysis patients revisited by bone histomorphometry: A new insight into an old problem. *Kidney Int.* **2006**, *69*, 1852–1857. [CrossRef]
177. Tousen, Y.; Matsumoto, Y.; Nagahata, Y.; Kobayashi, I.; Inoue, M.; Ishimi, Y. Resistant Starch Attenuates Bone Loss in Ovariectomised Mice by Regulating the Intestinal Microbiota and Bone-Marrow Inflammation. *Nutrients* **2019**, *11*, 297. [CrossRef]
178. McCabe, L.; Britton, R.A.; Parameswaran, N. Prebiotic and Probiotic Regulation of Bone Health: Role of the Intestine and its Microbiome. *Curr. Osteoporos. Rep.* **2015**, *13*, 363–371. [CrossRef]
179. Kasahara, K.; Krautkramer, K.A.; Org, E.; Romano, K.A.; Kerby, R.L.; Vivas, E.I.; Mehrabian, M.; Denu, J.M.; Backhed, F.; Lusis, A.J.; et al. Interactions between Roseburia intestinalis and diet modulate atherogenesis in a murine model. *Nat. Microbiol.* **2018**, *3*, 1461–1471. [CrossRef]

180. Lampe, J.W.; Navarro, S.L.; Hullar, M.A.; Shojaie, A. Inter-individual differences in response to dietary intervention: Integrating omics platforms towards personalised dietary recommendations. *Proc. Nutr. Soc.* **2013**, *72*, 207–218. [CrossRef]
181. Derrien, M.; Veiga, P. Rethinking Diet to Aid Human-Microbe Symbiosis. *Trends Microbiol.* **2017**, *25*, 100–112. [CrossRef] [PubMed]

© 2020 by the authors. Licensee MDPI, Basel, Switzerland. This article is an open access article distributed under the terms and conditions of the Creative Commons Attribution (CC BY) license (http://creativecommons.org/licenses/by/4.0/).

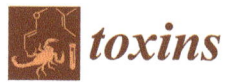

Review

Chronodisruption: A Poorly Recognized Feature of CKD

Sol Carriazo [1,2], Adrián M Ramos [1,2], Ana B Sanz [1,2], Maria Dolores Sanchez-Niño [1,2], Mehmet Kanbay [3] and Alberto Ortiz [1,2,*]

1. IIS-Fundacion Jimenez Diaz, Department of Medicine, Universidad Autonoma de Madrid, Fundacion Renal Iñigo Alvarez de Toledo-IRSIN, 28040 Madrid, Spain; sol.carriazo@quironsalud.es (S.C.); amramos@fjd.es (A.MR.); asanz@fjd.es (A.BS.); mdsanchez@fjd.es (M.D.S.-N.)
2. Red de Investigación Renal (REDINREN), 28040 Madrid, Spain
3. Division of Nephrology, Department of Medicine, Koc University School of Medicine, 34010 Istanbul, Turkey; drkanbay@yahoo.com
* Correspondence: aortiz@fjd.es; Tel.: +34-655538941

Received: 30 January 2020; Accepted: 20 February 2020; Published: 28 February 2020

Abstract: Multiple physiological variables change over time in a predictable and repetitive manner, guided by molecular clocks that respond to external and internal clues and are coordinated by a central clock. The kidney is the site of one of the most active peripheral clocks. Biological rhythms, of which the best known are circadian rhythms, are required for normal physiology of the kidneys and other organs. Chronodisruption refers to the chronic disruption of circadian rhythms leading to disease. While there is evidence that circadian rhythms may be altered in kidney disease and that altered circadian rhythms may accelerate chronic kidney disease (CKD) progression, there is no comprehensive review on chronodisruption and chronodisruptors in CKD and its manifestations. Indeed, the term chronodisruption has been rarely applied to CKD despite chronodisruptors being potential therapeutic targets in CKD patients. We now discuss evidence for chronodisruption in CKD and the impact of chronodisruption on CKD manifestations, identify potential chronodisruptors, some of them uremic toxins, and their therapeutic implications, and discuss current unanswered questions on this topic.

Keywords: chronodisruption; chronodisruptor; circadian rhythm; internal clock; chronic kidney disease

Key Contribution: Chronodisruption refers to the chronic disruption of circadian rhythms leading to disease. We now review evidence for chronodisruption, its causes (chronodisruptors) and consequences in chronic kidney disease (CKD).

---

1. Introduction: The Growing Global Health Burden of Chronic Kidney Disease

Chronic kidney disease (CKD) is currently defined as abnormalities of kidney structure or function, present for longer than 3 months, with implications for health [1]. The abnormalities of kidney structure or function may be recognized by several criteria. Just one of these criteria is enough to diagnose CKD. The most commonly used criteria are the ones that characterize CKD categories: An abnormal function defined by a decreased glomerular filtration rate (GFR, <60 mL/min/1.73 m^2, that is, G categories G3–G5) or evidence of kidney damage such as albuminuria (albumin excretion rate ≥ 30 mg/24 h; urinary albumin creatinine ratio ≥ 30 mg/g, that is, A categories A2 or A3). As for the concept of "implications for health", it reflects the fact that CKD is associated with an increased risk of all-cause or cardiovascular death, of CKD progression and of development of acute kidney injury (AKI). In this regard, the contribution of CKD to the global disease burden has increased sharply in recent decades. CKD is estimated to become the fifth global cause of death by 2040 and in countries with long life expectancies, it has been projected to become one of the two top causes of death before the end of the century [2,3]. The increasing contribution of CKD to the global burden of disease can be traced to several causes. On one hand, age-adjusted mortality for some key causes of death is actually decreasing. On the other, the longer life expectancy of the population and the increasing prevalence of risk factors for CKD such as obesity, diabetes and hypertension, together with the underdeveloped therapeutic armamentarium, are driving up the prevalence and impact of CKD. There is hope in the recent characterization of a dramatic nephroprotective impact of sodium-glucose transport protein 2 (SGLT2) inhibitors when added on top of renin angiotensin system (RAS) blockade for diabetic kidney disease and potentially other kidney diseases [4–6]. However, data from the hypertension field have clearly demonstrated that the availability of effective drugs is not enough, especially in polymedicated populations, where guidelines now emphasize measures to facilitate compliance [7]. In any case, the increasing burden of CKD at a time when other major causes of death are decreasing should be viewed in the context of the paucity of new therapeutic options that have become available in recent years, when compared, for example, with the cancer field [8]. This points towards major deficiencies in our understanding of the pathogenesis of CKD and of the pathophysiology of the CKD-associated increase in cardiovascular risk and premature aging. A key feature of advanced CKD is accumulation of uremic toxins that are no longer excreted by damaged kidneys, although in some instances increased toxin production also contributes to CKD manifestations [9–11]. However, this would not explain why there is already an increased risk of death when GFR is preserved, i.e., in patients in whom CKD is diagnosed because of abnormally high albuminuria yet GFR is still above 60 mL/min/1.73 m^2. Additional pathogenic events have been recently identified in these patients, such as loss of the kidney production of the anti-aging factor Klotho [12]. A long-recognized feature of CKD is an alteration of well characterized circadian rhythms, including circadian changes in blood pressure and urine concentrating ability. The widespread use of 24 h ambulatory blood pressure monitoring has familiarized physicians with the concept of the sleep time dip of blood pressure and the lack of such dip in CKD patients: CKD patients are characteristically non-dippers [13]. However, the molecular basis of this altered blood pressure circadian rhythm and the existence of other altered rhythms as well as the consequences of these altered rhythms for CKD progression and CKD-associated morbidity and mortality are less well known. We now review the basics of internal clocks and circadian rhythms, the concept of chronodisruption and how this concept applies to CKD leading to the identification of kidney and central chronodisruptors characteristic of the CKD situation and how this may change our approach to CKD management.

2. Biological Rhythms

Exposure to periodic environmental changes during evolution is thought to have driven the development of adaptive biological rhythms of which the best known are the circadian rhythms, which have a period length of around 24 h. However, there are also ultradian rhythms (>24 h) and infradian rhythms (<24 h) [14,15]. Biological rhythms allow the adaptation to changing environments, from the light-night cycle, to the seasons or feed-fast cycles. However, current 24/7 lifestyles dim the environmental differences between day and night, resulting in weak zeitgebers (weak day light, absence of darkness during night, constant environmental temperature, sedentarism and frequent snacking), which may impair the circadian system [16].

The central circadian clock lies in the suprachiasmatic nucleus in the anterior hypothalamus and coordinates peripheral clocks, including the kidney circadian clock which, in turn, coordinate local physiologic functions with patterns of activity and/or feeding [17]. Several signals contribute to coordinate peripheral circadian rhythms, including hormone secretion (e.g., production of the melatonin hormone by the pineal gland during nighttime, circadian production of aldosterone), neuronal activity (including physical activity and feeding) and body temperature. In addition, canonical clock genes (e.g., *Clock, Bmal1, Rev-erbα, Cry1, Cry2, Per1, Per2*) are expressed and/or active in a cyclical manner within cells, driving cell autonomous circadian rhythms [14,15]. In the most basic regulatory loop, *Clock* and *Bmal1* are transcription factors that promote *Cry* and *Per* gene expression, and *Cry* and *Per* in turn suppress *Clock/Bmal1* induction of their own transcription [18] (Figure 1). On top of this basic regulatory loop, associated elements account for the circadian regulation of 13% of kidney expressed genes. Furthermore, posttranslational modifications (e.g., phosphorylation, acetylation) are also responsible for circadian changes in protein activity. Functional circadian molecular clockwork evolves in the late fetal and early postnatal kidney. During the nursing period, oscillations are entrained by nutritional cues [19].

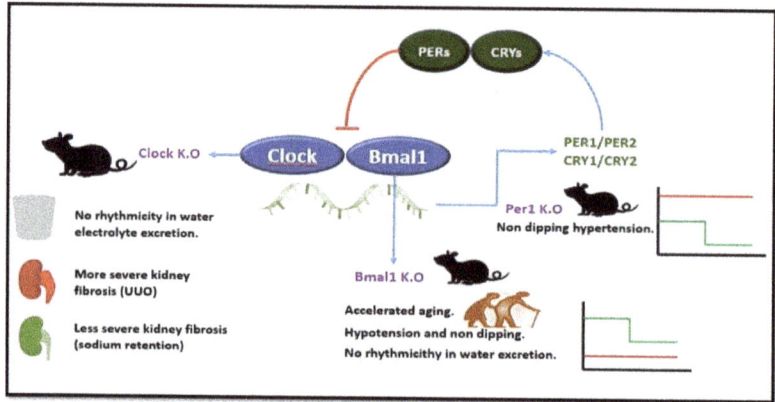

Figure 1. Canonical clock genes and the basic regulatory loop: impact on the kidney of genetic defects. In the most basic regulatory loop, *Clock* and *Bmal1* are transcription factors that promote *Cry* and *Per* gene expression, and *Cry* and *Per* proteins, in turn, suppress *Clock/Bmal1* induction of their *Cry* and *Per* transcription. Genetic disruption of some canonical clock genes has yielded renal-hypertension phenotypes as illustrated above for *Clock*, *Bmal1*, and *Per1* in mice. *Clock* KO mice display loss of water and electrolyte excretion rhythmicity as well as differential responses to induction of kidney fibrosis, which appears specific of the driver of fibrosis (worse unilateral ureteral obstruction (UUO)-induced fibrosis but milder sodium overload-induced fibrosis). *Bmal1* KO mice display accelerated aging, loss of rhythmicity of water excretion as well as non-dipping hypotension (red line) as compared to the normal blood pressure circadian rhythm (green line). *Per1* KO mice display non-dipping hypertension (red line) as compared to the normal blood pressure circadian rhythm (green line).

Kidney function has circadian rhythms (Table 1). The amplitude of circadian oscillations in GFR and renal plasma flow are around 50%, while water and electrolyte (sodium, potassium, calcium, magnesium, and phosphate) excretion may be several fold higher during the active phase and this is paralleled by circadian changes in kidney oxygenation and the corticomedullary interstitial osmolarity gradient and in the expression of genes involved in its regulation (e.g., vasopressin receptors V1aR, V2R, urea transporter UT-A2 and water channel Aqp2) [14]. Changes in kidney oxygenation modulate HIF-1α activation and erythropoietin levels, which display an amplitude of more than 10-fold under constant darkness and normoxia in mice [15]. Blood pressure peaks early in the beginning of the active period of both diurnal and nocturnal animals [20]. Molecular clocks regulate sodium balance, sympathetic function and vascular tone, all contributing to blood pressure regulation. Altered kidney circadian rhythms have been associated with the development of hypertension, chronic kidney disease, and kidney stones (reviewed in [14]).

Table 1. Some examples of kidney functions which have circadian rhythms.

Glomeruli	Circulation and Interstitial	Tubular
Glomerular filtration rate	Renal plasma flow	Water and electrolyte (sodium, potassium, calcium, magnesium, phosphate) excretion and corticomedullary interstitial osmolarity gradient
	Kidney oxygenation and erythropoietin production	H^+ excretion

Insights into the circadian regulation of kidney functions is derived from genetic defects in clock genes [14] (Figure 1). Thus, *Per1* KO mice develop non-dipping hypertension under conditions of sodium retention while *Clock* KO mice lose the circadian rhythmicity in urinary water and electrolyte excretion and develop more severe kidney fibrosis upon ureteral obstruction but were protected from kidney fibrosis driven by sodium retention conditions [14]. Additionally, *Clock* mutants had some features suggesting increased severity of adenine-induced CKD, such as higher blood pressure and expression as some gelatinase genes, but there were no differences in kidney fibrosis or serum creatinine [21]. *Bmal1* KO mice develop accelerated aging, hypotension and a non-dipping blood pressure pattern and lose the circadian variations in interstitial medullary osmolarity suggesting a role of circadian clocks in the control of urine volume beyond dietary clues [14,22]. Kidneys from conditional nephron-specific *Bmal1* deletion mice exhibited a decrease in NAD+-to-NADH ratio, increase in plasma urea and creatinine and a reduced capacity of the kidney to secrete anionic drugs (furosemide) paralleled by changes in the expression of tubule transporters such as organic anion transporter 3 (SLC22a8) [23]. Na+-H+ exchanger 3 (NHE3) activity also has rhythmic oscillations causing daily fluctuations in Na+ and water transport of the proximal tubule cell.

3. Concept of Chronodisruption

The concept of chronodisruption was coined in 2003 by Thomas C. Erren, Russel J. Reiter and Claus Piekarski from the University of Cologne [24] (Figure 2). The term was meant to go beyond the concept of chronodisturbance, a general term they proposed to refer to modulations of rhythms over time that are not necessarily deleterious since physiological compensations may prevent the development of chronic disease resulting from altered rhythms. Chronodisturbance itself was a conceptual leap from more common concepts such as "circadian disruption" or "disruption of circadian rhythms" that suggest that rhythms over 24 h can become desynchronized and that this may have adverse health effects, since these common terms may be more limited in time scope than chronodisturbance which may have a decade scope. Thus, circadian disruption may be caused by travel across several time zones, however, within a limited period of time within this new time zone, adaptation of the circadian rhythms to the new time zone occurs and there are no long-term consequences. By contrast, chronic work in night shifts will lead to chronodisturbance, that is to persistent desynchronization between time and activity. In 2009, they further elaborated on the chronodisruption concept, stating that "chronodisruption can be understood as a critical loss of time order, i.e., a disorder or chaos of an otherwise physiological timing at different organizational levels, including the gene expression levels in individual cells" and thus, it is "a breakdown of phasing internal biological systems appropriately relative to the external, i.e., environmental changes, which leads to chronobiological disorders" [25]. Following with the chronic night shift example, this would be considered chronodisturbance as long as there are no adverse consequences for health, and chronodisruption if this leads to adverse consequences for health. Furthermore, they characterized chronodisruptors as "exogenous and endogenous exposures or effectors which are chronobiologically active and can thus disrupt the timing and order, i.e., the temporal organization of physiologic functions and hierarchies" [25]. A clear example of a chronodisruptor is the use of artificial light or backlit screens during the night. They additionally proposed that assessment of melatonin levels in saliva, urine and blood may be a robust biomarker of chronodisruption. While in some fields the concept was immediately grasped (In 2007, the International Agency for Research on Cancer classified shift-work that involves circadian disruption as probably carcinogenic to humans), it was not until 2013 that the term chronodisruption was used in the context of CKD [26] and only in 2019 was a second manuscript published on the topic [27].

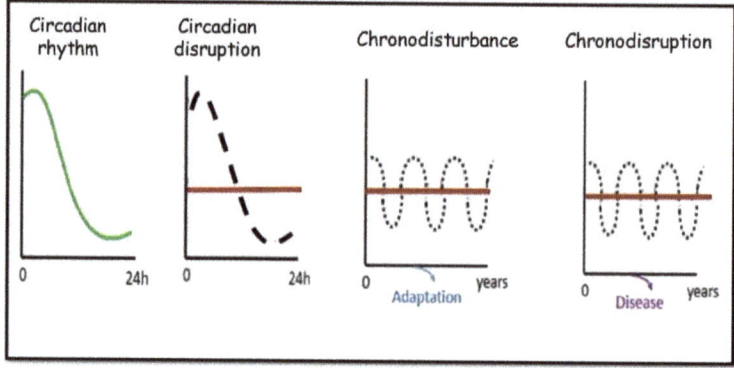

Figure 2. Concepts of circadian disruption, chronodisturbance and chronodisruption. As compared to a normal circadian rhythm, circadian disruptions are characterized by altered circadian rhythm that may be short or long lived. Chronodisturbance is a chronic disruption of circadian rhythms that somehow leads to adaptive phenomena that limit its negative impact. Chronodisruption is a chronic disruption of circadian rhythms that results in disease. Chronodisruptors (not shown) are the factors driving chronodisruption. The normal circadian rhythm is shown as a green line in the left panel and as a discontinuous line in the other panels. A red line represents the altered circadian rhythm in the three left panels. Please note the different timelines shown in the horizontal axis, with chronodisturbance and chronodisruption implying chronicity.

While this is surprising given the chronic nature of CKD, its similarities with aging and the widely known fact that circadian rhythms may be disturbed in CKD, it does not mean that the nephrological community is not aware of disruption of circadian rhythms in CKD. Indeed, very active research is going on as attested by recent reviews [14,15,26,28,29]. However, CKD researchers may benefit from a wider use of the terms and concepts of chronodisruption and chronodisruptor. Thus, the mere concept of chronodisruptor may facilitate the search of chronodisruptors involved in CKD manifestations. These may potentially be abnormal levels of uremic toxins or abnormally low levels of uremia-related factors, among others.

4. Chronodisruption in CKD

Several alterations of circadian rhythms are well characterized in CKD patients and there is accumulating evidence that at least some of them may adversely affect health, thus fulfilling criteria to be considered chronodisruption. These include disordered sleep, non-dipping hypertension, failure to properly concentrate urine at night and the circadian pattern of proteinuria in patients with nephrotic syndrome: Peak protein excretion occurs at around 16.00 h and the nadir at 03.00 h and is independent of GFR [14]. Ultradian rhythms have also been described in CKD. For example, in patients with end-stage renal disease treated with hemodialysis, blood pressure varies seasonally, with higher values in the winter and lower values in the summer [30]. However, this pattern has not been directly compared to that of non-CKD individuals. Of the diverse altered circadian rhythms in CKD, the ones best characterized with adverse consequences for health, meeting the criterion to define chronodisruption are disordered sleep and non-dipping hypertension and will be discussed more extensively.

Sleep timing, quality and/or duration are frequently disturbed in CKD patients and this can be reproduced by subtotal nephrectomy in rats [26] or in mice with adenine-induced CKD [21]. In patients with mild to moderate CKD, lower eGFR was associated with shorter sleep duration (−1.1 mL/min/1.73 m^2 per hour less sleep), greater sleep fragmentation (−2.6 mL/min/1.73 m^2 per 10% higher fragmentation) and later timing of sleep (−0.9 mL min/1.73 m^2 per hour later). Higher proteinuria was also associated with greater sleep fragmentation (approximately 28% higher per 10% higher fragmentation) [31]. However, from these studies, potential causality and direction of the association is unclear, since CKD may cause chronodisruption but chronodisruption may theoretically lead to CKD progression. The nocturnal melatonin peak appears to be preserved just in nocturnal hemodialysis patients but not in patients on other dialysis modalities. In this regard, exogenous melatonin may improve intrarenal renin angiotensin system activation and renal injury in experimental CKD [32]. Specific conditions associated to CKD may contribute to disrupted sleep patterns. These include nocturia elated to decreased urine concentration capacity and obstructive sleep apnea. The prevalence of obstructive sleep apnea increases as kidney function declines and is higher among patients with ESRD. obstructive sleep apnea may contribute to higher nocturnal blood pressure and to pulmonary hypertension and these may improve on continuous positive airway pressure (CPAP) [33–35].

In CKD patients, the prevalence of reverse dipping (night-time blood pressure peak) for systolic blood pressure and episodes of hypotension during daytime is doubled, independently of blood pressure control [36]. Uninephrectomy by itself interfered with blood pressure rhythms. Albuminuria in hypertensive patients is also accompanied by quantitatively striking higher nighttime systolic blood pressure, particularly in patients with diabetes with very high albuminuria and low eGFR [37]. Although studies regarding causality are needed, this observation may point out to a CKD A2/A3-dependent altered clock: That is, albuminuria itself may potentially be a chronodisruptor, even when global kidney function (GFR) is preserved, on top of any potential chronodisruptor activity of uremic toxins that accumulate when GFR falls. Further supporting a potential role of albuminuria itself, in minimal change nephrotic syndrome patients with overall preserved GFR (around 75 mL/min/1.73 m^2), sleeping/waking systolic and diastolic blood pressure ratios were higher than in healthy controls and this was reversed by remission of proteinuria [38].

Non-dipping is a recognized cardiovascular risk factor. In the general population, there is a linear relationship between the nocturnal decline in blood pressure and cardiovascular mortality. On average, each 5% decrease in the decline in nocturnal systolic/diastolic blood pressure was associated with an approximately 20% greater risk of cardiovascular mortality and this was observed even when 24-h blood pressure values were within the normal range (average 118/69 mmHg), diminished nocturnal decreases [39]. In CKD patients this may be magnified, as they have higher systolic blood pressure during the night-time and greater prevalence of non-dipping. Indeed, nocturnal systolic blood pressure correlated more strongly with cardiac organ damage [40]. In hemodialysis patients, increased short-term nighttime pulse pressure variability but not ambulatory blood pressure levels were significantly predictive of long-term all-cause mortality [41].

Several individual contributors to the circadian regulation of blood pressure have been identified and these include local kidney molecular clocks, whose local expression may be potentially altered by kidney disease mediators. Thus, *Bmal1* deficiency in juxtaglomerular renin-secreting granular cells resulted in polyuria, changes in the circadian rhythm of urinary sodium excretion, increased GFR, and lower plasma aldosterone levels and lower blood pressure [42]. The sodium-chloride cotransporter (NCC, SLC12A3) in distal convoluted tubules contributes to sodium balance and blood pressure regulation. Disturbing this rhythm induces "nondipping" blood pressure. Both mineralocorticoids and glucocorticoids regulate NCC activity. Mineralocorticoid receptor activation maintains the NCC protein pool while glucocorticoid receptor activation regulates NCC phosphorylation and the diurnal rhythm of NCC activity [43]. ATP1B1 encodes the β1 subunit of the Na$^+$/K$^+$-ATPase. Atp1b1 mRNA and protein levels in mouse kidney have a circadian rhythm that was antiphasic to the blood pressure rhythm. In *Dec1*-deficient mice, kidney Atp1b1 expression was increased and blood pressure was lower. In contrast, in *Clock*-mutant mice, Atp1b1 expression was low and blood pressure high [44]. The expression of both NCC and ATP1B1 is altered in kidney injury, potentially linking kidney injury to an altered expression of kidney circadian genes regulating blood pressure [45,46].

The location of disrupted timekeeping in CKD merits further study. In murine adenine-induced CKD, in vivo disrupted timekeeping could be dissociated in vitro into a suprachiasmatic nucleus pacing, which remained uncompromised, and a kidney clock that became a less robust circadian oscillator with a longer period, suggesting that the kidney contributes to overall circadian timekeeping and that there is local kidney disruption of circadian rhythms during CKD [47]. By contrast, in vivo exploration of mice with adenine-induced CKD disclosed low amplitude PER2:luciferase rhythms in their central suprachiasmatic nucleus circadian clock and in intact kidney, liver, and submandibular gland, as well as altered expression patterns of circadian genes including canonical clock genes and kidney genes such as Hif, Aqp2, and V2r [21]. Overall, these results point to interference of peripheral clocks with the central clock in CKD.

Failure to properly concentrate urine at night may further aggravate CKD-associated sleep disruption through nocturia. However, there are potentially more severe consequences. Thus, improper water excretion will promote the secretion of antidiuretic hormone (vasopressin, ADH). There is increasing evidence that overactivation of ADH may be detrimental. Specifically, the vasopressin 2 receptor (V2R) blocker tolvaptan slows the progression of autosomal dominant polycystic kidney disease (ADPKD) [48]. While this was initially thought to be related to kidney cyst specific intracellular signaling events, an adverse impact of ADH on glomerular hyperfiltration was later identified that may be a universal driver of CKD progression, not limited to ADPKD [49,50]. In this regard, circulating copeptin levels provide a better understanding of ADH activation that measuring ADH itself, which is short lived. Serum copeptin is increased in hypertension, CKD and cardiovascular disease, and ADH activation of V1R and/or V2R may be detrimental to the kidney and the cardiovascular system [51].

The altered circadian pattern of proteinuria may impact the assessment of the severity or proteinuria when different timed urine samples are assessed (12 h vs. 24 h vs. point collections), but whether this leads to any health consequence is currently unclear.

CKD has a bidirectional relationship with aging. On one hand, aging is associated with a progressive decrease in GFR. On the other, CKD causes accelerated aging and some of the factors responsible for this phenotype, such as decreased production of the anti-aging factor Klotho have been identified, as discussed below. Interestingly, aging is associated with altered central and peripheral circadian rhythms, and the sleep–wake cycle [52], leading to a phase advance, rhythm fragmentation and flattening [53]. This may in part be offset by regular physical activity [52]. Given the close association of CKD with aging, further studies are required that explore to what extent the age-associated loss of renal function contributes to age-associated circadian rhythm abnormalities and age-associated organ dysfunction and disease.

5. Chronodisruptors as Therapeutic Targets in CKD

A PubMed search for "chronodisruptors" in January 2020 resulted in only 5 hits, none of them related to CKD. This may relate to both limited understanding of chronodisruptors as with limited use of the term.

Identifying and targeting chronodisruptors may identify novel approaches to the prevention and therapy of CKD. Potential chronodisruptors include diet, the light–dark cycle, inflammatory mediators, uremic toxins, HIF abnormalities, and physical inactivity. We will briefly discuss examples of all of these (summarized in Table 2). While diet, light clues and inflammation may be active at all stages of CKD, even before GFR decreases, accumulation or uremic toxins would be expected to be active only after significant decrease of GFR has taken place, i.e., after significant loss of kidney mass.

Table 2. Examples of potential chronodisruptors in chronic kidney disease (CKD) patients.

Diet	Other Lifestyle Factors	Endogenous Factors
Dietary components, e.g., sodium	Night shift work	Gut microbiota and microbiota-associated uremic toxins
Mistimed eating		Kidney inflammation, non-canonical NFκB activation and RelB
		Mediators of kidney fibrosis such as Smad3

5.1. Dietary Clues

There is some evidence that dietary lipids and sodium may behave as chronodisruptors and, more specifically, that salt may be a chronodisruptor in CKD. Indeed, salt loading aggravates the inverse relationship between melatonin secretion, assessed as urinary levels of its metabolite 6-sulfatoxymelatonin (aMT6s) and albuminuria in CKD patients [54]. High salt feeding led to region-specific alterations in circadian clock components within the kidney and caused a 5.5-h phase delay in the peak expression of *Bmal1* and suppressed *Cry1* and *Per2* expression in the renal inner medulla, but not the renal cortex, of control rats. The phase delay in *Bmal1* expression appears to be mediated by endothelin-1 because this phenomenon was not observed in endothelin receptor B (ETB)-deficient rats. Thus, high salt feeding leads to intrarenal circadian dyssynchrony in part through activation of ETB receptors within the renal inner medulla [55]. There is less information on the molecular mechanisms engaged by dietary lipids to influence circadian kidney rhythms. One possibility is through epigenetic regulation of gene expression. Thus, dietary lipids modulate the expression of miR-107, a miRNA that regulates the circadian system [56].

An area of research is focused on altering circadian rhythms by time-related dietary approaches (chrononutrition) or pharmacological substances (chronobiotics) [57]. In a randomized clinical trial, short chronotype-adjusted diet was more effective than the traditional hypocaloric diet in decreasing BMI, and waist circumference [58]. In a further trial, eating late was associated with decreased resting-energy expenditure, decreased fasting carbohydrate oxidation, decreased glucose tolerance and blunted daily profile in free cortisol concentrations [59]. In this regard, it is widely recognized that chronodisruption and mistimed eating have deleterious effects on metabolic health that may exceed those of eating an unbalanced diet, during the normal active phase [60]. How CKD may affect these relationships and to what extent chronotype-adjusted diets may provide any advantages to CKD patients is, at this point, unclear.

Diet may also influence the gut microbiota. Gut bacteria modulate host rhythms via microbial metabolites such as butyrate and others, and amines and disturbed microbiome rhythms have been proposed to at least partially contribute to an increased risk of obesity and metabolic syndrome associated with chronodisruption [61]. Although there is little information on microbiota and chronodisruption in CKD, both obesity and metabolic syndrome increase the risk of CKD. Conversely, CKD has been associated with altered microbiota patterns and metabolites accumulated in CKD may modulate the gut microbiota and butyrate production [62–64].

5.2. Light Clues

In June 2019, a working group convened by the International Agency for Research on Cancer (IARC) concluded that "night shift work" is probably carcinogenic to humans and considered a Group 2A carcinogen [65]. There is very little information on night shift work and CKD. However, in a Korean study, the risk of CKD was two-fold higher in female shift workers than in female non-shift workers, although there were no differences in males [66]. In experimental animals, maternal chronic photoperiod shifting during gestation led to kidney gene expression changes in the offsprings, including the expression of sodium handling genes subject to circadian rhythms, and higher blood pressure values [27].

5.3. Kidney Inflammation

Kidney inflammation is a feature of both AKI and CKD. TWEAK is a proinflammatory cytokine of the TNF superfamily that promotes AKI and CKD [67,68]. A key feature of the TWEAK cytokine is that, contrary to TNF, it recruits the NIK-mediated, non-canonical pathway for activation of the NFκB transcription factor in kidney cells on top of the canonical pathway for NFκB activation [69–73]. NFκB is a key proinflammatory transcription factor that also downregulates kidney protective molecules [74]. Non-canonical NFκB is characterized by the nuclear translocation of RelB/NFκB2 p52 heterodimers [75]. Interestingly, the RelB subunit of NFκB directly binds *BMAL1* and acts as a negative regulator of circadian gene expression [76]. TWEAK also downregulates the kidney production of Klotho, an antiaging factor that is mainly expressed in the kidney, thus, potentially contributing to the accelerated aging of CKD [77,78]. Although the decrease in Klotho is mediated by the canonical NFκB pathway, it is nonetheless integrated within the cell response to TWEAK characterized by downregulation of tissue protective factors, as is a decrease in the mitochondrial biogenesis master regulator PGC1α [79,80]. In his regard, RelB also couples with the bioenergy NAD (+) sensor sirtuin 1 (SIRT1) to modulate cell metabolism and mitochondrial bioenergetics [81].

Kidney fibrosis sis very tightly linked to inflammation. In this regard, Smad3, a key signaling effector for the profibrotic cytokine TGFβ1, has circadian expression and modulates the expression of circadian rhythm genes such as *Dec1, Dec2,* and *Per1* [82].

5.4. Uremic Toxins

A key feature of advanced CKD is the accumulation of uremic retention solutes, molecules usually excreted by the kidneys that accumulate in the circulation when GFR decreases [11]. Some of these uremic retention solutes have a clear adverse impact on pathophysiological processes, promoting CKD progression and manifestations, they are the so-called uremic toxins. When kidneys fail, renal function is replaced by dialysis or eventually by a kidney graft. Unfortunately, while dialysis prevents acute uremic death, it provides only a very limited capacity to clear uremic toxins, especially those of gut origin that circulate bound to serum proteins, which may be of special interest from the point of view of chronodisruption. Thus, several gut-derived uremic toxins bind and activate the Aryl Hydrocarbon Receptor (AhR). These include uremic toxins derived from tryptophan, some of gut microbiota origin, such as indolic uremic toxins (indoxyl sulfate, indole-3 acetic acid, and indoxyl-β-d-glucuronide) and uremic toxins from the kynurenine pathway (kynurenine, kynurenic acid, anthranilic acid, 3-hydroxykynurenine, 3-hydroxyanthranilic acid, and quinolinic acid) [83,84]. Interestingly, AhR exhibits a rhythmic expression and time-dependent sensitivity to activation by AhR agonists and in response to at least some ligands, AhR forms a heterodimer with *Bmal1* and inhibits *Clock/Bmal1* activity, modulating amplitude and phase of rhythms in circadian clock genes [85,86]. In this regard, AhR deficiency enhanced behavioral responses to changes in the light–dark cycle, increased rhythmic amplitude of circadian clock genes in the liver, and altered glucose and insulin rhythms [86].

Kidney proximal tubule cells sense elevated endogenous, gut microbiome-derived, uremic retention solutes which elicit a compensatory response consisting of up-regulating the organic anion transporter-1 (OAT1), thus increasing metabolite secretion in urine [87]. This was clearly illustrated for indoxyl sulfate which induced OAT1 expression via AhR and EGFR signaling, controlled by miR-223 [87]. AhR protein expression was additionally positively associated with plasma levels of another indolic uremic toxin, indole-3 acetic acid (IAA) [88]. IAA is responsible for some adverse effects potentially related to the increased cardiovascular risk of CKD patients, such as increasing the expression of tissue factor in human vascular cells via the AhR [89]. However, up to now it is unknown to what extent the circadian expression of AhR is disrupted in CKD, what role might uremic toxins and the microbiota have in this phenomenon and what the consequences in any alterations in this system circadian regulation might be for CKD patients.

5.5. Disrupted HIF Activation and EPO Production

Hypoxia-inducible factor (HIF) are a family of transcription factors that protect from hypoxia both at the local, autocrine/paracrine level and by driving erythropoietin production, also through an endocrine mediator of kidney origin. Thus, the kidney has the lowest pO_2 in the body, a consequence of the existence of two consecutive capillary networks (glomerular and peritubular) and of the high metabolic rate of tubular cells which spend huge amounts of energy in recovering filtered molecules. This is the likely reason for the kidney location of erythropoietin-producing cells, a key defense mechanism against hypoxia that modulates hemoglobin availability and, thus, oxygen transport capacity by red blood cells.

The expression of a key HIF protein, HIF1α, is under circadian rhythm control. CRY1 reduces HIF-1α half-life and HIF binding to target gene promoters and abrogation of CRY1/2 stabilized HIF1α in response to hypoxia [90] while PER2 activates HIF-1α and facilitates its recruitment to promoter regions of its downstream genes. HIF-1α activation by PER2 was related to keeping the asparagine residue at position 803 of HIF-1α (HIF-1α N803) unhydroxylated by hypoxic stimulation in the absence of changes in HIF-1α protein levels [91]. In murine heart ischemia, *Per2* was required for Hif-1α stabilization [92]. This may be exploited therapeutically. Thus, *Per2* stabilization through adenosine activation of Adora2b or by exposure to intense light modified HIF-dependent cardiac metabolism, resulting in the transcriptional induction of glycolytic enzymes and *Per2*-dependent protection from ischemia [92]. So far, no such experiments have been reported for kidney disease. By contrast, BMAL1 deficiency increased HIF1α protein levels under hypoxic conditions. Induction of clock and HIF1α target genes in response to strenuous exercise varied according to the time of day in wild-type mice. Thus, interactions between circadian and HIF pathways influence metabolic adaptation to hypoxia [93].

Circadian transgenic zebrafish cells simulating a repressed or an overstimulated circadian clock, resulted in altered gene transcription levels of oxygen-regulated genes such as *EPO* and altered the hypoxia-induced increase in Hif-1α protein concentration. The amount of Hif-1α protein accumulated during the hypoxic response depended on the time of the day, with one maximum during the light phase and a second one during the dark phase [94].

The positive effects of HIF prolyl hydroxylase inhibitors (that is, HIF activators) over anemia and other cardiovascular risk parameters in CKD patients [95] raises the possibility that downregulation of HIF activation righter than loss of renal mass is a key driver of uremic anemia and may allow the exploration of the chronodisruption impact of uremic anemia itself.

5.6. Physical Inactivity

Both the drivers (e.g., obesity) and consequences (e.g., anemia, cardiovascular disease, malnutrition) of CKD may be associated to physical inactivity and this may act as a chronodisruptor. The impact of regular physical activity on kidney functions circadian misalignment should be studied, since regular endurance exercise appears to entrain peripheral clocks in muscle and heart [52].

5.7. Integration of Several Chronodisruptors

It is likely that the end result of the impact of several chronodisruptors relates to the integration of the different signaling events. In this regard, there is evidence that chronodisruptors potentially associated with CKD interact between them. Thus, RelB directly binds to the AhR and AhR interacts with dietary clues [81,96]. AhR-deficient mice are protected from high fat diet-induced disruption in metabolic rhythms, exhibiting enhanced insulin sensitivity and glucose tolerance [96].

6. The Way Forward

Table 3 summarizes some key answered questions regarding chronodisruption, chronodisruptors and CKD. A key to the clinical translation of the current state of knowledge regarding chronodisruption in CKD, beyond preventing and treating CKD itself, is to identify targetable chronodisruptors.

Table 3. Some key answered questions regarding chronodisruption, chronodisruptors and CKD.

When Does Chronodisruption Start in CKD Natural History?	What Are the Key Chronodisruptors in CKD and What Are Their Targets? Can Chronodisruptors Be Targeted Therapeutically?	Other Questions
Before or after the current GFR threshold to define CKD?	Can chronodisruptors be modified by altering the diet or timing of meals?	Is basic research in CKD tainted by chronodisruption resulting from performing mouse and rat experiments during daytime, which should be their inactive period?
Is a decreased GFR needed to trigger CKD-associated chronodisruption?	Or by altering the microbiota?	To what extent the age-associated loss of renal function contributes to age-associated circadian rhythm abnormalities?
Or is pathological albuminuria sufficient to trigger chronodisruption?	Or by drugs modulating their signaling pathways?	
	Does therapeutic targeting of CKD-related chronodisruptors improve outcomes?	
	Has melatonin any role in managing CKD?	
	Has chronopharmacology a role in CKD?	

An issue frequently overlooked by researchers is that the most common laboratory animals used to study kidney disease are rats and mice, which are nocturnal animals. Thus, essentially all experiments are performed during their inactive period and manipulation during this period risks creating chronodisruption which may have an unknown impact on experimental results [20]. This emphasizes the need for human studies. However, clinical research into CKD-related chronodisruption would require easy access to non-invasive techniques that allow monitoring of biological rhythms beyond blood pressure. Wrist skin temperature has been proposed as a new index for evaluating circadian system status [97]. Development of chronodisruption scores [98] and computational model of the renal circadian clock [99] would also facilitate clinical research. Longitudinal studies and ideally, interventional trials, would provide information on the causality and direction in the clinical association of disturbed sleep (a likely manifestation of chronodisruption) and CKD. In this regard, in a prospective cohort study of over 4000 participants from the Nurses' Health Study, shorter sleep duration was prospectively and independently associated with faster decline in renal function [100].

Chronopharmacology studies how biological rhythms influence pharmacokinetics, pharmacodynamics, and toxicity, and determines whether time-of-day administration modifies the pharmacological characteristics of the drug. Chronotherapy applies chronopharmacological studies to clinical treatments, determining the best biological time for dosing [101]. Well known examples in CKD patients include phosphate binders. In addition, there is a school of thought supported by meta-analyses results and clinical trials emphasizing the benefits of nighttime administration of anti-hypertensive medication [14].

In a recent clinical trial in hypertensive patients without CKD, ingestion of at least one blood pressure-lowering medication at bedtime resulted in improved ambulatory blood pressure control with a significant further decrease of asleep blood pressure and reduced risk of incident CKD than early morning administration [102].

While this may be initially viewed as CKD prevention, it is likely that it may additionally represent slowing of CKD progression, Thus, current diagnostic criteria for CKD are late events and patients who progressed to meet the diagnostic criteria for CKD during the trial likely had baseline subclinical CKD, maybe as cause of hypertension [103]. New upcoming drugs may also benefit from chronopharmacology studies. Thus, HIF activators were recently approved for clinical use in China and are expected to be soon available worldwide to treat uremic anemia [104]. Whether chronopharmacology may optimize timing of administration is currently unknown. Finally, cardiovascular and nephroprotective effects have been described for melatonin [105].

Author Contributions: All authors have contributed and read and agreed to the published version of the manuscript.

Funding: This work was funded by FIS CP14/00133, PI16/02057, PI18/01366, PI19/00588, PI19/00815, DTS18/00032, ERA-PerMed-JTC2018 (KIDNEY ATTACK AC18/00064 and PERSTIGAN AC18/00071, National Institute of Health (2R01AI063331), ISCIII-RETIC REDinREN RD016/0009 Fondos FEDER, FRIAT, Sociedad Española de Nefrología, Comunidad de Madrid B2017/BMD-3686 CIFRA2-CM, Miguel Servet MS14/00133 to MDSN and ABS. IIS-Fundacion Jimenez Diaz Biobank, part of the Spanish Biobanks Platform (PT17/0015/0006). The APC was funded by PI19/00815.

Conflicts of Interest: The authors declare no conflict of interest.

References

1. Perez-Gomez, M.V.; Bartsch, L.A.; Castillo-Rodriguez, E.; Fernandez-Prado, R.; Fernandez-Fernandez, B.; Martin-Cleary, C.; Gracia-Iguacel, C.; Ortiz, A. Clarifying the concept of chronic kidney disease for non-nephrologists. *Clin. Kidney J.* **2019**, *12*, 258–261. [CrossRef]
2. Foreman, K.J.; Marquez, N.; Dolgert, A.; Fukutaki, K.; Fullman, N.; McGaughey, M.; Pletcher, M.A.; Smith, A.E.; Tang, K.; Yuan, C.W.; et al. Forecasting life expectancy, years of life lost, and all-cause and cause-specific mortality for 250 causes of death: Reference and alternative scenarios for 2016-40 for 195 countries and territories. *Lancet* **2018**, *392*, 2052–2090. [CrossRef]
3. Ortiz, A.; Sanchez-Niño, M.D.; Crespo-Barrio, M.; De-Sequera-Ortiz, P.; Fernández-Giráldez, E.; García-Maset, R.; Macía-Heras, M.; Pérez-Fontán, M.; Rodríguez-Portillo, M.; Salgueira-Lazo, M.; et al. The Spanish Society of Nephrology (SENEFRO) commentary to the Spain GBD 2016 report: Keeping chronic kidney disease out of sight of health authorities will only magnify the problem. *Nefrologia* **2019**, *39*, 29–34. [CrossRef]
4. Fernandez-Fernandez, B.; Fernandez-Prado, R.; Górriz, J.L.; Martinez-Castelao, A.; Navarro-González, J.F.; Porrini, E.; Soler, M.J.; Ortiz, A. Canagliflozin and Renal Events in Diabetes with Established Nephropathy Clinical Evaluation and Study of Diabetic Nephropathy with Atrasentan: What was learned about the treatment of diabetic kidney disease with canagliflozin and atrasentan? *Clin. Kidney J.* **2019**, *12*, 313–321. [CrossRef]
5. Sarafidis, P.; Ferro, C.J.; Morales, E.; Ortiz, A.; Malyszko, J.; Hojs, R.; Khazim, K.; Ekart, R.; Valdivielso, J.; Fouque, D.; et al. SGLT-2 inhibitors and GLP-1 receptor agonists for nephroprotection and cardioprotection in patients with diabetes mellitus and chronic kidney disease. A consensus statement by the EURECA-m and the DIABESITY working groups of the ERA-EDTA. *Nephrol. Dial. Transplant.* **2019**, *34*, 208–230. [CrossRef]
6. Herrington, W.G.; Preiss, D.; Haynes, R.; von Eynatten, M.; Staplin, N.; Hauske, S.J.; George, J.T.; Green, J.B.; Landray, M.J.; Baigent, C.; et al. The potential for improving cardio-renal outcomes by sodium-glucose co-transporter-2 inhibition in people with chronic kidney disease: A rationale for the EMPA-KIDNEY study. *Clin. Kidney J.* **2018**, *11*, 749–761. [CrossRef] [PubMed]
7. Williams, B.; Mancia, G.; Spiering, W.; Agabiti Rosei, E.; Azizi, M.; Burnier, M.; Clement, D.; Coca, A.; De Simone, G.; Dominiczak, A.; et al. 2018 Practice Guidelines for the management of arterial hypertension of the European Society of Hypertension and the European Society of Cardiology: ESH/ESC Task Force for the Management of Arterial Hypertension. *J. Hypertens.* **2018**, *36*, 2284–2309. [CrossRef] [PubMed]
8. Sanchez-Niño, M.D.; Sanz, A.B.; Ramos, A.M.; Ruiz-Ortega, M.; Ortiz, A. Translational science in chronic kidney disease. *Clin. Sci. (Lond.)* **2017**, *131*, 1617–1629. [CrossRef]
9. Fernandez-Prado, R.; Esteras, R.; Perez-Gomez, M.V.; Gracia-Iguacel, C.; Gonzalez-Parra, E.; Sanz, A.B.; Ortiz, A.; Sanchez-Niño, M.D. Nutrients Turned into Toxins: Microbiota Modulation of Nutrient Properties in Chronic Kidney Disease. *Nutrients* **2017**, *9*, 489. [CrossRef] [PubMed]

10. Castillo-Rodríguez, E.; Pizarro-Sánchez, S.; Sanz, A.B.; Ramos, A.M.; Sanchez-Niño, M.D.; Martin-Cleary, C.; Fernandez-Fernandez, B.; Ortiz, A. Inflammatory Cytokines as Uremic Toxins: "Ni Son Todos Los Que Estan, Ni Estan Todos Los Que Son". *Toxins* **2017**, *9*, 114.
11. Duranton, F.; Cohen, G.; De Smet, R.; Rodriguez, M.; Jankowski, J.; Vanholder, R.; Argiles, A. European Uremic Toxin Work Group. *Norm. Pathol. Conc. Urem. Toxins J. Am. Soc. Nephrol.* **2012**, *23*, 1258–1270. [CrossRef] [PubMed]
12. Fernandez-Fernandez, B.; Izquierdo, M.C.; Valiño-Rivas, L.; Nastou, D.; Sanz, A.B.; Ortiz, A.; Sanchez-Niño, M.D. Albumin downregulates Klotho in tubular cells. *Nephrol. Dial. Transplant.* **2018**, *33*, 1712–1722. [CrossRef]
13. Rossignol, P.; Massy, Z.A.; Azizi, M.; Bakris, G.; Ritz, E.; Covic, A.; Goldsmith, D.; Heine, G.H.; Jager, K.J.; Kanbay, M.; et al. The double challenge of resistant hypertension and chronic kidney disease. *Lancet* **2015**, *386*, 1588–1598. [CrossRef]
14. Firsov, D.; Bonny, O. Circadian rhythms and the kidney. *Nat. Rev. Nephrol.* **2018**, *14*, 626–635. [CrossRef] [PubMed]
15. Firsov, D.; Bonny, O. Circadian regulation of renal function. *Kidney Int.* **2010**, *78*, 640–645. [CrossRef] [PubMed]
16. Martinez-Nicolas, A.; Madrid, J.A.; Rol, M.A. Day-night contrast as source of health for the human circadian system. *Chronobiol. Int.* **2014**, *31*, 382–393. [CrossRef]
17. Zhang, D.; Pollock, D.M. Diurnal Regulation of Renal Electrolyte Excretion: The Role of Paracrine Factors. *Annu. Rev. Physiol.* **2019**, *82*, 343–363. [CrossRef]
18. Chiou, Y.Y.; Yang, Y.; Rashid, N.; Ye, R.; Selby, C.P.; Sancar, A. Mammalian Period represses and de-represses transcription by displacing CLOCK-BMAL1 from promoters in a Cryptochrome-dependent manner. *Proc. Natl. Acad. Sci. USA* **2016**, *113*, E6072–E6079. [CrossRef]
19. Mészáros, K.; Pruess, L.; Szabó, A.J.; Gondan, M.; Ritz, E.; Schaefer, F. Development of the circadian clockwork in the kidney. *Kidney Int.* **2014**, *86*, 915–922. [CrossRef]
20. Becker, B.K.; Zhang, D.; Soliman, R.; Pollock, D.M. Autonomic nerves and circadian control of renal function. *Auton. Neurosci.* **2019**, *217*, 58–65. [CrossRef]
21. Motohashi, H.; Tahara, Y.; Whittaker, D.S.; Wang, H.B.; Yamaji, T.; Wakui, H.; Haraguchi, A.; Yamazaki, M.; Miyakawa, H.; Hama, K.; et al. The circadian clock is disrupted in mice with adenine-induced tubulointerstitial nephropathy. *Kidney Int.* **2020**. [CrossRef]
22. Hara, M.; Minami, Y.; Ohashi, M.; Tsuchiya, Y.; Kusaba, T.; Tamagaki, K.; Koike, N.; Umemura, Y.; Inokawa, H.; Yagita, K. Robust circadian clock oscillation and osmotic rhythms in inner medulla reflecting cortico-medullary osmotic gradient rhythm in rodent kidney. *Sci. Rep.* **2017**, *7*, 1–9. [CrossRef] [PubMed]
23. Nikolaeva, S.; Ansermet, C.; Centeno, G.; Pradervand, S.; Bize, V.; Mordasini, D.; Henry, H.; Koesters, R.; Maillard, M.; Bonny, O.; et al. Nephron-Specific Deletion of Circadian Clock Gene Bmal1 Alters the Plasma and Renal Metabolome and Impairs Drug Disposition. *J. Am. Soc. Nephrol.* **2016**, *27*, 2997–3004. [CrossRef] [PubMed]
24. Erren, T.C.; Reiter, R.J.; Piekarski, C. Light, timing of biological rhythms, and chronodisruption in man. *Naturwissenschaften* **2003**, *90*, 485–494. [CrossRef] [PubMed]
25. Erren, T.C.; Reiter, R.J. Defining chronodisruption. *J. Pineal Res.* **2009**, *46*, 245–247. [CrossRef]
26. Bonny, O.; Vinciguerra, M.; Gumz, M.L.; Mazzoccoli, G. Molecular bases of circadian rhythmicity in renal physiology and pathology. *Nephrol. Dial. Transplant.* **2013**, *28*, 2421–2431. [CrossRef]
27. Mendez, N.; Torres-Farfan, C.; Salazar, E.; Bascur, P.; Bastidas, C.; Vergara, K.; Spichiger, C.; Halabi, D.; Vio, C.P.; Richter, H.G. Fetal Programming of Renal Dysfunction and High Blood Pressure by Chronodisruption. *Front. Endocrinol.* **2019**, *10*, 362. [CrossRef]
28. Wuerzner, G.; Firsov, D.; Bonny, O. Circadian glomerular function: From physiology to molecular and therapeutical aspects. *Nephrol. Dial. Transplant.* **2014**, *29*, 1475–1480. [CrossRef]
29. Firsov, D.; Tokonami, N.; Bonny, O. Role of the renal circadian timing system in maintaining water and electrolytes homeostasis. *Mol. Cell. Endocrinol.* **2012**, *349*, 51–55. [CrossRef]
30. Argilés, A.; Mourad, G.; Mion, C. Seasonal changes in blood pressure in patients with end-stage renal disease treated with hemodialysis. *N. Engl. J. Med.* **1998**, *339*, 1364–1370. [CrossRef]

31. Knutson, K.L.; Lash, J.; Ricardo, A.C.; Herdegen, J.; Thornton, J.D.; Rahman, M.; Turek, N.; Cohan, J.; Lawrence, J.; Bazzano, L.; et al. Habitual sleep and kidney function in chronic kidney disease: The Chronic Renal Insufficiency Cohort study. *J. Sleep Res.* **2018**, *27*, 281–289. [CrossRef] [PubMed]
32. Ohashi, N.; Ishigaki, S.; Isobe, S. The pivotal role of melatonin in ameliorating chronic kidney disease by suppression of the renin-angiotensin system in the kidney. *Hypertens. Res.* **2019**, *42*, 761–768. [CrossRef]
33. Voulgaris, A.; Marrone, O.; Bonsignore, M.R.; Steiropoulos, P. Chronic kidney disease in patients with obstructive sleep apnea. *Narrat. Rev. Sleep Med. Rev.* **2019**, *47*, 74–89. [CrossRef] [PubMed]
34. Sarafidis, P.A.; Persu, A.; Agarwal, R.; Burnier, M.; de Leeuw, P.; Ferro, C.J.; Halimi, J.M.; Heine, G.H.; Jadoul, M.; Jarraya, F.; et al. Hypertension in dialysis patients: A consensus document by the European Renal and Cardiovascular Medicine (EURECA-m) working group of the European Renal Association-European Dialysis and Transplant Association (ERA-EDTA) and the Hypertension and the Kidney working group of the European Society of Hypertension (ESH). *Nephrol. Dial. Transplant.* **2017**, *32*, 620–640. [PubMed]
35. Bolignano, D.; Rastelli, S.; Agarwal, R.; Fliser, D.; Massy, Z.; Ortiz, A.; Wiecek, A.; Martinez-Castelao, A.; Covic, A.; Goldsmith, D.; et al. Pulmonary hypertension in CKD. *Am. J. Kidney Dis.* **2013**, *61*, 612–622. [CrossRef] [PubMed]
36. Di Daniele, N.; Fegatelli, D.A.; Rovella, V.; Castagnola, V.; Gabriele, M.; Scuteri, A. Circadian blood pressure patterns and blood pressure control in patients with chronic kidney disease. *Atherosclerosis* **2017**, *267*, 139–145. [CrossRef]
37. Ruiz-Hurtado, G.; Ruilope, L.; De la Sierra, A.; Sarafidis, P.; De la Cruz, J.; Gorostidi, M.; Segura, J.; Vinyoles, E.; Banegas, J. Association between High and Very High Albuminuria and Nighttime Blood Pressure: Influence of Diabetes and Chronic Kidney Disease. *Diabetes Care* **2016**, *39*, 1729–1737. [CrossRef]
38. Ando, D.; Yasuda, G. Circadian Blood Pressure Rhythm Is Changed by Improvement in Hypoalbuminemia and Massive Proteinuria in Patients with Minimal Change Nephrotic Syndrome. *Cardiorenal. Med.* **2016**, *6*, 209–215. [CrossRef]
39. Ohkubo, T.; Hozawa, A.; Yamaguchi, J.; Kikuya, M.; Ohmori, K.; Michimata, M.; Matsubara, M.; Hashimoto, J.; Hoshi, H.; Araki, T.; et al. Prognostic significance of the nocturnal decline in blood pressure in individuals with and without high 24-h blood pressure: The Ohasama study. *J. Hypertens.* **2002**, *20*, 2183–2189. [CrossRef]
40. Fedecostante, M.; Spannella, F.; Cola, G.; Espinosa, E.; Dessì-Fulgheri, P.; Sarzani, R. Chronic kidney disease is characterized by "double trouble" higher pulse pressure plus night-time systolic blood pressure and more severe cardiac damage. *PLoS ONE* **2014**, *9*, e86155. [CrossRef]
41. Huang, J.T.; Cheng, H.M.; Yu, W.C.; Lin, Y.P.; Sung, S.H.; Chen, C.H. Increased Nighttime Pulse Pressure Variability but Not Ambulatory Blood Pressure Levels Predicts 14-Year All-Cause Mortality in Patients on Hemodialysis. *Hypertension* **2019**, *74*, 660–668. [CrossRef] [PubMed]
42. Tokonami, N.; Mordasini, D.; Pradervand, S.; Centeno, G.; Jouffe, C.; Maillard, M.; Bonny, O.; Gachon, F.; Gomez, R.A.; Sequeira-Lopez, M.L. Local renal circadian clocks control fluid-electrolyte homeostasis and BP. *J. Am. Soc. Nephrol.* **2014**, *25*, 1430–1439. [CrossRef] [PubMed]
43. Ivy, J.R.; Jones, N.K.; Costello, H.M.; Mansley, M.K.; Peltz, T.S.; Flatman, P.W.; Bailey, M.A. Glucocorticoid receptor activation stimulates the sodium-chloride cotransporter and influences the diurnal rhythm of its phosphorylation. *Am. J. Physiol. Renal Physiol.* **2019**, *317*, F1536–F1548. [CrossRef] [PubMed]
44. Nakashima, A.; Kawamoto, T.; Noshiro, M.; Ueno, T.; Doi, S.; Honda, K.; Masaki, T.; Higashi, Y.; Kato, Y. Dec1 and CLOCK Regulate Na. *Hypertension* **2018**, *72*, 746–754. [CrossRef]
45. Valiño-Rivas, L.; Cuarental, L.; Agustin, M.; Husi, H.; Cannata-Ortiz, P.; Sanz, A.B.; Mischak, H.; Ortiz, A.; Sanchez-Niño, M.D. MAGE genes in the kidney: Identification of MAGED2 as upregulated during kidney injury and in stressed tubular cells. *Nephrol. Dial. Transplant.* **2019**, *34*, 1498–1507. [CrossRef]
46. Gil, R.B.; Ortiz, A.; Sanchez-Niño, M.D.; Markoska, K.; Schepers, E.; Vanholder, R.; Glorieux, G.; Schmitt-Kopplin, P.; Heinzmann, S. Increased urinary osmolyte excretion indicates chronic kidney disease severity and progression rate. *Nephrol. Dial. Transplant.* **2018**, *33*, 2156–2164. [CrossRef]
47. Myung, J.; Wu, M.Y.; Lee, C.Y.; Rahim, A.R.; Truong, V.H.; Wu, D.; Piggins, H.D.; Wu, M.S. The Kidney Clock Contributes to Timekeeping by the Master Circadian Clock. *Int. J. Mol. Sci.* **2019**, *20*, 2765. [CrossRef]
48. Gansevoort, R.; Arici, M.; Benzing, T.; Birn, H.; Capasso, G.; Covic, A.; Devuyst, O.; Drechsler, C.; Eckardt, K.U.; Emma, F.; et al. Recommendations for the use of tolvaptan in autosomal dominant polycystic kidney disease: A position statement on behalf of the ERA-EDTA Working Groups on Inherited Kidney Disorders and European Renal Best Practice. *Nephrol. Dial. Transplant.* **2016**, *31*, 337–348. [CrossRef]

49. Torres, V.E.; Chapman, A.B.; Devuyst, O.; Gansevoort, R.T.; Perrone, R.D.; Koch, G.; Ouyang, J.; McQuade, R.D.; Blais, J.D.; Czerwiec, F.S.; et al. Tolvaptan in Later-Stage Autosomal Dominant Polycystic Kidney Disease. *N. Engl. J. Med.* **2017**, *377*, 1930–1942. [CrossRef]
50. Montero, D.; Diaz-Canestro, C.; Oberholzer, L.; Lundby, C. The role of blood volume in cardiac dysfunction and reduced exercise tolerance in patients with diabetes. *Lancet Diabetes Endocrinol.* **2019**, *7*, 807–816. [CrossRef]
51. Parizadeh, S.M.; Ghandehari, M.; Parizadeh, M.R.; Ferns, G.A.; Ghayour-Mobarhan, M.; Avan, A.; Hassanian, S. The diagnostic and prognostic value of copeptin in cardiovascular disease, current status, and prospective. *J. Cell. Biochem.* **2018**, *119*, 7913–7923. [CrossRef] [PubMed]
52. Schmitt, E.E.; Johnson, E.C.; Yusifova, M.; Bruns, D.R. The renal molecular clock: Broken by aging and restored by exercise. *Am. J. Physiol. Renal Physiol.* **2019**, *317*, F1087–F1093. [CrossRef]
53. Batinga, H.; Martinez-Nicolas, A.; Zornoza-Moreno, M.; Sánchez-Solis, M.; Larqué, E.; Mondéjar, M.T.; Moreno-Casbas, M.; García, F.J.; Campos, M.; Rol, M.A.; et al. Ontogeny and aging of the distal skin temperature rhythm in humans. *Age* **2015**, *37*, 29. [CrossRef] [PubMed]
54. Ohashi, N.; Ishigaki, S.; Isobe, S.; Matsuyama, T.; Sato, T.; Fujikura, T.; Tsuji, T.; Kato, A.; Yasuda, H. Salt Loading Aggravates the Relationship between Melatonin and Proteinuria in Patients with Chronic Kidney Disease. *Intern. Med.* **2019**, *58*, 1557–1564. [CrossRef] [PubMed]
55. Speed, J.S.; Hyndman, K.A.; Roth, K.; Heimlich, J.B.; Kasztan, M.; Fox, B.M.; Johnston, J.G.; Becker, B.K.; Jin, C.; Gamble, K.L.; et al. High dietary sodium causes dyssynchrony of the renal molecular clock in rats. *Am. J. Physiol. Renal Physiol.* **2018**, *314*, F89–F98. [CrossRef] [PubMed]
56. Daimiel-Ruiz, L.; Klett-Mingo, M.; Konstantinidou, V.; Micó, V.; Aranda, J.F.; García, B.; Martínez-Botas, J.; Dávalos, A.; Fernández-Hernando, C.; Ordovás, J.M. Dietary lipids modulate the expression of miR-107, a miRNA that regulates the circadian system. *Mol. Nutr. Food Res.* **2015**, *59*, 1865–1878. [CrossRef]
57. Laermans, J.; Depoortere, I. Chronobesity: Role of the circadian system in the obesity epidemic. *Obes. Rev.* **2016**, *17*, 108–125. [CrossRef]
58. Galindo Muñoz, J.S.; Gómez Gallego, M.; Díaz Soler, I.; Barberá Ortega, M.C.; Martínez Cáceres, C.M.; Hernández Morante, J.J. Effect of a chronotype-adjusted diet on weight loss effectiveness: A randomized clinical trial. *Clin. Nutr.* **2019**. [CrossRef]
59. Bandín, C.; Scheer, F.A.; Luque, A.J.; Ávila-Gandía, V.; Zamora, S.; Madrid, J.A. Meal timing affects glucose tolerance, substrate oxidation and circadian-related variables: A randomized, crossover trial. *Int. J. Obes.* **2015**, *39*, 828–833.
60. Challet, E. The circadian regulation of food intake. *Nat. Rev. Endocrinol.* **2019**, *15*, 393–405. [CrossRef]
61. Parkar, S.G.A.; Cheeseman, J.F. Potential Role for the Gut Microbiota in Modulating Host Circadian Rhythms and Metabolic Health. *Microorganisms* **2019**, *7*, 41. [CrossRef] [PubMed]
62. Aguilera-Correa, J.-J.; Madrazo-Clemente, P.; Martínez-Cuesta, M.D.C.; Peláez, C.; Ortiz, A.; Sánchez-Niño, M.D.; Esteban, J.; Requena, T. Lyso-Gb3 modulates the gut microbiota and decreases butyrate production. *Sci. Rep.* **2019**, *9*, 1–10. [CrossRef] [PubMed]
63. Perna, A.F.; Glorieux, G.; Zacchia, M.; Trepiccione, F.; Capolongo, G.; Vigorito, C.; Anishchenko, E.; Ingrosso, D. The role of the intestinal microbiota in uremic solute accumulation: A focus on sulfur compounds. *J. Nephrol.* **2019**, *32*, 733–740. [CrossRef] [PubMed]
64. Joossens, M.; Faust, K.; Gryp, T.; Nguyen, A.T.L.; Wang, J.; Eloot, S.; Schepers, E.; Dhondt, A.; Pletinck, A.; Vieira-Silva, S.; et al. Gut microbiota dynamics and uraemic toxins: One size does not fit all. *Gut* **2019**, *68*, 2257–2260. [CrossRef]
65. Erren, T.C.; Morfeld, P.; Groß, J.V.; Wild, U.; Lewis, P. IARC 2019: "Night shift work" is probably carcinogenic: What about disturbed chronobiology in all walks of life? *J. Occup. Med. Toxicol.* **2019**, *14*, 29. [CrossRef]
66. Uhm, J.Y.; Kim, H.R.; Kang, G.H.; Choi, Y.G.; Park, T.H.; Kim, S.Y.; Chang, S.S.; Choo, W.O. The association between shift work and chronic kidney disease in manual labor workers using data from the Korea National Health and Nutrition Examination Survey (KNHANES 2011–2014). *Ann. Occup. Environ. Med.* **2018**, *30*, 69. [CrossRef]
67. Sanz, A.B.; Ruiz-Andres, O.; Sanchez-Niño, M.D.; Ruiz-Ortega, M.; Ramos, A.M.; Ortiz, A. Out of the TWEAKlight: Elucidating the Role of Fn14 and TWEAK in Acute Kidney Injury. *Semin. Nephrol.* **2016**, *36*, 189–198. [CrossRef]

68. Sanz, A.B.; Izquierdo, M.C.; Sanchez-Niño, M.D.; Ucero, A.C.; Egido, J.; Ruiz-Ortega, M.; Ramos, A.M.; Putterman, C.; Ortiz, A. TWEAK and the progression of renal disease: Clinical translation. *Nephrol. Dial. Transplant.* **2014**, *29* (Suppl. 1), i54–i62. [CrossRef]
69. Valiño-Rivas, L.; Vaquero, J.J.; Sucunza, D.; Gutierrez, S.; Sanz, A.B.; Fresno, M.; Ortiz, A.; Sanchez-Niño, M.D. NIK as a Druggable Mediator of Tissue Injury. *Trends Mol. Med.* **2019**, *25*, 341–360. [CrossRef]
70. Valiño-Rivas, L.; Gonzalez-Lafuente, L.; Sanz, A.B.; Ruiz-Ortega, M.; Ortiz, A.; Sanchez-Niño, M.D. Non-canonical NFκB activation promotes chemokine expression in podocytes. *Sci. Rep.* **2016**, *6*, 28857. [CrossRef]
71. Sanz, A.B.; Sanchez-Niño, M.D.; Izquierdo, M.C.; Jakubowski, A.; Justo, P.; Blanco-Colio, L.M.; Blanco-Colio, L.M.; Ruiz-Ortega, M.; Selgas, R.; Egido, J.; et al. TWEAK activates the non-canonical NFkappaB pathway in murine renal tubular cells: Modulation of CCL21. *PLoS ONE* **2010**, *5*, e8955. [CrossRef] [PubMed]
72. Ortiz, A.; Husi, H.; Gonzalez-Lafuente, L.; Valiño-Rivas, L.; Fresno, M.; Sanz, A.B.; Mullen, W.; Albalat, A.; Mezzano, S.; Vlahou, T.; et al. Mitogen-Activated Protein Kinase 14 Promotes AKI. *J. Am. Soc. Nephrol.* **2017**, *28*, 823–836. [CrossRef]
73. Cuarental, L.; Sucunza-Sáenz, D.; Valiño-Rivas, L.; Fernandez-Fernandez, B.; Sanz, A.B.; Ortiz, A.; Vaquero, J.J.; Sanchez-Niño, M.D. MAP3K kinases and kidney injury. *Nefrologia* **2019**, *39*, 568–580. [CrossRef] [PubMed]
74. Sanz, A.B.; Sanchez-Niño, M.D.; Ramos, A.M.; Moreno, J.A.; Santamaria, B.; Ruiz-Ortega, M.; Mullen, W.; Albalat, A.; Mezzano, S.; Vlahou, T.; et al. NF-kappaB in renal inflammation. *J. Am. Soc. Nephrol.* **2010**, *21*, 1254–1262. [CrossRef] [PubMed]
75. Poveda, J.; Tabara, L.C.; Fernandez-Fernandez, B.; Martin-Cleary, C.; Sanz, A.B.; Selgas, R.; Ortiz, A.; Sanchez-Niño, M.D. TWEAK/Fn14 and Non-Canonical NF-kappaB Signaling in Kidney Disease. *Front. Immunol.* **2013**, *4*, 447. [CrossRef]
76. Bellet, M.M.; Zocchi, L.; Sassone-Corsi, P. The RelB subunit of NFκB acts as a negative regulator of circadian gene expression. *Cell Cycle* **2012**, *11*, 3304–3311. [CrossRef] [PubMed]
77. Poveda, J.; Sanz, A.B.; Carrasco, S.; Ruiz-Ortega, M.; Cannata-Ortiz, P.; Sanchez-Niño, M.D.; Ortiz, A. Bcl3: A regulator of NF-κB inducible by TWEAK in acute kidney injury with anti-inflammatory and antiapoptotic properties in tubular cells. *Exp. Mol. Med.* **2017**, *49*, e352. [CrossRef]
78. Moreno, J.A.; Izquierdo, M.C.; Sanchez-Niño, M.D.; Suárez-Alvarez, B.; Lopez-Larrea, C.; Jakubowski, A.; Blanco, J.; Ramirez, R.; Selgas, R.; Ruiz-Ortega, M.; et al. The inflammatory cytokines TWEAK and TNFα reduce renal klotho expression through NFκB. *J. Am. Soc. Nephrol.* **2011**, *22*, 1315–1325. [CrossRef]
79. Ruiz-Andres, O.; Sanchez-Niño, M.D.; Moreno, J.A.; Ruiz-Ortega, M.; Ramos, A.M.; Sanz, A.B.; Ortiz, A. Downregulation of kidney protective factors by inflammation: Role of transcription factors and epigenetic mechanisms. *Am. J. Physiol. Renal Physiol.* **2016**, *311*, F1329–F1340. [CrossRef]
80. Ruiz-Andres, O.; Suarez-Alvarez, B.; Sánchez-Ramos, C.; Monsalve, M.; Sanchez-Niño, M.D.; Ruiz-Ortega, M.; Egido, J.; Ortiz, A.; Sanz, A.B. The inflammatory cytokine TWEAK decreases PGC-1α expression and mitochondrial function in acute kidney injury. *Kidney Int.* **2016**, *89*, 399–410. [CrossRef]
81. Millet, P.; McCall, C.; Yoza, B. RelB: An outlier in leukocyte biology. *J. Leukoc. Biol.* **2013**, *94*, 941–951. [CrossRef]
82. Sato, F.; Otsuka, T.; Kohsaka, A.; Le, H.T.; Bhawal, U.K.; Muragaki, Y. Smad3 Suppresses Epithelial Cell Migration and Proliferation via the Clock Gene Dec1, Which Negatively Regulates the Expression of Clock Genes Dec2 and Per1. *Am. J. Pathol.* **2019**, *189*, 773–783. [CrossRef] [PubMed]
83. Sallée, M.; Dou, L.; Cerini, C.; Poitevin, S.; Brunet, P.; Burtey, S. The aryl hydrocarbon receptor-activating effect of uremic toxins from tryptophan metabolism: A new concept to understand cardiovascular complications of chronic kidney disease. *Toxins* **2014**, *6*, 934–949. [CrossRef]
84. Castillo-Rodriguez, E.; Fernandez-Prado, R.; Esteras, R.; Perez-Gomez, M.V.; Gracia-Iguacel, C.; Fernandez-Fernandez, B.; Kanbay, M.; Tejedor, A.; Lazaro, A.; Ruiz-Ortega, M.; et al. Impact of Altered Intestinal Microbiota on Chronic Kidney Disease Progression. *Toxins* **2018**, *10*, 300. [CrossRef] [PubMed]
85. Tischkau, S.A. Mechanisms of circadian clock interactions with aryl hydrocarbon receptor signalling. *Eur. J. Neurosci.* **2019**, *51*, 379–395. [CrossRef]
86. Jaeger, C.; Khazaal, A.Q.; Xu, C.; Sun, M.; Krager, S.L.; Tischkau, S.A. Aryl Hydrocarbon Receptor Deficiency Alters Circadian and Metabolic Rhythmicity. *J. Biol. Rhythms* **2017**, *32*, 109–120. [CrossRef] [PubMed]

87. Jansen, J.; Jansen, K.; Neven, E.; Poesen, R.; Othman, A.; van Mil, A.; Sluijter, J.; Sastre Torano, J.; Zaal, E.A.; Berkers, C.R.; et al. Remote sensing and signaling in kidney proximal tubules stimulates gut microbiome-derived organic anion secretion. *Proc. Natl. Acad. Sci. USA* **2019**, *116*, 16105–16110. [CrossRef] [PubMed]
88. Brito, J.S.; Borges, N.A.; Anjos, J.S.D.; Nakao, L.S.; Stockler-Pinto, M.B.; Paiva, B.R.; Cardoso-Weide, L.C.; Cardozo, L.F.M.F.; Mafra, D. Aryl Hydrocarbon Receptor and Uremic Toxins from the Gut Microbiota in Chronic Kidney Disease Patients: Is There a Relationship between Them? *Biochemistry* **2019**, *58*, 2054–2060. [CrossRef]
89. Addi, T.; Poitevin, S.; McKay, N.; El Mecherfi, K.E.; Kheroua, O.; Jourde-Chiche, N.; de Macedo, A.; Gondouin, B.; Cerini, C.; Brunet, P.; et al. Mechanisms of tissue factor induction by the uremic toxin indole-3 acetic acid through aryl hydrocarbon receptor/nuclear factor-kappa B signaling pathway in human endothelial cells. *Arch. Toxicol.* **2019**, *93*, 121–136. [CrossRef]
90. Dimova, E.Y.; Jakupovic, M.; Kubaichuk, K.; Mennerich, D.; Chi, T.F.; Tamanini, F.; Oklejewicz, M.; Hänig, J.; Byts, N.; Mäkelä, K.A.; et al. The Circadian Clock Protein CRY1 Is a Negative Regulator of HIF-1α. *iScience* **2019**, *13*, 284–304. [CrossRef]
91. Kobayashi, M.; Morinibu, A.; Koyasu, S.; Goto, Y.; Hiraoka, M.; Harada, H. A circadian clock gene, PER2, activates HIF-1 as an effector molecule for recruitment of HIF-1α to promoter regions of its downstream genes. *FEBS J.* **2017**, *284*, 3804–3816. [CrossRef] [PubMed]
92. Eckle, T.; Hartmann, K.; Bonney, S.; Reithel, S.; Mittelbronn, M.; Walker, L.A.; Lowes, B.D.; Han, J.; Borchers, C.H.; Buttrick, P.M.; et al. Adora2b-elicited Per2 stabilization promotes a HIF-dependent metabolic switch crucial for myocardial adaptation to ischemia. *Nat. Med.* **2012**, *18*, 774–782. [CrossRef] [PubMed]
93. Peek, C.B.; Levine, D.C.; Cedernaes, J.; Taguchi, A.; Kobayashi, Y.; Tsai, S.J.; Bonar, N.A.; Mc, M.R.; Ramsey, K.M.; Bass, J. Circadian Clock Interaction with HIF1α Mediates Oxygenic Metabolism and Anaerobic Glycolysis in Skeletal Muscle. *Cell Metab.* **2017**, *25*, 86–92. [CrossRef] [PubMed]
94. Egg, M.; Köblitz, L.; Hirayama, J.; Schwerte, T.; Folterbauer, C.; Kurz, A.; Fiechtner, B.; Möst, M.; Salvenmoser, W.; Sassone, P.; et al. Linking oxygen to time: The bidirectional interaction between the hypoxic signaling pathway and the circadian clock. *Chronobiol. Int.* **2013**, *30*, 510–529. [CrossRef]
95. Chen, N.; Hao, C.; Liu, B.C.; Lin, H.; Wang, C.; Xing, C.; Liang, X.; Jiang, G.; Liu, Z.; Li, X.; et al. Roxadustat Treatment for Anemia in Patients Undergoing Long-Term Dialysis. *N. Engl. J. Med.* **2019**, *381*, 1011–1022. [CrossRef] [PubMed]
96. Jaeger, C.; Xu, C.; Sun, M.; Krager, S.; Tischkau, S.A. Aryl hydrocarbon receptor-deficient mice are protected from high fat diet-induced changes in metabolic rhythms. *Chronobiol. Int.* **2017**, *34*, 318–336. [CrossRef]
97. Martinez-Nicolas, A.; Ortiz-Tudela, E.; Rol, M.A.; Madrid, J.A. Uncovering different masking factors on wrist skin temperature rhythm in free-living subjects. *PLoS ONE* **2013**, *8*, e61142. [CrossRef]
98. Corbalán-Tutau, M.D.; Gómez-Abellán, P.; Madrid, J.A.; Canteras, M.; Ordovás, J.M.M. Toward a chronobiological characterization of obesity and metabolic syndrome in clinical practice. *Clin. Nutr.* **2015**, *34*, 477–483. [CrossRef]
99. Wei, N.; Gumz, M.L.; Layton, A.T. Predicted effect of circadian clock modulation of NHE3 of a proximal tubule cell on sodium transport. *Am. J. Physiol. Renal Physiol.* **2018**, *315*, F665–F676. [CrossRef] [PubMed]
100. McMullan, C.J.; Curhan, G.C.; Forman, J.P. Association of short sleep duration and rapid decline in renal function. *Kidney Int.* **2016**, *89*, 1324–1330. [CrossRef]
101. De Lavallaz, L.; Musso, C.G. Chronobiology in nephrology: The influence of circadian rhythms on renal handling of drugs and renal disease treatment. *Int. Urol. Nephrol.* **2018**, *50*, 2221–2228. [CrossRef] [PubMed]
102. Hermida, R.C.; Ayala, D.E.; Mojón, A.; Fernández, J.R. Risk of incident chronic kidney disease is better reduced by bedtime than upon-awakening ingestion of hypertension medications. *Hypertens. Res.* **2018**, *41*, 342–353. [CrossRef] [PubMed]
103. Sanchez-Niño, M.D.; Sanz, A.B.; Ramos, A.M.; Fernandez-Fernandez, B.; Ortiz, A. Clinical proteomics in kidney disease as an exponential technology: Heading towards the disruptive phase. *Clin. Kidney J.* **2017**, *10*, 188–191. [CrossRef] [PubMed]

104. Chen, N.; Hao, C.; Peng, X.; Lin, H.; Yin, A.; Hao, L.; Tao, Y.; Liang, X.; Liu, Z.; Xing, C. Roxadustat for Anemia in Patients with Kidney Disease Not Receiving Dialysis. *N. Engl. J. Med.* **2019**, *381*, 1001–1010. [CrossRef]
105. Asfar, B.; Asfar, R.; Sag, A.; Kanbay, A.; Korkmaz, H.; Cipolla-Neto, J.; Covic, A.; Ortiz, A.; Kanbay, M. Sweet Dreams: Therapeutic Insights, Targeting Imaging and Physiologic Evidence Linking Sleep, Melatonin, and Diabetic Nephropathy. *Clin. Kidney J.* **2019**. accepted.

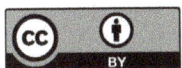

© 2020 by the authors. Licensee MDPI, Basel, Switzerland. This article is an open access article distributed under the terms and conditions of the Creative Commons Attribution (CC BY) license (http://creativecommons.org/licenses/by/4.0/).

MDPI
St. Alban-Anlage 66
4052 Basel
Switzerland
Tel. +41 61 683 77 34
Fax +41 61 302 89 18
www.mdpi.com

Toxins Editorial Office
E-mail: toxins@mdpi.com
www.mdpi.com/journal/toxins

www.ingramcontent.com/pod-product-compliance
Lightning Source LLC
LaVergne TN
LVHW070654100526
838202LV00013B/963